NUTRITION IN PREGNANCY AND CHILD BIRTH

C000116792

Making good nutritional choices can mean women optimise the outcomes of their birthing experience and offer their babies the best possible start in life. To support this, all health professionals who work with women during pregnancy, birth and the postnatal period need to have an appropriate knowledge of nutrition, healthy eating and other food related issues.

This evidence-based text provides an informative and accessible introduction to nutrition in pregnancy and childbirth. As well as allowing readers to recognise when nutritional deficiency may be creating challenges, it explores the psychosocial and cultural context of food and considers their relevance for women's eating behaviour. Finally, important emerging issues, such as eating during labour, food supplements and maternal obesity, are discussed.

An important reference for health professionals working in midwifery or public health contexts especially, this book is also the ideal companion for a course on nutrition in pregnancy and childbirth.

Lorna Davies is a principal Lecturer in Midwifery at Christchurch Polytechnic Institute of Technology, NZ and a part time lecturer for the New Zealand College of Midwives.

Ruth Deery is Professor in Maternal Health at the University of the West of Scotland, UK. She holds a joint appointment with the University of the West of Scotland and NHS Ayrshire & Arran.

PREGNANCY: Nutrition   27308

NUTRITION IN PREGNANCY AND CHILD BIRTH

Davies L.

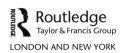

Routledge
Taylor & Francis Group

LONDON AND NEW YORK

2014

First published 2014
by Routledge

Simultaneously published in the USA and Canada
by Routledge
711 Third Avenue, New York, NY 10017

Routledge is an imprint of the Taylor & Francis Group, an informa business

The right of the editor to be identified as the author of the editorial
material, and of the authors for their individual chapters, has been
asserted in accordance with sections 77 and 78 of the
Copyright, Designs and Patents Act 1988.

All rights reserved. No part of this book may be reprinted or reproduced
or utilised in any form or by any electronic, mechanical, or other means,
now known or hereafter invented, including photocopying and recording,
or in any information storage or retrieval system, without permission in
writing from the publishers.

Trademark notice: Product or corporate names may be trademarks or
registered trademarks, and are used only for identification and
explanation without intent to infringe.

British Library Cataloguing in Publication Data
A catalogue record for this book is available from the British Library

Library of Congress Cataloging in Publication Data
   Nutrition in pregnancy and childbirth : food for thought /
   edited by Lorna Davies and Ruth Deery.—First edition
   p. ; cm.
   Includes bibliographical references.
   ISBN 978–0–415–53605–9 (hardback)—
   ISBN 978–0–415–53606–6 (pbk)—
   ISBN 978–0–203–11190–1 (ebook)
   I. Davies, Lorna, editor of compilation. II. Deery, Ruth
   (Professor in maternal health), editor of compilation.
   [DNLM: 1. Prenatal Nutritional Physiological Phenomena.
   2. Maternal Nutritional Physiological Phenomena.
   3. Nutrition Assessment. 4. Nutritional Requirements—physiology.
   5. Nutritive Value. WQ 175]
   RG559
   6618.2'42—dc23
   2013022374

Typeset in Times New Roman
by Swales & Willis Ltd, Exeter, Devon

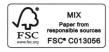

Printed and bound in Great Britain by
TJ International Ltd, Padstow, Cornwall

CONTENTS

ILLUSTRATIONS

Figures

Tables

Boxes

CONTRIBUTORS

Lucy Aphramor PhD, RD is director of the social enterprise Well Founded Ltd. To bring Health At Every Size (HAES) to communities and practitioners, Lucy pioneered the use of a health at every size approach in the UK National Health Service through the HAES course, Well Now, uniquely addressing the impact of self-care and social justice on well-being. She is an honorary research fellow at Glyndwr University, has published widely in the field of critical weight science and is active in the new Critical Dietetics movement, where her research spans issues of ethics, equity and embodied knowledge in the dietetics profession.

Jennifer Brady is a PhD candidate in the School of Kinesiology and Health Studies at Queen's University in Ontario, Canada. Her dissertation asks, 'what roles can and should we expect health professionals to play in advancing social justice?' To explore answers to this question she will conduct a critical history of the dietetic profession and its evolving, and sometimes fraught, relationship with home economics and feminism. Her other research interests include feminist theory, visual and embodied research methods, oral history, food, critical perspectives of fatness and the scholarship of teaching and learning. Jennifer recently won a student award from the Canadian Association for Food Studies for a paper in which she described a novel research method called 'cooking as inquiry'. She intends to further explore cooking as a method of creative scholarly inquiry.

Penny Champion, RM, RGN, ADM, MSc (Advanced Midwifery Practice), PG Dip (Learning and teaching) has been a midwife since 1991 and has worked in many areas of practice, including hospital and community settings. She currently holds a caseload in Essex, UK, supporting women in their birth choices. Penny has worked in midwifery education and continues to work there on a part-time basis, teaching on modules which develop midwives' skills for emergency care for mothers and babies. Her interest in eating and drinking in labour began whilst undertaking an MSc in Advanced Midwifery Practice. She has written a book entitled *Eating and Drinking in Labour*.

Rea Daellenbach, BA (Hons) PhD (Sociology) became active in the Home Birth Association in the mid-1980s and, as a consumer representative, was involved in the establishment of the New Zealand College of Midwives. At the same time, she completed a PhD in Sociology about the home birth movement in New Zealand. In 2004 she was appointed as a 'lay person' to the inaugural Midwifery Council of New Zealand. Rea has written and co-written chapters for several textbooks and was the co-editor of *Sustainability, Midwifery and Birth*. She is frequently invited to sit on maternity-related groups and committees in order to offer a consumer perspective. Currently, she is a lecturer in the School of Midwifery at the Christchurch Polytechnic Institute of Technology, New Zealand.

Lorna Davies (editor), RN, RM, BSc (Hons), PGCEA, MA, PhD candidate, is a UK-qualified midwife who has worked in midwifery education for the last two decades. She has published extensively in midwifery journals and texts and has edited three midwifery titles in recent years. She has been interested in food-related issues relating to maternal and newborn health for some time and is particularly interested in exploring this area through the lens of sustainability. Lorna is currently a principal lecturer in Midwifery at Christchurch Polytechnic Institute of Technology in New Zealand and a part-time lecturer for the New Zealand College of Midwives. She also carries a small caseload as a self-employed midwife and is a childbirth educator. She is presently undertaking a doctoral thesis exploring midwifery practice within a framework of sustainability.

Ruth Deery (editor), PhD, BSc (Hons), ADM, RM, FHEA is Professor in Maternal Health, holding a joint appointment with the University of the West of Scotland and NHS Ayrshire & Arran. She has a particular interest in applying sociological and political theory, action research and implementation science to the organisational culture of midwifery in the National Health Service in the UK. Her main research has been in the maternity services, with particular interests in organisational culture and change, public policy, emotions and care and critical obesity. Ruth is a member of the international editorial board for *Midwifery* and a Fellow of the Higher Education Academy. Ruth is also co-author of *Emotions in Midwifery and Reproduction* (Palgrave) and lead author of *Tensions and Barriers to Maternity Services: the story of a struggling birth centre* (Radcliffe). Currently she is lead editor for *Sociology for Midwives* (Polity Press).

Emma Derbyshire, PhD, PGCAP, RNutr is a Senior Lecturer in Nutritional Physiology at Manchester Metropolitan University and a Registered Nutritionist. She has written over 60 peer-reviewed reviews and research papers, several book chapters and two books, mainly within the field of maternal nutrition and public health nutrition, with her main areas of expertise being fertility, iron deficiency and functional foods and health. She is also a peer reviewer for several international academic and medical journals and has recently developed a smartphone technology application called Nutriprompt™ Planning for Pregnancy, with the intention of improving nutrition in the periconceptual period.

Jacqui Gingras, PhD, RD is an Associate Professor in the School of Nutrition at Ryerson University. Her research involves theoretical and experiential explorations of critical dietetics epistemology (how knowing in dietetics is defined and positioned), and engages feminist autoethnographic, narrative and arts-informed methods as a means for situated and particular understandings of dietetic theory, education and practice. She is the author of *Longing for Recognition: The Joys, Complexities, and Contradictions of Practicing Dietetics* (2009) and has co-authored chapters in several other textbooks and has published many journal articles. Her full CV is available at www.jacquigingras.ca. She is the recipient of Ryerson University's Research (2010) and Teaching (2009) Awards and she is a member of the College of Dietetics of Ontario. She is the founding editor of the *Journal of Critical Dietetics*, an online, peer-reviewed, open-access journal at www.criticaldietetics.org.

Colin R. Martin RN, BSc, PhD, MBA, YCAP, CPsychol, AFBPsS, CSci is Professor of Mental Health at Buckinghamshire New University, Middlesex, UK. He is a Registered

Mental Health Nurse, Chartered Health Psychologist and a Chartered Scientist. He also trained in analytical biochemistry. He has published or has in press approximately 200 research papers and book chapters. He is a keen book author and editor and his outputs include the seminal five-volume magnum opus, *Handbook of Behavior, Food and Nutrition (2011),* and the recently published prophetic insight into the treatment of neurological disease, *Nanomedicine and the Nervous System* (2012). He also has a long-standing interest in perinatal health and developmental psychology and is editor of the influential *Journal of Reproductive and Infant Psychology.* He is involved in collaborative international research with many European and non-European countries.

Ruth Martis, RM, RGON, Adv Dpl Nrsg, Grad Dip Tchg, BA (Soc. Sci) MA (Midwifery), IBCLC has practised as a midwife for over thirty years in a variety of settings, including home births. She has been involved in research, particularly in South-East Asia, and midwifery education for a number of years. Ruth is currently a full-time senior midwifery lecturer at Christchurch Polytechnic Institute of Technology (CPIT), New Zealand. Ruth is a fledging Cochrane Systematic Review author and interested in transferring knowledge into practice. Her master's thesis focused on her other passion, young pregnant women and their antenatal education needs. Food and nutrition has become a recent interest of hers through noticing the rise of gestational diabetes and the lack of information to share with women during their pregnancy.

Clara Miriam is a practising midwife. Supporting friends through death and birth made her realise, at the age of 30, that she was supposed to be a midwife. Witnessing the work of Becky Reed and the Albany midwives provided a touchstone for her aspirations. She learned from women, midwives and University of Bradford, West Yorkshire and now continues to learn daily from the women and midwives of Stroud, Gloucestershire, where she works in the community and at Stroud's 60-year-old midwife-led birth unit. Inspired by her Granny's stories of using 'psychoprophylaxis' in the 1950s, Clara has trained as a HypnoBirthing practitioner. Her interests include propagating equality, connectedness and empowerment through midwifery practice. She also loves midwifery books and is very pleased to be contributing to one.

Victoria Hall Moran, BSc (Hons), RM, MSc, PhD is an Associate Professor in Maternal and Child Nutrition in the Maternal and Infant Nutrition and Nurture Unit (MAINN) at the University of Central Lancashire, UK. Her research has focused on the infant feeding experiences and nutritional needs of adolescents during pregnancy and lactation. Recent work includes a review of dietary zinc requirements and associated health outcomes within the European Commission funded 'Eurreca' Network of Excellence. This network is designed to harmonise the approach to setting European micronutrient recommendations with specific focus on vulnerable populations such as infants, pregnant and lactating women and the elderly. She is a senior editor of the Wiley-Blackwell journal Maternal & Child Nutrition.

Anne Mullen, BSc, PhD, RD is a Lecturer in Nutritional Sciences at King's College London and a Registered Dietitian. She studied Human Nutrition and Dietetics in the Dublin Institute of Technology and Trinity College Dublin and obtained her PhD in Molecular Nutrition from Trinity College Dublin. Anne worked as a research fellow on an infant feeding project in Zambia with the London School of Hygiene and Tropical Medicine. She now teaches on nutrition, dietetic, biomedical science and dentistry courses at King's

College London, and her area of research interest is how nutrients and the immune system interact in non-communicable chronic diseases such as obesity, atherosclerosis, diabetes and lipodystrophy syndromes such as that associated with HIV. Anne uses cellular and molecular, clinical and public health studies in her research.

Gill Rapley, RGN, RM, HV, MSc has practised as a health visitor, midwife and voluntary breastfeeding counsellor. She qualified as a lactation consultant in 1994. From 1996 to 2010 she worked for the UNICEF UK Baby Friendly Initiative, focusing on breastfeeding but pursuing her interest in solid feeding in her spare time. For her master's degree, Gill undertook a small piece of research that showed that babies of six months and older could feed themselves with solid foods, rather than needing to be spoon fed, and she subsequently pioneered the approach known as baby-led weaning (BLW). Since then she has collaborated on a small series of videos and developed a successful writing partnership with Tracey Murkett. She is currently studying for a PhD in the area of infant feeding.

Lydia Jade Turner, BA (Psych), PG Dip (Psych), PG Dip (Pr) is the Managing Director and Psychologist at eating disorders clinic BodyMatters Australasia (www.bodymatters.com.au), specialising in eating disorders and unhealthy weight loss practices. BodyMatters provides a range of services for the treatment and prevention of disordered eating, including counselling, education, consultancy and advocacy using individual counselling and family-based therapy. Lydia regularly presents at conferences across Australia, New Zealand and the US, and speaks in schools, tertiary institutions, public hospitals and NGOs about eating pathology. As a freelance writer she has had her work published in a number of national Australian newspapers, including the *Sydney Morning Herald*, *The Age* and the *National Times*. In 2013 Lydia published a chapter in the book *Raising Girls* by psychologist Steve Biddulph. Lydia is regularly quoted and interviewed in the Australian media.

Jade Wratten, RM, BM, PG Dip, GCTLT is a registered and practising midwife in New Zealand. She graduated from Massey University, Wellington with a Bachelor of Midwifery and also holds a post-graduate diploma in midwifery and a certificate of tertiary teaching and learning from Otago Polytechnic. Jade is a lecturer in Midwifery for Otago Polytechnic's Bachelor of Midwifery programme and has a keen interest in nutrition in pregnancy; she coordinates the Nutrition for Childbearing undergraduate course. Currently Jade works in the Manawatu area of New Zealand as a community-based case-loading midwife and has extensive experience also working as a staff midwife and associate charge midwife at Mid-Central Health hospital.

ACKNOWLEDGEMENTS

We would like to thank all our contributors for sharing their knowledge and expertise and, in doing so, making this book a reality. We are grateful to them for writing their chapters in and amongst their other work and family commitments. We especially thank Jade Wratten, who stepped in at the last minute to help out.

Lorna would particularly like to pay tribute to Alex, who has taught her many things with his passion for food in his role as a philosphically sound chef and confirmed locavore. She would also like to acknowledge Tom, who has worked tirelessly against all odds to establish Mt Pleasant Farmers Market for the people who lost their food shops in the Christchurch earthquake of 2011. In so doing he has created a social space that is so much more than a local place to buy food.

We would like to say thank you to our editing team at Routledge, especially Grace and James for their flexibility and patience and for their support during the writing of the book through to production, and to the anonymous reviewers for their encouraging and constructive comments.

FOREWORD

This book reminds me yet again, as if I needed any reminding, of why I – a sociologist – so value midwifery. Of course I value midwives, as any feminist would, for their 'with women' stance. But it is the sociological imagination that midwives so often bring to their work that shines through this book, which particularly pleases me.

C. Wright Mills defined the sociological imagination as focusing not on individual 'troubles,' but on social issues, not on individual biography, but the historical context in which that life is lived. Clinicians, entirely appropriately but so very unlike sociologists, tend to focus on the highly individualized – the needs of individual bodies. Sadly, too much of what we call 'public health' has come to mean simply the 'massification' of individual advice, more about public education programs than about social change. Let's take a non-food example for a start: large-scale environmental changes have made the rays of the sun ever more dangerous, especially for fair-skinned people. If an individual – any given human body – wants to protect himself, herself, or his or her children, from these dangerous rays, they need to cover up the fair skin. Stay inside? Wear long sleeves? Slather on sunscreen? A combination of all of these? Of course. But we must never forget that these are individual solutions to a social problem. Skin cancer is trouble, big trouble. But the hole in the ozone layer, the environmental issues – those are social issues, not solvable by individual adherence to the sunscreen guidelines. All of the slathering of sunscreen in the world won't solve the larger problem. The problem will only get worse and individual solutions will need to get ever more drastic and complex.

Public Health, as it first started, tried to look at the level of the larger social problems. Individuals were getting sick because of an unclean water supply? Well then, let's clean up the water! Close down the infected sources and bring clean water down to our central cities. It was a massive social undertaking. I look at what is going on in much of the world of Public Health these days and think that, with today's approach, the solution would have been a massive public awareness campaign about using bottled water. Bottled water is, of course, expensive, and so only available to people of some privilege. And the very bottling processes will themselves contribute to the larger social problem of environmental degradation. For that matter, I imagine that all the processing of plastic sunscreen packages and the creams and ointments themselves aren't doing the ozone layer any good.

When we turn to the world of food, it is that individualizing, clinical mindset that we mostly see at work these days. Getting fat are you? Eat more lean meat, more seafood, more fresh greens and healthy fruits. Obesity is a problem in pregnancy? Solve it! For yourself, for your pregnancy and for the health of your child. Not getting enough Vitamin D? Well, you could get it from the sun, but no, never mind, that's not safe. Hard to get enough Vitamin D out of the typical diet? Let's do research on the efficacy of supplements. And – not irrelevantly in a capitalist world – that's the place where somebody can make some money. That's where most of what I read these days seems to stop.

But it is where this book starts. There are structural causes, larger social patterns, that shape the nutritional status of individual women, factors far beyond their own food choices. Yes, of course, as a clinician, as a provider of healthcare services, the midwife absolutely must look at individual women's Vitamin D status, body mass index, and dozens of other 'risk factors' that exist in her body and for her pregnancy, and counsel her intelligently about her risks and how to lower them. But the midwife who reads this book will also be made to think about the larger structural factors that shape available food choices. What is it about the way we organize our societies that makes women susceptible to eating disorders? How can a midwife help a woman to deal with her depression, her drug use, her anorexia, her binge-eating, her obesity, in ways that are not just 'victim blaming'? How can she help to sort out what are real problems, actual physical threats to a healthy body and a healthy pregnancy, and what are stigma-igniters, flags for others to begin harassment or blame?

Partly it is done via that midwifery stance of being with the woman – on her side, respectfully listening, open to her needs and her concerns. Look her straight in the eye, an author counsels, when asking the hard questions about drug use – and so we might say about dietary questions of women who daily confront the constant demeaning label of 'fat.' The midwife isn't there to judge; she is there to help. Feeling 'scrutinized, exposed, humiliated, abused, ignored or in any way emotionally unsafe may,' Clara Miriam reminds the reader, 'inhibit the oxytocin system.' Too often, the humiliating, scrutinizing, abusive 'care' that women get can inhibit the very behaviors that the caregivers are trying to bring about. Eating well is very much dependent on what food the environment offers, its true availability and affordability, but it is also dependent on a woman's feelings of strength, deservedness, and comfort in her environment.

It is all unthinkably complex, and I admire the way that the authors have each and all attempted to address the complexity respectfully, not oversimplifying complex systems of interaction into simple statements of causation. That is true in their written analyses of the data on nutrition in pregnancy and childbirth, and also in their suggestions for working with and helping the women in their care. Women do not need yet another printed guideline of what to eat and what to avoid – they need so much more. They need a safe and generous world. Midwives cannot give them that. But they can give them the time it takes to explore their food worlds, to think and talk and listen and work through what would help, what would enable them to do the best they can to manage their individual troubles in the face of the larger social issues.

It is indeed, as the final piece concludes, time for a conversation about food. But not just one conversation – not just the clinical conversation that shapes biography. We are also in the midst of a larger social conversation about our food worlds – we are shaping our history now, and midwifery is an important part of the conversation.

Professor Barbara Katz Rothman
The City University of New York

We would like to express our gratitude to the Brazilian artist Itaiana Battoni for her generosity in sharing her wonderful image for the cover of the book. The image represents the world of food and birth in a simple analogous way that words would not be able to achieve. The context in which Itaiana works is significant because birth for many Brazilian women means an induction of labour or a caesarean section. However, this is the case in many other countries too. We hope that the wonderful birth images created by Itaiana will serve to raise consciousness and perhaps help to lead to a change in birth philosophy, so that the peach is indeed allowed to ripen instead of being plucked prematurely from the tree.

Part I

HEALTHY EATING AND NUTRITION IN CHILDBIRTH

1

SO WHAT'S FOR DINNER?

Ruth Deery

Food is an important commodity in all our lives because, nutritionally, we have to eat to survive. Pregnancy and birth are also known to be extremely energy-demanding processes, with the ingestion of food a crucial part of this process (Davies *et al.*, 2013). However, food has much more than a biological function, as there are cultural and emotional connotations associated with disease, death, emotion and pleasure. Culturally, food is also about a person's interaction with their environment and community: having 'multi-sensorial properties of taste, touch, sight, sound, and smell . . . it has the ability to communicate . . . and constitutes a form of language' (Counihan and Van Esterik, 2013: 10). Therefore the individual, social and cultural significances of food are as important as its nutritional factor. From a midwifery and pregnant woman's perspective, food and nutrition are two important cornerstones in determining the outcome of pregnancy and birth. As midwives, we need to understand the different connotations of food in human life, particularly so within the context of pregnancy and birth.

The chapters in this book address food and nutrition in pregnancy, during birth and in the postnatal period from some of the different perspectives highlighted above. The book takes an interdisciplinary and cross-cultural perspective to nutrition and food but is not a complete meal. It is not meant to be a deeply theoretical book. Rather, it is an appetizer, meant to introduce midwives and other health professionals to the variety of intellectual dishes now available and developing around food and nutrition in health. It is highly appropriate for midwives and other health professionals who connect with women during pregnancy, birth and the postnatal period to have a sound cross-cultural knowledge of nutrition, healthy eating and other food-related issues, given the multicultural and interdisciplinary nature of our work as midwives. This will enable us to recognize when nutritional deficiency or attitudinal and behavioural issues (for example, the adage 'eating for two') towards food may be creating challenges for midwives and women. Such challenges might be differing attitudes to food, the meaning and reason for preferences of certain foods, ambivalence to foods, and attitudes, behaviours and beliefs about the relationship between diet and health (see Chapter 13). These challenges are not specific to pregnant women. As midwives, we too need to be challenged to address our own values and beliefs so that we can provide compassionate, person-centred care for pregnant women and their families.

Increasingly we are seeing food-related issues playing a significant role in clinical practice situations. For example, we are now concerned with excess food consumption and there is an alarming concern over increasing obesity rates (Unnithan-Kumar and Tremayne, 2011). In midwifery, obesity in pregnancy has had a considerable impact for women with a high BMI both in terms of choices around childbirth and their qualitative experience of our maternity services (see Chapters 12 and 13; Deery, 2011). 'Obesogenic organisms' have been described as living in environments where routine and everyday circumstances encourage them to eat less and exercise more (Hanlon *et al.*, 2012: 90). Whilst environmentally this might be ideal, using 'eating less and exercising more' as a mantra for losing excess weight is not helpful because it does not take account of the different ways in which individuals 'use' food, culturally and emotionally. For example, excess body fat is valued in some cultures because it is a sign of health and wealth (Belasco, 2008; Brown, 1993), attainable only by those of higher socio-economic standing. Other individuals use food as a means of dealing with the stresses of everyday life (Orbach, 1986). However, these viewpoints have shifted over time, with fatness/obesity now seen in Western society as being deviant, ugly and as a disease (Lupton, 2012). Fatless bodies have now become something for Western women to emulate, although boundaries have become blurred as to what actually constitutes acceptable thinness. Thus we have seen an increase in eating disorders such as anorexia nervosa and bulimia (Bordo, 2013; see also Chapter 6). Susie Orbach's words describing the pressures some women feel when striving for thinness are as relevant today as they were in 1986:

> Diet, deprive, deny is the message women receive, or – even more sinister – they must pretend that cottage cheese and melon is as pleasurable as a grilled cheese sandwich for lunch. For a woman, then, food is an object of an entirely different character. It is a potential enemy and a threat. A cardinal rule of femininity, from young women in their teens through women in their fifties, is that they should be desirable. Desirability is linked with an ever-diminishing body size, which is attainable by most women only through severe restrictions on their food intake. And because the 'right size' for women has been decreasing yearly since 1965, so women have been encouraged to decrease their food intake yearly.
>
> (Orbach, 1986: 65)

Food as a 'potential enemy and a threat' can describe the way in which some people 'use' food (sparingly and to excess) to deal with the stresses of life. The manner in which people use food in this way is a neglected area of research and one that is rarely taken into account when midwives are giving nutritional advice. An edited text by Unnithan-Kumar and Tremayne (2011) addresses some of these less well-understood motivations relating to body weight in different social, economic and cultural contexts.

The dominant bio-medical discourses around pregnant women and their behaviours are understood primarily as risks to their contained fetus (Davies *et al.*, 2013). As such, issues of nutrition and feeding in pregnancy, including food scarcity and obesity as well as specific food taboos, present us with an 'ingenuity gap' (Homer-Dixon, 2000; Hanlon *et al.*, 2012) – a gulf between the above challenges and our capacity as midwives to provide and devise effective solutions with women. Midwifery has the potential to offer an interconnected approach, encouraging healthy eating in the interests of the mother–fetus dyad (Davies *et al.*, 2013; see Chapter 13).

As midwives, we are in a privileged position to be connecting with women when they are at a vulnerable time in their lives – a time that gives us the opportunity to work in partnership with them. As Leap (2000: 4) has stated,

> At every stage of our interactions with childbearing women, as midwives, we should be adopting behaviours that will ensure that women can take up the power that will

enable them to lead fulfilling lives as individuals and as mothers. The process of empowerment may have far reaching consequences in terms of women's feelings of self worth and confidence.

As midwives, we know pregnant women who come from communities with low levels of social capital may be particularly at risk from a fragmented midwifery approach. As Putnam (1995: 67) has stated, '"social capital" refers to features of social organization such as networks, norms and social trust that facilitate coordination and cooperation for mutual benefit'. However, maternity services have been criticized, especially in the UK, as providing services that are unconnected, too complex and fragmented (Kirkham, 2010) and not inclusive, facilitative, or user friendly (Feldman, 2013). Disconnected services are not conducive to the provision of effective and equitable maternity services for women and in the UK we now read about women who make choices to opt out of our services (Edwards and Kirkham, 2012). We also know that lower socio-economic status seems to be a risk factor for increased levels of obesity, particularly among women and members of ethnic minorities (Wilkinson and Pickett, 2010). Environment may also be related to the accessibility of healthy food, although proximity to appropriate shops does not necessarily make healthy food accessible to everyone. Financial resources, mobility and expertise in cooking are also factors to take into account (Wilkinson and Pickett, 2010).

As Kirkham (2010) highlights, we live in a highly technologized society where problems are defined and solved by experts with specialist knowledge. As midwives, we tend to create a dependency culture, wanting to 'make things better' and 'work problems out' in a solution-focused way for women. Despite efforts in public health to move from this type of approach to making more changes to our physical and social environment, a healthier approach to individual lifestyle (especially around nutrition) does not seem to have taken place (Hanlon *et al.*, 2012). In midwifery particularly we seem to have adopted an approach that can reproach women for eating poorly and thus placing their babies/children at risk as a result. This blame becomes most obvious in the dilemma of obesity, and I use this as an example here.

The issue of obesity, weight gain and pregnancy within a conventional weight-based paradigm has attracted enormous attention in recent years (Aphramor, 2005; see Chapter 13). Pregnant women using maternity services often receive clear messages that if they are obese they have a greater risk of developing a range of complications in pregnancy and childbirth (Deery and Wray, 2009). Obesity has become increasingly medicalized, with its relationship to poor neonatal outcome often misstated as cause rather than a correlation (Davies *et al.*, 2013). In this respect the 'black box, junk in; junk out' scenario comes into play – inconclusive, incorrect evidence is deposited into the box, and reappears at the other side of the black box as legitimate conclusions (Fleck, 1979). As a result the media and health professionals often leap to conclusions that any possible health risks (e.g. hypertension, diabetes, heart disease and cancers) are caused by obesity. When behavioural variables are strongly favoured, other legitimate forms of evidence simply do not enter into the public domain for discussion and debate; the regurgitated 'junk' is merely asserted without reference to evidence that demonstrates otherwise, or questions the credibility of the findings (Aphramor, 2005). Increasingly, health professionals are taught to view obese women as 'a statistic waiting to happen' (Vireday, 2002), when in fact not all obese women will present as problematic. The degree of risk will vary, with clear differences between a well-nourished and an under-nourished pregnant woman, and weight/fat alone does not capture that distinction (Davies *et al.*, 2013).

When midwives focus on women's problems and needs a deficits model comes into play. When we do this we define communities and women in terms of what they cannot do, do wrong, or do not possess (McLean, 2011). Indeed, as described above, we encourage women to depend on midwives as well as on hospital and welfare services. Therein is the potential to disempower women who are the intended beneficiaries of our maternity services. As discussed earlier, women who are not seen by some midwives and obstetricians to be making adaptive changes towards health are labelled and stigmatized (Deery, 2011; see also Chapters 12 and 13). Such an approach also prevents midwives from asking questions about the promotion of health, well-being and nutrition from the perspective of the woman using maternity services.

Policy development has also focused too much on the failure of individuals and local communities to avoid disease, rather than on their potential to create and sustain health and continued development (Morgan and Ziglio, 2007). Alternatively, in public health approaches, and especially in midwifery, we are increasingly realizing that many of the solutions to the challenges, such as education around good nutrition, need to be much more rooted in local circumstances and communities. Failure to do this has resulted in current approaches to public health not making the anticipated improvement in health outcomes (Hanlon et al., 2012). The gap between the affluent and the deprived in society continues to increase, and whilst there is a vast amount of information claiming which groups and populations suffer the worst health there is less information about how best to reduce the gap and improve health (Wilkinson and Pickett, 2010). An asset-based approach has the potential to revitalize not only the evidence base for public health (McLean, 2011) but our clinical practice as midwives.

An 'asset-based approach' to food and nutrition

Nutrition and food provide good examples of the way in which an asset-based approach can be effective for midwives. This approach builds on the assets and strengths of specific communities (pregnant, birthing and postnatal women, in this case) and engages women and their families in taking action. It is often cost-effective, since it provides a link for the resources of individuals, charities or social enterprises to complement the work of local service providers such as maternity services. Given the current global growing pressure on government finances and lack of resources in our health systems and maternity units, these are important benefits.

An asset-based model has the potential to reframe our approach to one of more positivity when engaging with women to discuss not only food and nutrition but all other aspects of care. An asset-based approach is based on salutogenic thinking (Antonovsky, 1987), which is about creating positive health, focusing on a person's existing strengths and capabilities. Salutogenesis focuses on the discovery and use of personal resources (assets in this case) within a person or environment that help to maintain a healthy status (McLean, 2011). In particular, salutogenesis can explain why some people become ill under stressful conditions and others do not. In midwifery there are implications here for the way we understand particular events in women's lives, e.g. why some women continue to smoke when pregnant and others abuse drugs or alcohol, thus neglecting adequate nutrition.

Eriksson and Lindström (2005) describe a salutogenic approach as a deeply personal way of being, thinking and acting, a feeling of inner trust that our lives will be in order, independently of whatever happens. According to McLean (2011), the core salutogenic concepts are Generalised Resistance Resources (GRRs) and a Sense of Coherence (SoC). For example,

GRRs are the biological, material and psychosocial factors which would make it easier for pregnant women to understand and structure their lives. They include factors such as money, social support, knowledge, experience, intelligence and traditions. When communities have these sorts of resources available, the likelihood of being able to deal with the challenges of life increases (Eriksson and Lindström, 2005). As McLean (2011) points out, GRRs identify important 'ingredients' and an SoC provides the capability to use them.

The SoC framework is a useful theory for taking a salutogenic approach to a positive way of looking at life, alongside an ability to successfully manage the many stresses encountered throughout life. McLean (2011) describes a SoC as a mediator between a GRR (or asset) and an outcome of improved health and well-being, coping and control – an ideal mediator for midwifery practice. SoC may therefore be the part of self-awareness that releases a woman's health assets. Midwives are in an ideal situation to be able to help women release their health assets. According to Antonovsky (1993), three types of life experiences shape an individual's SoC:

- comprehensibility (life has a certain predictability and can be understood)
- manageability (resources are enough to meet personal demands)
- meaningfulness (life makes sense, problems are worth investing energy in).

More recently, a fourth concept has been added: emotional closeness, which refers to the extent to which a person has emotional bonds with others and feels part of their community (Sagy and Antonovsky, 2000).

A recent systematic review came to the conclusion that a salutogenic model is a health promoting resource because it defines the means by which individual resilience may be improved and people may be helped to feel physically and mentally healthy, with a good quality of life and sense of well-being (Eriksson and Lindström, 2006). However, while the salutogenic approach provides us with a lens through which we can understand how health comes about and can be maintained, there is little evidence at present of how salutogenic concepts can be put to good use in policies to help women, their families and communities in midwifery.

Downe (2010) has proposed a vision for 21st-century midwifery that is based on a salutogenic approach, combining expert practice with wisdom, skilled practice and enacted vocation. Combinations of the following are suggested:

- a coherent humanist realist philosophy
- effective clinical and interpersonal skills
- comprehensive knowledge
- positive appreciative relationships
- facilitative health system, organizational context
- societal/community buy-in.

(Downe, 2010: 294)

Taking the above into account, midwives could take the opportunity to help to define communities and pregnant women in terms of the resources they have to stay healthy. They could encourage women to take control of their own health during pregnancy and birth and encourage women to help and support each other. We have successful examples of this in midwifery in terms of peer support and breastfeeding (Dykes, 2005; Kirkham et al., 2006).

Key to the above is that an asset-based approach promotes self-esteem and the ability to cope with life.

Resilience is also key to an asset-based approach in midwifery. Resilience is a dynamic process whereby individuals display positive adaptation despite having experienced significant adversity or trauma (Rutter, 1999). From a midwifery perspective, greater resilience means women being better able to access and use resources, including public resources such as our maternity systems and services. However, we know that excluded or disadvantaged groups often have limited networks and this restricts their access to resources/assets and their associated benefits (Edwards and Kirkham, 2012; Feldman, 2013). Connections and networks are essential aspects of resilience because they enable people and communities to give support and get resources. Again, midwifery has good examples of peer support and breastfeeding as well as clinical supervision as a support mechanism to help sustain midwives when their practice becomes challenging and too stressful (Deery, 2005; Derbyshire, 2000).

In summary there is little doubt that a nutritionally rich diet with a sensible balance of both macro- and micronutrients offers the best possible start in life (see Chapters 2 and 3). Suboptimal nutrition may adversely affect the growth of the fetus, and impaired fetal growth is associated with increased perinatal morbidity and mortality as well as infant mortality and childhood morbidity. There appears to be a lack of knowledge amongst midwives and health professionals of the social, psychological and economic effects that influence obesity as well as personal well-being. This knowledge deficit adversely influences access to maternity services, quality of care, health equity and outcomes of care for women who are more vulnerable and disadvantaged (Davies *et al.*, 2013). Using an asset-based approach to facilitate communication and relationship building between women and midwives could contribute to improving health and reducing health inequalities.

So what is for dinner . . .?

Overview of the chapters

This book is divided into four parts. Each chapter is meant to facilitate further thought and encourage an increased understanding of food and nutrition in pregnancy, childbirth and the postnatal period. The first part, 'Healthy eating and nutrition in childbirth', starts with Ruth Deery (this chapter) providing an introduction to food and nutrition through a public health approach. She introduces salutogenesis and an asset-based approach that could be used by midwives when they discuss nutrition, food and diet with women.

In Chapter 2 Anne Mullen, Colin R. Martin and Lorna Davies explore the significance and influence of macronutrients on the body, both generally and specifically, on the health of the mother and the fetus/baby. The chapter explores the complexity of the interactions with other food components and the metabolic processes of macronutrients. We know from numerous research studies that when maternal nutrition is sub-optimal, the growth and development of the fetus may be adversely affected. Whilst macronutrients yield energy, micronutrients do not; they assist with regulating growth and facilitating the release of energy. In Chapter 3 Anne Mullen, Colin R. Martin and Jade Wratten take a cross-cultural perspective, examining how micronutrients nourish the mother in pregnancy and are responsible for vital life processes such as DNA synthesis and cell division.

In Chapter 4 Victoria Hall Moran explores nutritional needs for lactation, drawing our attention to the fact that breastfeeding is one of the most nutritionally demanding times of a woman's life; a time when nutritional requirements increase to support newborn and infant growth and development. She highlights recent research that is providing new knowledge on the nutrient requirements of breastfeeding women. Now that there is wide variation in breastfeeding practices across the world, making nutritional recommendations for lactating women has become challenging. Hall Moran emphasizes the importance of examining the cultural practices within and across populations. She urges us to avoid making assumptions that when we provide women with the 'correct' information about nutritional requirements during lactation this will lead them to make the 'right choices' in terms of their own nutrition and the patterns and practices of breastfeeding.

Part II, 'Context and cultural issues', begins with Rea Daellenbach examining insights from archaeology and food psychology about the genetic human predispositions related to food consumption. She then goes on to pose a question for midwives about the cultural values and expectations that shape women's relationship with food. An exploration of three interlinked aspects that describe the cultural landscape of food follows in the chapter; the economy and the polity, the household and the individual. The chapter concludes with a focus on women's special relationship with food within the household and food choices as expressions of individuality, health and ethical commitments.

In Chapter 6 Lydia Jade Turner explores caring for women with eating disorders. She acknowledges that the etiology of eating disorders is complex and multifactorial and that eating disorders may strike at any time during a woman's life. Pregnancy can be a vulnerable time for relapse or even the onset of an eating disorder. In vulnerable women, the hormonal changes that take place during pregnancy may enhance an existing low self-esteem. Turner draws our attention to those women who may not have developed effective coping strategies, in which case pregnancy may act as a trigger for the development of an eating disorder.

Emma Derbyshire addresses the increasingly popular dietary choices of vegetarianism and veganism in Chapter 7. She explains which nutrients, if any, are most likely to be lacking from vegetarians' diets. She encourages a varied diet including a range of different foods groups, i.e. protein, dairy substitute and fresh fruits and vegetables and supplements where appropriate. She suggests that women may benefit from taking a specially formulated pregnancy supplement containing the essential nutrients needed during this important time. She concludes the chapter with some key messages for women and midwives.

In Chapter 8 Ruth Martis explores the way in which midwives can engage with young pregnant women when talking about food and nutrition. She highlights evidence indicating that adolescents have very specific nutrient requirements, especially calcium and iron, not because of pregnancy but because of the rapid growth and physiological changes that occur during this time. Working with young pregnant women and teenage mothers is a rewarding experience but can also be challenging. Ruth Martis contends that establishing a relationship grounded in trust and respect, incorporating a psycho-social development approach (that of adolescent, not adulthood) and understanding the need for teenage women to emotionally 'regrow' enables effective food talk with young pregnant women. She identifies, and encourages the use of, HEADDS (Home, Health, Education, Employment, Activities, Drugs, Depression and Safety) as a useful tool to guide and support midwives and other health professionals.

Part III, 'Debates and controversies', starts with Lorna Davies taking a look at sustainability, food and childbirth in Chapter 9, where she aims to stimulate thought and discussion around the significance of food and nutrition during the childbearing period in relation to the concept of sustainability. She highlights the complexity of the subject area at both local and global levels, exposing the challenging nature of some of the problems. As midwives, this can leave us with more questions than answers, but Lorna Davies stresses the importance of engaging with the issues at stake because they are increasingly likely to influence our own lives and those of the women and families that we attend. The chapter begins with an overview establishing the generic relationship between food and sustainability from environmental, economic and social perspectives and then proceeds to make links with childbirth. Davies encourages us to reflect on what we could do within our own clinical practice to make positive changes for the women and babies that we work with.

Gill Rapley introduces baby-led weaning in Chapter 10, explaining the nature of baby-led feeding and why it makes sense to support parents to implement this type of approach. Baby-led weaning is described as being as old as baby-led breastfeeding but has tended to be practised in secret, for fear that the (experienced) mother will be exposed as a lazy or undisciplined woman. However a baby-led approach to the continuum of infant feeding is now being seen as logical and natural by increasing numbers of parents, and an increasing number of health professionals are now willing and able to support it. Just as most adults appreciate being able to choose what to eat, how to eat, how often, how much and how quickly, so too, infants probably feel the same way, particularly if their instincts and abilities are driving them to want to make these decisions for themselves. Rapley contends that research strongly suggests that denying the very young the opportunity to make feeding choices has the potential to lead to serious consequences and that health professionals need to be wary of interfering in matters about which babies probably do know best.

In Chapter 11 Penny Champion explores nutrition and birth and the issues which surround eating and drinking in labour. She provides an exploration of the ways in which midwives impose restrictions and limitations on women's oral intake in labour, the physiology relating to labour and birth and appetite. She highlights how the interventions that we use as midwives can affect the physiology of birth and adaptation of the newborn, and how midwives can facilitate evidence-based practice and woman-led eating and drinking around the time of birth. Champion concludes that the decision about whether or not to eat and drink in labour must be made on an individual basis, using the evidence we have but with an overriding emphasis on the woman's choice as to what feels right for her at the time.

Clara Miriam provides an exploration of anti-fat prejudice, connecting the medical model of childbirth and social control of women, in Chapter 12. She provides some socio-cultural context to the medicalized idea of obesity and introduces the current critique of obesity science, going on to take a critical look at national guidelines that influence maternity care. She explores what she terms big-bodied women's experiences of maternity care. She reports stories that reveal their perceptions of the impact of healthcare professionals' attitudes on women's physical and mental well-being. Miriam concludes the chapter by suggesting how the power of compassion may be one of the most useful midwifery tools for relieving shame and improving outcomes in this group of women.

In Chapter 13 Jennifer Brady, Lucy Aphramor and Jacqui Gingras highlight that nutritional advice given by midwives can be inconsistent and prescriptive, reflecting professional, personal and social mores about fat and food. As dieticians, they have witnessed the harm that has been inflicted on fat bodies. They explore alternative possibilities for midwifery care that are respectful of, and compassionate toward, all bodies of any size. They propose a Health at Every Size® (HAES®) approach informed by relational-cultural theory (RCT) as one such alternative. They outline the principles of HAES as they understand them before exploring RCT and how this connects to HAES. They then compare and contrast pregnancy-related guidelines for health practitioners involved in the care of pregnant women that are published by the National Health Service in the UK and Health Canada.

In Part IV the final chapter, which could be considered to be a micro-section of the book, information from the other chapters is brought together, to discuss the findings and their application to midwifery practice. The chapter critically explores how nutritional assessment may be carried out as part of antenatal care and encourages the reader to consider which tools can be used to encourage an on-going discussion with the woman around her nutritional status and how to plan for the future.

References

Antonovsky, A. (1987) *Unravelling the Mystery of Health: How People Manage Stress and Stay Well*, California: Jossey-Bass.

Antonovsky, A. (1993) The structure and properties of the sense of coherence scale, *Social Science & Medicine*, 36 (6): 725–733.

Aphramor, L. (2005) Is a weight-centred health framework salutogenic? Some thoughts on unhinging certain dietary ideologies, *Social Theory & Health*, (4): 315–340.

Belasco, W. (2008) *Food, The Key Concepts*, Oxford: Berg.

Bordo, S. (2013) Not just 'a white girl's thing': the changing face of food and body image problems. In: Counihan, C. and Van Esterik, P. (Eds) *Food and Culture: A Reader* (3rd edn), London: Routledge.

Brown, P.J. (1993) Cultural perspectives on the etiology and treatment of obesity. In: Stunkard, A.J. and Wadden, T.A. (Eds) *Obesity: Theory and Therapy* (2nd edn), New York: Raven Press.

Counihan, C. and Van Esterik, P. (2013) *Food and Culture: A Reader* (3rd edn), London: Routledge.

Davies, L., Deery, R. and Katz Rothman, B. (2013) Pregnancy and food. In: Thompson, P. and Kaplan, D. (Eds) *Encyclopedia of Food and Agricultural Ethics*, Springer Reference (www.springerreference.com). Berlin and Heidelberg: Springer-Verlag. DOI: 10.1007/SpringerReference_334988 2013–01–03 08:16:43 UTC.

Deery, R. (2005) An action research study exploring midwives' support needs and the effect of group clinical supervision, *Midwifery*, 21 (2): 161–176.

Deery, R. (2011) 'Obesing' pregnant women: by whom, and for what reasons? *AIMS Journal*, 23 (4): 12–13.

Deery, R. and Wray, S. (2009) 'The hardest leap': acceptance of diverse body size in midwifery, *The Practising Midwife*, 12 (10): 14–16.

Derbyshire, F. (2000) Clinical supervision within midwifery. In: M. Kirkham (Ed.) *Developments in the Supervision of Midwives*, Manchester: Books for Midwives Press.

Downe, S. (2010) Towards salutogenic birth in the 21st century. In: Walsh, D. and Downe, S. (Eds) *Essential Midwifery Practice Intrapartum Care*, pp. 289–295, Wiley-Blackwell: Blackwell Publishing Ltd.

Dykes, F. (2005) Government funded breastfeeding peer support projects: implications for practice, *Maternal & Child Nutrition*, 1 (1): 21–31.

Edwards, N. and Kirkham, M. (2012) Why women might not use NHS maternity services, *Essentially MIDIRS*, 3 (9): 17–21.

Eriksson, M. and Lindström, B. (2005) Validity of Antonovsky's sense of coherence scale: a systematic review, *Journal of Epidemiology and Community Health*, 59 (6): 460–466.

Eriksson, M. and Lindström, B. (2006) Antonovsky's sense of coherence scale and the relation with health: a systematic review, *Journal of Epidemiology and Community Health*, 60 (5): 376–381.

Feldman, R. (2013) *When Maternity Doesn't Matter, Dispersing Pregnant Women Seeking Asylum*, London: Refugee Council.

Fleck, L. (1979) *Genesis and Development of a Scientific Fact*. London: University of Chicago Press.

Hanlon, P., Carlisle, S., Hannah, M. and Lyon, A. (2012) *The Future Public Health*, Berkshire: McGraw Hill, Open University Press.

Homer-Dixon, T. (2000) *The Ingenuity Gap: Facing the Economic, Environmental, and Other Challenges of an Increasingly Complex and Unpredictable Future*, New York: Vintage Books.

Kirkham, M. (ed.) (2010) *The Midwife–Mother Relationship*, London: Palgrave Macmillan.

Kirkham, M., Sherridan, A., Thornton, D., Smale, M., Moran, V.H. and Dykes, F. (2006) 'Breast-friends' Doncaster: the story of our peer support project. In Moran, V.H. and Dykes, F. (Eds) *Maternal and Infant Nutrition and Nurture: Controversies and Challenges*, London: MA Healthcare Limited, Quay Books Division.

Leap, N. (2010) The less we do the more we give. In: Kirkham, M. (ed.) *The Midwife–Mother Relationship*, London: Palgrave Macmillan.

Lupton, D. (2012) *Fat*. Routledge.

McLean, J. (2011) *Asset-based Approaches for Health Improvement: Redressing the Balance*, Glasgow: Glasgow Centre for Population Health.

Morgan, A. and Ziglio, E. (2007) Revitalising the evidence base for public health: an assets model, *Promotion & Education*, 14 (2 suppl.), 17–22.

Orbach, S. (1986) *Hunger Strike: The Anorectic's Struggle as a Metaphor for Our Age*, New York: Avon.

Putnam, R. (1995) Bowling alone: America's declining social capital, *Journal of Democracy*, 6 (1): 65–79.

Rutter, M. (1999) Resilience, concepts and findings: Implications for family therapy, *Journal of Family Therapy*, 21, 119–144.

Sagy, S. and Antonovsky, H. (2000) The development of the sense of coherence: a retrospective study of early life experiences in the family, *International Journal of Aging and Human Development*, 51 (2): 155.

Unnithan-Kumar, M. and Tremayne, S. (2011) *Fatness and the Maternal Body, Women's Experiences of Corporeality and the Shaping of Social Policy*, Oxford: Berghahn Books.

Vireday, P. (2002) Are you a size friendly midwife? *Midwifery Today*, Spring: 28–32.

Wilkinson, R. and Pickett, K. (2010) *The Spirit Level, Why Equality Is Better for Everyone*, London: Penguin Books.

2

MACRONUTRIENTS IN PRECONCEPTION AND PERINATAL HEALTH

Anne Mullen, Colin R. Martin and Lorna Davies

Introduction

Food, food products and food metabolism are essential to the health of the developing foetus and the newborn. A macronutrient, as its name suggests, is a nutrient that is required in relatively large amounts for normal growth and development. The macronutrients, protein, fat and carbohydrate, represent the chemical compounds that not only are essential to life and homeostasis but, importantly, provide the vast majority of bulk energy – energy that necessarily must be stored, utilised and synthesised through complex processes of metabolism. A critical understanding of the properties of macronutrients is crucial to determining the role of these chemical compounds to development and growth, both *in utero* and following birth. The focus of this chapter is to describe the fundamental features of macronutrients and then to highlight their role in the metabolic process for women during the childbearing continuum.

Carbohydrates

The main function of carbohydrates is to supply energy for normal bodily functions and levels of physical activity. Because of their significant importance for effective cellular function, blood glucose levels must be kept relatively constant, and carbohydrates assist in the regulation of blood glucose. They also play a part in the breaking down of fatty acids, thus helping to avoid ketosis. Carbohydrates include a diverse range of foods within the diet, including sugars, cereals, breads, beans, potatoes, bran, rice, pasta and fruits.

In 1991, the Department of Health (DoH) produced the Dietary Reference Values for Food Energy and Nutrients for the UK that outlined the recommended nutritional intakes for the UK population within the framework of Dietary Reference Values (DRV). The document stated that 50 per cent of food energy should be from carbohydrate sources, with no more than 11 per cent from non-milk extrinsic sugars (NMES), which are sugars that are not present in the cellular structure of food, such as added sugar or honey (COMA, 1991). The Estimated Average Requirements (EARs) of energy for women throughout their life course are presented in Table 2.1.

Structure and metabolism

The molecular unit of the carbohydrate is the monosaccharide, which is a simple union of carbon, hydrogen and oxygen. The major dietary monosaccharides or simple sugars are

Table 2.1 Estimated Average Requirements (EARs) of energy for women

Age	EAR kcal/day
0–3 months	515
4–6 months	645
7–9 months	765
10–12 months	865
1–3 years	1165
4–6 years	1545
7–10 years	1740
11–14 years	1845
15–18 years	2110
19–50 years	1940
51–59 years	1900
60–64 years	1900
65–74 years	1900
75+ years	1810
Pregnancy (last trimester only)	+200
Lactation:	
1 month	+450
2 months	+530
3 months	+570
4–6 months (Group 1)	+480
4–6 months (Group 2)	+570
> 6 months (Group 1)	+240
> 6 months (Group 2)	+550

Source: Adapted from COMA (1991).

glucose, fructose (fruit sugar) and galactose (milk sugar). Monosaccharide units sometimes combine to form disaccharides. Disaccharides include sucrose (glucose + fructose), maltose (glucose + glucose) and lactose (glucose + galactose). Complex carbohydrates are defined as oligosaccharides or polysaccharides and are made of three or more linked saccharides. Oligosaccharides are chains of monosaccharides up to seven in length and polysaccharides are even longer chains. These form the 'starches' that are found in plant-based foods such as grains, root vegetable and legumes.

Another form of carbohydrate is derived from the non-starch polysaccharides (NSP) which are collectively known as dietary fibre. NSP may be soluble (fruits and vegetables, legumes and oats) or non-soluble (whole grains). The body does not have the enzymes that are required to break down dietary fibre into saccharides and so it passes through the body in an undigested state (Elias and Gibbons 2010). NSPs are required to regulate bowel function, increase satiety and control blood glucose levels.

The data elicited from the National Diet and Nutrition Survey (NDNS; Henderson *et al.*, 2003) found that the mean total carbohydrate intakes for women aged 19–64 formed 48.5 per cent of their total food energy. The survey results also identified that the mean intake of dietary added sugars for women aged 19–64 years was 11.9 per cent of food energy and the mean NSP intake for women in this age group was 12.6g; cereal and cereal products contributed about 45 per cent; potatoes and savoury snacks about 12 per cent; sugars, preserves and confectionary about 10 per cent and drinks about 11 per cent of carbohydrate intake. The recommended daily intake of NSP is 18g/day.

Glycaemic index and load

It may be useful at this stage to introduce the concepts of the glycaemic index (GI) and glycaemic load (GL). The concept of glycaemic index (GI) was developed by Jenkins *et al.* (1981) and has become a very popular tool in recent years, particularly in relation to the management of both type 1 and type 2 diabetes. In simple terms, the GI indicates how quickly and how high a particular food can raise blood glucose levels. A food with a low GI will typically prompt a moderate rise in blood glucose, while a food with a high GI may cause the blood glucose level to increase above the optimal level. Figure 2.1 shows the principle of how high and low GI foods relate to blood glucose. Table 2.2 shows glycaemic indices of common foods as measured by Jenkins *et al.* (1981). The glycaemic load (GL) is the product of the GI and carbohydrate content (g) divided by 100. A low GL ranges from 1 to 10; medium GL is 11–19; and a high GL has values of 20 or greater (McGowan and McAuliffe, 2010).

To understand more about the glycaemic index and how energy is derived from carbohydrate, as well as the other physiological functions of carbohydrates, we need to consider the digestion, absorption and utilisation of carbohydrates in the body.

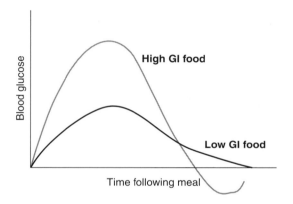

Figure 2.1 Glycemic index of Jenkins *et al.* (1981)

Table 2.2 Glycemic indices (GI) of commonly consumed foods

Food	GI
Bread, white	69
Bread, wholemeal	72
Rice, white	66
Rice, brown	72
Potatoes, new	70
Carrots	92
Beans, baked, tinned	40
Milk, whole	34
Apple, Golden Delicious	39
Banana	62
Glucose	100
Sucrose	59
Fructose	20

In humans, the digestion of carbohydrates begins in the mouth with the action of salivary amylase enzyme breaking down food during mastication. In the stomach, the digestion of carbohydrates is mechanical (the churning motions of the stomach) and chemical (hydrochloric acid produced by the parietal cells of the stomach), and much of the polysaccharide and oligosaccharide is broken down into shorter-chain dextrins. Salivary amylase is inactivated by the pH of the stomach. The digestion of carbohydrates largely occurs in the upper small intestine. Chyme (the acidic fluid generated from gastric juices and partly digested food) enters the duodenum through the constricted pyloric sphincter muscle of the stomach under high pressure. The pancreas liberates its enzymes into the duodenum and the acidic pH of the stomach contents neutralises the buffering effect of sodium bicarbonate, activating pancreatic amylase, which continues the process of hydrolysing the bonds between glycosidic residues. The brush border membrane enzymes, along with the microvilli – hair-like projections of the jejunum and ileum – complete the digestion of carbohydrate by the cells of the intestine. Glucose is absorbed across the enterocyte, or gut cell, in a sodium-dependent manner. Fructose is absorbed without sodium dependence. Monosaccharides and disaccaharides enter the portal vein after food has been ingested, and leakage of glucose from the portal vein causes a rise in glucose concentration, typically peaking 15–30 minutes after the consumption of carbohydrate. Insulin secretion from the B-cells of the pancreas is stimulated by cellular glucose sensing, and thus the peak of insulin, postprandially, closely follows that of glucose. Glucose may be stored in the liver and skeletal muscle as glycogen. The reserve in the liver is largely used for maintaining blood sugar levels, whilst the stores in skeletal muscle are used for energy.

Carbohydrate in pregnancy and the perinatal period

Focus on: glycaemic index

Carbohydrate derived from the maternal diet and hepatic stores provides significant energy for intrauterine growth (Moses et al., 2006). All pregnancies result in a degree of altered metabolism, and a dynamic state exists whereby the woman can become resistant to the uptake of ingested fuel such that the developing foetus benefits. Insulin secretion doubles throughout the course of pregnancy, and insulin resistance appears to be a normal physiological response whereby maternal glucose uptake is compromised to allow for uptake by the growing baby. However, the state of insulin resistance is a subtle mechanism, and if equilibrium is not achieved the pathophysiological condition of 'gestational diabetes' can result, causing sustained maternal hyperglycemia, which increases the risk of macrosomia and neonatal hypoglycaemia. Parretti et al. (2001), as reviewed by McGowan and McAuliffe (2010), have demonstrated that when a woman has blood glucose levels outside the normal range expected in pregnancy, her baby may lay down excessive fat cells in utero that may lead to increased adiposity throughout life. Macrosomia is related to higher risk of adverse obstetric and neonatal outcomes, and babies that are other than those who are constitutionally large for gestational age (LGA) may be at greater risk of childhood obesity and obesity-related adult diseases such as cardiovascular disease, type 2 diabetes and hypertension (McGowan and McAuliffe, 2010). GI has been recognised as having a role in the management of maternal plasma glucose concentrations and, hence, regulation of energy supply to the intrauterine environment in the less controlled metabolic state of late pregnancy.

Moses et al. (2006) randomised 70 healthy pregnant women to either a high GI or low GI diet comprised of 55 per cent energy from carbohydrate and 30 per cent energy from fat. Although there was no difference in weight gain between the groups of mothers, babies born to women in the high GI group tended to be heavier. A significantly higher proportion of babies born to women on the high GI diet were LGA and had a significantly higher ponderal index (measure of body fatness) compared to the babies of women on the low GI diet. There was no effect of the low GI on the proportion of those within the accepted weight range at birth or those born small for gestational age. The ROLO study (Walsh *et al.*, 2012) randomised 800 women believed to have babies that were LGA to either receive a lower GI dietary advice or standard antenatal care. There was no significant difference between birth weight or ponderal index among the babies, and no significant difference in the incidence of LGA delivery. The rate of glucose intolerance was significantly lower among women in the intervention arm. Scholl *et al.* (2004) investigated associations between dietary GI and neonatal growth amongst 1082 women from a relatively deprived urban background in the United States. In this study, women in the lowest 20 per cent of GI were associated with reduced infant birth weight and were twice as likely to give birth to a growth-restricted baby. High GI did not affect birth weight in this study. However, in a study where the Danish National Birth Cohort data were used (Knudsen *et al.*, 2006), there were no discernible differences in the birth weights of babies born to mothers who had taken diets within a broad GI range.

Fat

Gram for gram, fats can be viewed as the most efficient source of food energy providing, 9g of energy per gram of fat. We would need to consume a large amount of carbohydrate or protein in order to produce the same amount of energy. Fats provide insulation and assist in thermoregulation. They also assist in the absorption of fat-soluble vitamins, which prevents deficiencies of these vitamins. The slower metabolism of fat means that it increases satiety and staves hunger (Cecil *et al.*, 1999). There is some evidence that suggests that the orosensory stimulation of fat in the diet may activate β-endorphin neurons, which promotes β-endorphin release (Matsumura *et al.*, 2012) This may stimulate a 'feel good' effect, which may in turn reduce food cravings.

Structure and metabolism

There are three types of fatty acids: short chain fatty acids (SCFA), which are water soluble; medium chain fatty acids (MCFA), which are not a common feature of diet; and long chain fatty acids (LCFA), which are of most pertinence to the human diet. Fatty acids with single bonds between all carbons are called saturated fatty acids (SFA). These fatty acids tend to be solid at room temperature and are, more often than not, of animal origin, such as butter and lard. Fatty acids with one double bond in the carbon chain are called monounsaturated fatty acids (MUFA) and food sources for these include avocado, nuts and seeds, olives and the oils derived from them (Figure 2.2). These fatty acids tend to confer relative liquidity to the food product at room temperature but become cloudy when refrigerated. It is believed that foods containing monounsaturated fats may have the ability to reduce low-density lipoprotein (LDL) cholesterol and to increase high-density lipoprotein (HDL) cholesterol. However, this currently remains a subject of debate.

Fatty acids with more than one double bond in the carbon chain are called polyunsaturated fatty acids (PUFA). In a natural state these remain liquid even when refrigerated. When polyunsaturated fatty acids in the form of vegetable oil are partially hydrogenated or

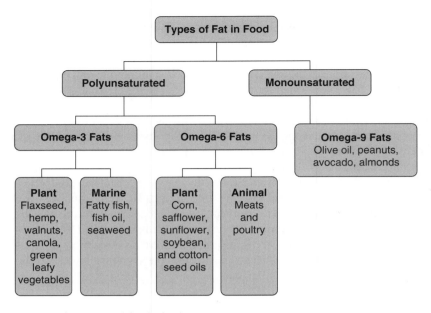

Figure 2.2 Types of unsaturated fats in food

'hardened' during industrial processing to create spreads such as margarine or cooking fats for deep-frying, this leads to the formation of trans-fats. It is hypothesised that trans-fats raise the levels of LDLs and lower levels of HDLs. There are also naturally occurring trans-fats which are found in some animal products, including butter, cheese and meat, and some trans-fats are also formed during high-temperature cooking. The roles of fats and fatty acids in human health have recently been reviewed by a Food and Agricultural Organisation expert consultation (FAO, 2010). The report from the consultation concludes that there is increasing evidence that partially hydrogenated vegetable oils are related to an increase in coronary heart disease, and that there is an association with metabolic syndrome components and diabetes. These fats are most commonly found in highly processed manufactured foods, including biscuits, ice-cream and snack foods and fast foods such as burgers, but are not commonly found in food in the EU and the UK because of strict legislation.

The Committee on Medical Aspects of Food, in the DRV report, recommend that adults in the UK consume no more than 35 per cent of dietary energy from fat, with no more than 11 per cent from saturated, 13 per cent from monounsaturated and 6.5 per cent from polyunsaturated fats (Department of Health, 1991). The recommendation for trans-fats is no more than 2 per cent. The NDNS published the intake of fats among the UK population and indicated that women aged 19 to 64 were receiving 34.9 per cent of food energy from fats (Henderson *et al.*, 2003). Saturated fat represented 13.2 per cent of the total food energy for women; monounsaturated represented 11.5 per cent; n-3 PUFA (omega-3) 1 per cent; n-6 PUFA (omega-6) 5.3 per cent and trans-fats 1.2 per cent.

The digestion of fat in humans begins in the stomach with mechanical digestion. The pancreas produces lipase and co-lipase enzymes, buffered in sodium bicarbonate, which enter the digestive tract at the duodenum in response to cholecystokinin (CCK). The secretion of bile from the gall bladder has a detergent effect, emulsifying fats and creating fine lipid droplets called micelles. The micelles diffuse across the brush border membrane and within the enterocyte are repackaged into the lipoprotein particle called the chylomicron (CM). The CM enters the lymphatic circulation and manifests in the circulation 3–6 hours postprandially as the lymphatic system drains into the subclavian vein. CM delivers fat and apolipoproteins (proteins that bind to lipids) to extra-hepatic tissue, before being assimilated by the liver as the CM remnant, and subsequent repackaging of fats and apolipoproteins as low-density lipoproteins.

Fats in pregnancy and the perinatal period

Fats play a significant role during pregnancy as an available energy source. Fats provide the fat-soluble vitamins A, D, E and K and polyunsaturated fats (particularly linoleic acid and n-3 PUFA (omega-3) fat and alpha-linoleic acid, an n-3 PUFA (omega-6 fat) that are necessary for foetal growth and development. Polyunsaturated fats are essential in the production of eicosanoids, which are hormone-like substances that play a significant role in homeostasis. They are of particular significance in the childbearing continuum, as they help to maintain blood pressure and haemostasis and may therefore play a part in pregnancy induced hypertension and post-partum haemorrhage (Olafsdottir *et al.*, 2006).

Focus on: long chain omega-3 polyunsaturated fatty acids

In a review on lipid metabolism in pregnancy, Ghio *et al.* (2011) stated that from 12 weeks' gestation, phospholipid, cholesterol and, particularly, triglyceride concentrations increase, providing fuel and building material for the developing foetus. Although absolute concentrations of the long chain n-3 PUFA fatty acids increase in the maternal plasma pool, relative concentrations of other fatty acids decrease (Larqué *et al.*, 2012). This depletion in maternal n-3 PUFA is probably due to selective maternal–foetal transfer of these fatty acids across the placenta for the visual and neuronal development of the foetus (Larqué *et al.*, 2012). Both omega-3 and omega-6 appear to play a role in preventing hypertension and in controlling haemostasis, and low levels during pregnancy are associated with preterm birth. There is evidence to suggest that a diet rich in seafood, and in particular oily fish, may result in fewer preterm births (Olsen *et al.*, 2007; Fei *et al.*, 2007). However, this information has been shadowed by warnings about the high methylmercury levels found in fish, with the potential for poor cognitive development in children. Such information led to recommendations in the USA that women should eat no more than 340g of fish per week (Food and Drug Administration, 2004). However, more recently it has been contested that consumption of seafood by women in pregnancy above 340g per week offered beneficial effects on child development and that advice to reduce intake could therefore be ill founded (Hibbeln *et al.*, 2007).

However, in practice the evidence is not strong enough to warrant a recommendation, and a role for n-3 PUFA in optimising a child's cognitive development is not currently supported by evidence (Mozurkewich and Klemens, 2012). Women who are concerned about increasing their seafood intake may be advised to supplement with omega-3 during pregnancy, as this may contribute to a reduction in premature birth and to higher birth weight, as well as potentially offering an immunological effect towards reducing food allergy risk (Larqué *et al.*, 2012; Mozurkewich and Klemens, 2012).

Protein

Protein, like carbohydrates and fats, is an energy source, but is a source that is used sparingly by the body in order to preserve this macronutrient for its many other specialist roles. In the body the amino acids are used to make new proteins, to convert into hormones such as adrenalin and to play a crucial part in maintaining the structural integrity of muscle, bone and connective tissue. Protein additionally safeguards the constancy of fluid balance within the body, which promotes homeostasis. Many of the foods that we eat contain protein, particularly flesh foods (chicken, beef, lamb and fish) and legumes like beans and lentils (Table 2.3)

Structure and metabolism

When proteins are digested they release amino acids, which are the molecular units of protein. There are 20 amino acids, and 9 of these are thought to be essential. Animal sources are understood to contain all of the amino acids, although plant sources are never fully complemented with all of these. As Table 2.3 illustrates, the protein content of plant-based foods is significantly lower than that of animal sources. This has implications for non-meat eaters, which are discussed in Chapter 7. The body appears to gather the amino acids over a 24-hour period and uses the amino acids as required.

The combustion of protein yields 4kcal per gram. The Committee on Medical Aspects of Food, in the 1991 DRVs (COMA, 1991), recommends a series of Reference Nutrient Intake (RNI) for proteins, presented in Table 2.4.

It is widely accepted that intakes of protein in the UK are adequate and above the RNIs. The NDNS (Henderson *et al.*, 2003) mentioned above indicated that average intake among women in the UK aged 19 and over was 63.7g/day.

Protein digestion begins in the stomach, where pepsinogen is converted to pepsin by the action of hydrochloric acid. Pancreatic enzymes secreted into the duodenum are trypsin, chymotrypsin and carboxypeptidases. These enzymes continue the breakdown and, as a result, most proteins are already reduced to a single amino acid or peptides of several amino acids

Table 2.3 Protein content of foods

Food	Protein (g)
1 grilled chicken breast (160g)	39.6
1 grilled lean beef fillet steak (135g)	38.2
1 can tuna in spring water (90g)	25.3
1 grilled pork leg steak (80g)	19.3
1 cup reduced fat milk (260ml)	9.1
1/4 can boiled red kidney beans (100g)	8.4
Tofu (100g)	8.1
1 pot plain, low fat yoghurt (150g)	7.2
1 boiled egg (50g)	6.4
1/4 can baked beans in tomato sauce (100g)	4.2
1 slice multigrain bread (45g)	3.6
1 slice white bread (40g)	3.1
10 almonds (10g)	2.5
2cm cube Edam cheese (10g)	2.1

Source: www.nutritionfoundation.org.nz/nutrition-facts/protein.

Table 2.4 Recommended a Reference Nutrient Intake (RNI) for proteins (adapted from the DRVs for protein)

Age	RNI g/day
0–3 months	12.5
4–6 months	12.7
7–9 months	13.7
10–12 months	14.9
1–3 years	14.5
4–6 years	19.7
7–10 years	28.3
11–14 years	41.2
15–18 years	45.0
19–50 years	45.0
50+ years	46.5
Pregnancy	+6
Lactation:	
0–4 months	+11
> 4 months	+8

Source: Adapted from the website of the Glaycaemic Index Foundation, www.gisymbol. com.au/aboutGI.php#5.

before they are absorbed in the small intestine. The small intestine itself takes about 90 per cent of glutamate and aspartate for its own use, which is called 'first pass metabolism'. The liver removes about two-thirds of amino acids absorbed and the other one-third reach peripheral tissue, including skeletal muscle, where they are an important source of energy and used for biosynthesis of other amino acids and proteins. The absorption rates of individual amino acids are highly dependent on the protein source. For milk proteins, about 50 per cent of the ingested protein is absorbed between the stomach and the jejunum and 90 per cent is absorbed by the time the digested food reaches the ileum.

Protein during pregnancy and postnatally

The requirement for dietary protein in pregnancy increases to accommodate the need for the tissue growth of both mother and baby.

Focus on: low-protein diets

The foetus has a remarkable capacity for adaptation to the *in utero* environment. The work of Godfrey and Barker (2001) and others has led to the concept of the foetal origins of adult disease, whereby restricted *in utero* conditions will induce adaptive mechanisms of the growing foetus, in which tissues such as the brain is spared at the expense of the trunk and abdominal viscera (Gallagher *et al.*, 2005). This programming *in utero* may predispose to chronic disease in adulthood. Godfrey and Barker (2001) associated low birth weight with increased rates of coronary heart disease.

Animal studies have shown that protein-restricted diets are associated with the development of hypertension and other cardiovascular risk factors in adulthood (Gao *et al.*, 2012) and that an inverse relationship exists between maternal protein intake and foetal fat deposition

(Sørensen *et al.*, 2008). Blumfield *et al.* (2012) analysed diets from 179 Australian women and measured foetal body composition. They found that low protein intake was associated with abdominal fat deposition in the neonate, and concluded that maternal macronutrient intake may play a role in the baby's risk of adult disease. Although low-protein diets are not a common feature of the Western diet, a number of population groups may be at risk, due to chronically low intakes of protein-rich foods.

Conclusion

This chapter has demonstrated the relevance, importance and impact of macronutrients for the developing foetus and the newborn baby. Some issues relating to preconception in terms of macronutrients have also been addressed. Understanding the role of carbohydrate, protein and the types of fats and the complexity of the interactions between these food components is important for midwives and other health professionals so that they are able to emphasise the subsequent impact on developmental processes. Against a background of complex metabolic processes, the role of macronutrients as the most quantitatively significant component of dietary intake cannot be underestimated. Consequently, the necessity for an appreciation of these food components and their underlying mechanisms of metabolism by midwives and others cannot be understated. Irrespective of their health profession, there is the potential for all those involved caring for women using the maternity services to be further empowered through their engagement and understanding of the contribution of macronutrients to health, well-being and normal development of the foetus.

References

Blumfield, M.L., Hure, A.J., Macdonald-Wicks, L., Smith, R. and Collins, C.E. (2012) Systematic review and meta-analysis of energy and macronutrient intakes during pregnancy in developed countries. *Nutritional Reviews* 70 (6): 322–336.

Cecil, J.E., Francis, J. and Read, N.W. (1999) Comparison of the effects of a high-fat and high-carbohydrate soup delivered orally and intragastrically on gastric emptying, appetite, and eating behaviour. *Physiology & Behavior*, 67: 299–306.

COMA (1991) *Report on Health and Social Subjects 41Dietary Reference Values (DRVs) for Food Energy and Nutrients for the UK*, Report of the Panel on DRVs of the Committee on Medical Aspects of Food Policy (COMA) 1991. London. The Stationery Office.

Department of Health (1991) *Dietary Reference Values for Food Energy and Nutrients for the United Kingdom*. London. HMSO.

Elias, S. and Gibbons, M. (2010) Nutritional foundation for pregnancy, childbirth and breastfeeding. In Pairman, S., Tracy, S., Thorogood, C. and Pincombe, J. (Eds) *Midwifery Preparation for Practice*, 2nd edition. Australia. Elsevier, pp. 415–430.

Fei, X., Holzman, C., Rahbar, M.H., Trosko, K. and Fischer, L. (2007) Maternal fish consumption, mercury levels, and risk of preterm delivery. *Environmental Health Perspectives* 115 (1): 42–47.

Food and Agricultural Organisation (FAO) (2010) *Fats and Fatty Acids in Human Nutrition. Report of an Expert Consultation*. Rome. FAO.

Food and Drug Administration (2004) What you need to know about mercury in fish and shellfish (Online) Available at: www.gov/downloads/Food/ResourcesForYou/Consumers/UCM182158.pdf [accessed 21 February 2013].

Gallagher, E.A., Newman, J.P., Green, L.R. and Hanso, M.A. (2005) The effect of low protein diet in pregnancy on the development of brain metabolism in rat offspring. *Journal of Physiology* 568 (2): 553–558.

Gao, H., Yallampalli, U. and Yallampalli, C. (2012) Gestational protein restriction reduces expression of Hsd17b2 in rat placental labyrinth. *Biology of Reproduction* 87 (3): 68.

Ghio, A., Bertolotto, A., Resi, V., Volpe, L. and Di Cianni, G. (2011) Triglyceride metabolism in pregnancy. *Advances in Clinical Chemistry* 55: 133–53.

Godfrey, K.M. and Barker, D.J. (2001) Fetal programming and adult health. *Public Health Nutrition* 4 (2B): 611–624.

Henderson, L., Gregory, J., Irving, K. and Swan, G. (2003) *The National Diet and Nutrition Survey: Adults aged 19 to 64 years*. Vol. 2. *Energy, Protein, Carbohydrate, Fat and Alcohol Intake*. London. The Stationery Office.

Hibbeln, J.R., Davis, J.M., Steer, C., Emmett, P., Rogers, I. *et al.* (2007) Maternal seafood consumption in pregnancy and neurodevelopmental outcomes in childhood (ALSPAC study): an observational cohort study. *Lancet* 369 (9561): 578–85.

Jenkins, D.J., Wolever, T.M., Taylor, R.H., Barker, H., Fielden, H. *et al.* (1981) Glycemic index of foods: a physiological basis for carbohydrate exchange. *American Journal of Clinical Nutrition* 34 (3): 362–366.

Knudsen, V.K., Orozova-Bekkevold, I.M., Mikkelsen, T.B., Wolff, S. and Olsen, S.F. (2008) Major dietary patterns in pregnancy and fetal growth. *European Journal of Clinical Nutrition*, 62, 463–470; doi:10.1038/sj.ejcn.1602745; published online 28 March 2007.

Larqué, E., Gil-Sánchez, A., Prieto-Sánchez, M.T. and Koletzko, B. (2012) Omega 3 fatty acids, gestation and pregnancy outcomes. *British Journal of Nutrition* 107 (Suppl. 2): S77-S84.

Matsumura, S., Eguchi, A., Okafuji, Y., Tatsu, S., Mizushige, T. *et al.* (2012) Dietary fat ingestion activates Œ≤-endorphin neurons in the hypothalamus. *Federation of the European Biochemical Societies Letters* 586: 1231–1235.

McGowan, C.A. and McAuliffe, F.M. (2010) The influence of maternal glycaemia and dietary glycaemic index on pregnancy outcome in healthy mothers. *British Journal of Nutrition* 104 (2): 153–159.

Moses, R.G., Luebcke, M., Davis, W.S., Coleman, K.J., Tapsell, L.C. *et al.* (2006) Effect of a low-glycemic-index diet during pregnancy on obstetric outcomes. *American Journal of Clinical Nutrition* 84 (4): 807–812.

Mozurkewich, E.L. and Klemens, C. (2012) Omega-3 fatty acids and pregnancy: current implications for practice. *Current Opinion in Obstetrics and Gynaecology* 24 (2): 72–77.

Olafsdottir, A.S., Skuladottir, G.V., Thorsdottir, I., Hauksson, A., Thorgeirsdottir, H. and Steingrimsdottir, L. (2006) Relationship between high consumption of marine fatty acids in early pregnancy and hypertensive disorders in pregnancy. *BJOG: An International Journal of Obstetrics and Gynecology* 113: 301–9.

Olsen, S.F., Østerdal, M.L., Salvig, J.D., Weber, T., Tabor, A. and Secher, N.J. (2007) Duration of pregnancy in relation to fish oil supplementation and habitual fish intake: a randomized clinical trial with fish oil, *European Journal of Clinical Nutrition* 61 (8): 976–985.

Scholl, T.O., Chen, X., Khoo, C.S. and Lenders, C. (2004) The dietary glycemic index during pregnancy: influence on infant birth weight, fetal growth, and biomarkers of carbohydrate metabolism. *American Journal of Epidemiology* 159 (5): 467–474.

Sørensen, A., Mayntz, D., Raubenheimer, D. and Simpson, S.J. (2008) Protein-leverage in mice: the geometry of macronutrient balancing and consequences for fat deposition. *Obesity* 16 (3): 566–571.

Walsh, J.M., McGowan, C.A., Mahony, R., Foley, M.E. and McAuliffe, F.M. (2012) Low glycaemic index diet in pregnancy to prevent macrosomia (ROLO study): randomized control trial. *British Medical Journal* 30 August, 345:e5605.

3

MICRONUTRIENTS IN PREGNANCY AND LACTATION

Anne Mullen, Colin R. Martin and Jade Wratten

Introduction

Micronutrients include vitamins and minerals and, as their name suggests, are small in both size and the amounts required by the body to function. Whilst macronutrients yield energy, micronutrients do not; they assist with regulating growth and facilitating the release of energy. In pregnancy, micronutrients nourish the mother and are responsible for vital life processes such as DNA synthesis and cell division. It is worth noting that conditions and diseases that occur later in life such as diabetes, obesity and cardiovascular disease may actually originate from, or at the very least be influenced by, the nutrition the fetus receives *in utero* (Barker, 1994). Ensuring a diet which adequately meets micronutrient requirements during pregnancy is therefore of utmost importance for pregnant women, their children and all future generations. It is true that requirements for micronutrients increase during pregnancy; however, in general so does the body's ability to meet these requirements, as physiological adaptations will occur in the pregnant woman to meet most of the increased need.

Understanding how specific micronutrients work within the body during pregnancy and lactation is valuable for midwives and health professionals; however, individuals eat food, not micronutrients, and so, whilst acknowledging micronutrients and their role, one must appreciate that they are only one part in the complex array of factors contributing to one's nutrition. Micronutrients also do not work alone or in isolation; their reactions and interactions within the body are complex and influenced by the many complexities of the human body, where they create a synergy that is not possible with isolated supplementation. Therefore the consumption of foods is generally much better than supplementation. It should be noted too that toxicity is rare from food consumption and is much more likely to occur from ingesting supplements. Pregnant and lactating women will therefore benefit from holistic individualised information based on the midwife's sound knowledge of micronutrients and the part they play in a well-balanced diet. This chapter will focus on micronutrients and their role in pregnancy and lactation, highlighting some of the more relevant nutrients, along with the consequences that can occur if required intakes are not met or are met in excess. Particular foods rich in the specific nutrients will be discussed and shown in the relevant tables within the chapter.

Classifications of micronutrients

How specific nutrients are absorbed, transported, utilised, stored and excreted in the body can give us more clues about them. We may generally be able to state how frequently they are required by the body, whether supplements can be toxic or not and what particular types of foods the nutrients may come from by grouping them. This can be achieved by classifying vitamins into either water- or fat-soluble vitamins. To review, water-soluble vitamins are consumed and enter the bloodstream where they freely move about and enter cells where they are required. The kidneys filter the blood for excess vitamins and excrete this excess in urine. In comparison, fat-soluble vitamins require a carrier and are transported into the lymph and then into the blood stream. Once in the blood stream, they are stored in the liver or in the adipose of the individual, where they can be used where and when required. Fat-soluble vitamins therefore will not be required to be consumed as frequently as water-soluble vitamins; also, because these vitamins are stored, excessive levels have the potential to become toxic. Fat-soluble vitamins include vitamins A, E, D and K and are contained generally and broadly within foods that contain fats and oils. Water-soluble vitamins include vitamin C and eight B vitamins: thiamin (B1), riboflavin (B2), niacin (B3), B6, B12, biotin, pantothenic acid and folate. Deficiencies of water-soluble vitamins can develop after only a few days of no intake, and generally speaking these vitamins can be found in more watery foods and substances such as fruits and vegetables. Foods-containing water soluble vitamins need to be handled and cooked with extreme care, as the vitamins can be damaged in the process of cooking. Consuming raw foods or a vegetable added to pre-boiled water and cooked quickly at moderate temperatures is ideal, as compared to prolonged cooking.

Minerals are naturally formed chemical elements. Major minerals include calcium, chloride, phosphorus, potassium, magnesium, sodium and sulphate, with trace minerals being chromium, copper, fluoride, iron, iodine, manganese, molybdenum, selenium and zinc (Whitney and Rolfes, 2008). Minerals themselves are not damaged by cooking; however, the mineral can leach out into the water during cooking, or from cast iron cookware, and therefore saving the water for reuse in cooking can be beneficial for maximum nutrient absorption.

Vitamin A

Vitamin A is a fat-soluble vitamin which is involved in growth, reproduction, immunity and for healthy eyes and vision, with a deficiency resulting in a failure to see in dim light (Thurnham, 2007). Vitamin A is complex and not simply made up from one compound, but of many retinoid and carotenoid compounds. Retinol, retinal and retinyl esters are found in foods of animal origin, whereas carotenoids, including beta-carotene, alpha-carotene, lycopene and lutein, are found mainly in plant sources. Retinol is readily absorbed in the human intestine, but carotenoid absorption is relatively low (Harrison, 2005), highlighting that deficiencies occur more frequently in those individuals who do not consume meat. A recent report showed that 12 per cent of the New Zealand female population over the age of 15 years had inadequate consumptions of vitamin A (Ministry of Health, 2011). A deficiency of vitamin A in pregnancy is related to stillbirths (Thurnham, 2007). Vitamin A is found in foods such as cod liver oil, liver, red meat, milk, cheese, butter, fortified margarines and coloured fruits and vegetables such as tomatoes and carrots. Pregnant and lactating women are not recommended to take supplements of vitamin A unless they live in regions where deficiency and night blindness occur in more than 5 per cent of the population (McGuire, 2012). This is due to the risk of vitamin A toxicity, which can lead to serious problems in pregnancy such as spontaneous miscarriage and abnormalities of the fetus, including those of the central nervous system, brain, heart, kidneys and face such as cleft lip and palate (Ackermans et al., 2011; Thurnham, 2007). Whilst toxicity of vitamin A exists, it is very rare for this to occur from food sources, with the exception of the consumption of liver. As up to 80 per cent of an animal's total vitamin A is stored in the liver, direct consumption of animal livers could potentially be toxic. High intakes of carotenoids such as carrot and pumpkin can cause a yellow discolouration of the skin, but this is not associated with any toxic effects (Thurnham, 2007). Infants are born with low stores of the vitamin, whereas colostrum and early breast milk has a relatively high vitamin A content, although this is dependent on the mother's intake, highlighting lactating women's requirements for more vitamin A in their diet.

Vitamin D

Vitamin D is a fat-soluble vitamin which assists with calcium absorption, bone health, cell differentiation and muscle function (Ministry of Health, 2013) and is required for the development of the fetal skeleton, the formation of tooth enamel and general growth in pregnancy (Wagner *et al.*, 2012). However, physiological adaptions in pregnancy do result in calcium working independently of vitamin D (Kovacs, 2008), and whilst it is rare for deficiencies to occur *in utero* which affect the fetus, the vitamin D status of the newborn is directly reflective of the mother's. Breast milk, whilst being beneficial for health, is relatively low in vitamin D, and deficiencies in neonates and in children are serious and lead to rickets and impaired growth. Approximately one-third of all women of child-bearing age in New Zealand are reportedly deficient in vitamin D (Ministry of Health, 2013) and, whilst population statistics and the definitions of optimal levels vary, the deficiency is reportedly extensive also in other income-rich countries like United States and Great Britain (Wagner *et al.*, 2012). Exposure to the sun provides the human body with the majority of its required vitamin D, with dietary vitamin D accounting for less than 10 per cent of the circulating volume; however, consuming dietary sources of vitamin D is still important, especially in pregnancy and lactation. Vitamin D can be found in foods such as oily fish, dairy products, mushrooms and fortified margarine and cereals (Wagner *et al.*, 2012). Vitamin D deficiencies, whilst not new, may be influenced by current lifestyle factors which trend towards people being more obese, working and playing indoors and using skin cancer preventions such as sunscreen (Hollis and Wagner, 2004).

The National Institute for Health and Care Excellence (NICE) is currently working on evidence-based recommendations to reduce vitamin D deficiency, but recommends that women should be provided with information about achieving adequate vitamin D stores during pregnancy by their healthcare professionals at their booking appointment (NICE, 2013). There are several risk factors that midwives should be aware of which may indicate a lack of vitamin D. Risk factors include having darker skin, as the pigment makes it more difficult for sunlight to penetrate the skin; also the use of sunscreen; the season of the year; and the geographic location one lives in, with populations living further from the equator having lowered levels of vitamin D; having little outdoor exposure; and the wearing of protective or full clothing such as veils and burkas (Ministry of Health, 2013). Women who are obese also appear to have less circulating vitamin D. Pregnant women in the United Kingdom are recommended to take 10µg per day of vitamin D; however, only in New Zealand are women with risk factors offered a supplement, which is taken monthly. Recent research associates vitamin D insufficiency with a range of immune conditions and non-communicable chronic diseases such as cancer and cardiovascular disease (Tsiaras and Weinstock, 2011); also, a recent meta-analysis found that women who were vitamin D deficient were at greater risk of developing gestational diabetes (Poel *et al.*, 2012). Furthermore, a review by Harris (2011) provides evidence of an association between vitamin D deficiency and bacterial vaginosis among pregnant women. However, whether these studies warrant a universal supplement to all pregnant women remains questionable. A 2012 Cochrane review concluded that the current research around vitamin D does not provide consistent results and, whilst vitamin D supplementation is shown to increase vitamin D levels in pregnant women, no clear causal relationship has been found to implement routine supplementation (Ministry of Health, 2013; De-Regil *et al.*, 2012). Routine testing of vitamin D levels in pregnancy is also not recommended unless there is a concern over severe deficiency (Ministry of Health, 2013; Truswell, 2007).

Vitamin E

Vitamin E, also known as Tocopherol, meaning 'to bring forth offspring', was highlighted by scientists when rats on diets low in vitamin E could not produce live babies (Ministry of Health, 2006; Skeaff, 2007). Vitamin E is known as a powerful antioxidant and is believed to 'quench' free radicals that cause tissue damage, particularly around the cell membrane. Being fat soluble, vitamin E is stored in the adipose, although toxicity from dietary sources is not reported (Ministry of Health, 2006). Foods in general have an abundance of vitamin E available. Plant-based foods which are naturally high in fat, such as wheat germ and polyunsaturated oils are the best sources of vitamin E (Skeaff, 2007). Other foods which are good sources of vitamin E include butter and margarine, fruit, alfalfa, lettuce, potatoes, kumara and almonds (Ministry of Health, 2006).

Vitamin K

Vitamin K mainly found as phylloquinone (vitamin K1) is produced by bacteria in the gut and has a role in blood clotting. Vitamin K is absorbed from the intestine with the help of bile and is found in relatively high concentrations in the liver, heart and bone (Greer, 2010). The dietary reference values (DRVs), dietary sources, UK adult intakes and symptoms of deficiency of the fat-soluble vitamins are presented in Table 3.1. Food sources for vitamin K include green leafy vegetables, kale, spinach, Brussels sprouts, broccoli, parsley, coriander, mint, cabbage, lettuce, alfalfa, kelp, whole-grain cereals, olive oil, soybean, wheat bran, cheese and milk.

A baby's gut is sterile at birth. Babies are therefore born with low levels of vitamin K and can be at risk of vitamin K deficiency bleeding (VKDB), formerly known as Hemorrhagic Disease of the Newborn (HDN). Whilst this is a rare complication, women are offered the choice of giving their baby a dose of vitamin K after birth for prophylactic intervention of this disease, by either an oral or an injectable route. Breastfeeding provides babies with vitamin K, and the mother's levels are dependent on her consumption of vitamin K-rich foods; however, it is not thought that dietary intake alone would eradicate the risk of VKDB (Women's Health Action Trust, 2010; Shearer, Fu and Booth, 2012).

B vitamins

Micronutrients do not produce energy; however, the B group vitamins are largely involved with reactions associated with energy metabolism. This group of vitamins generally has a high turnover and excretion rate, which means that our bodies require daily intakes, otherwise deficiencies can occur. With this in mind, deficiencies in B group vitamins often indicate multiple micronutrient deficiencies and inadequate food intake (Truswell, 2007).

Table 3.1 DRVs, intakes, signs of deficiency and dietary sources and deficiency symptoms of fat-soluble vitamins for females in the UK

Micronutrient	DRVs (women 11–50+ years, including pregnancy; Department of Health, 1991)	UK adult intakes (women 19–64 years; Henderson et al., 2003)	Signs of deficiency	Good dietary sources
Vitamin A	11–50+ years = 600µg/day pregnancy +100µg/day	671µg/day	Night blindness, xerophthalmia	Liver, milk, margarine, eggs, carrots, sweet potatoes, pumpkin, kale, spinach (Harrison, 2005).
Vitamin D	Pregnancy = 10µg/day	2.8µg/day	Rickets, osteomalacia	Dairy products, oily fish, mushrooms, fortified foods.
Vitamin E	3mg/day (safe intake)	8.1mg/day	Neuropathy, myopathy	Vegetables oils and lipid–rich plant products (Wong and Radhakrishnan, 2012).
Vitamin K	10µg/day (safe intake)		Defective blood clotting	Green leafy vegetables, beef liver.

Toxicity of B vitamins is rare, as amounts in excess of requirements are filtered through the kidneys and excreted in the urine.

Thiamin (B1) is mandatorily fortified in breads and cereals in the United Kingdom, United States and Australia and can be found in whole grains, nuts, wheat germ, yeast, pork, duck and other meats (Truswell, 2007). Deficiencies are rare, are seen in alcoholics and lead to beri-beri or Wernicke-Korsakoff syndromes. These are potentially fatal conditions that do, however, respond rapidly to treatment (Truswell, 2007). Riboflavin is found in milk and milk products, eggs and yeast, but it should be noted that it is sensitive to ultraviolet light, which can destroy the vitamin. Ariboflavinosis is a deficiency in riboflavin which causes inflammation of the lining of the mouth and wasting of the tongue. Niacin, also known as vitamin B3, was found to be consumed in adequate amounts throughout the entire population in New Zealand and provided mostly by foods such as poultry, bread, meat, potatoes, kumara, taro, fish and seafood (Ministry of Health, 2011). Cereals and cereal products (many of which are fortified with B group vitamins), peanuts, brans, pulses and wholemeal wheat are also good sources (Truswell, 2007). A deficiency in niacin, although rare in developed countries, can lead to pellagra, a condition in which the skin is inflamed, peels and cracks, specifically around the neck, and results also in diarrhoea and dementia (Truswell, 2007). Vitamin B6 has a role in protein metabolism and also in the process of converting and releasing glucose from glycogen stores (Truswell, 2007). Good intake of vitamin B6 can be achieved by consuming fruits and vegetables, potatoes, kumara, taro, cereals and meats (Ministry of Health, 2011). A deficiency in vitamin B6 can cause symptoms such as weariness, weakness and impaired immunity. A deficiency was seen in 1953 when an error occurred in failing to include vitamin B6 in infant formula, resulting in infants convulsing (Truswell, 2007).

Folate

Folate is a B vitamin. Its name stems from the Latin word for 'leaf'. It is required in much greater amounts during pregnancy, as it is needed for the closure of the neural tube. As the name suggests, food sources include leafy vegetables such as spinach, broccoli, cabbage, lettuce and asparagus. Vitamin C assists with the absorption of folate from foods, although it is important to remember that, being a water-soluble vitamin, folate is susceptible to being destroyed by prolonged cooking and therefore requires careful handling. Other foods such as beans, beetroot, bran, peanuts, yeast, avocados, bananas, whole grains and eggs are also good sources of folate (Truswell, 2007). It would be difficult for women to receive all of the folate that they need in order to achieve suitable levels of folate during pregnancy; therefore supplementation with the synthetic folic acid is recommended to women, ideally before they conceive and continued until well after the neural tube has closed (24 to 28 days post conception). However, it is estimated that 40 per cent of pregnancies in the United Kingdom are unplanned. Wider mandatory folic acid fortification of flour and bread has therefore been considered extensively, but it has not been legislated in either the United Kingdom or New Zealand. Voluntary fortification is allowed and some manufacturers add folic acid to their breads and cereals. Mandatory fortification of folate into foods has occurred since 1998 in the USA and Canada. Interestingly, the dosage recommended is not universal and the daily amount varies in individual countries. For example, in the UK the recommended dose is 400μg/day, whilst in New Zealand it is 800μg daily.

Vitamin B12

Vitamin B12 is an essential vitamin with indirect roles for DNA, myelin and bone marrow synthesis and is involved with the processes in the body which release energy (Pawlak *et al.*, 2013). Vitamin B12 is produced by bacteria in the stomachs of animals is therefore found mostly in meat and offal, with smaller amounts also in fish, poultry, eggs, cheese, yogurt and shellfish. This highlights specific implications for vegetarian and vegan women and their breastfed infants. A deficiency in vitamin B12, known as pernicious anaemia, was found, in a review of the literature, to occur in 62 per cent of pregnant vegetarian women regardless of age, ethnicity and type of vegetarian diet (Pawlak *et al.*, 2013). Women who consume a vegetarian and vegan diet would benefit from biological tests to assess their status, with supplementation recommended if dietary B12 is inappropriate (see Chapter 7). Breastfed infants from vitamin B12-deficient mothers are likely to also be deficient in the vitamin, and this has the potential to lead to serious neurological complications, therefore supplementation may be warranted (Truswell, 2007). Absorption of the vitamin from supplements requires B12 activity that may be present in only 60 per cent of the vitamin consumed or, surprisingly, only 20 per cent of the likes of marketed sources such as Spirilina (Truswell, 2007).

Vitamin C

Vitamin C, also known as ascorbic acid, is a water-soluble vitamin. A deficiency can result in the condition of scurvy. Vitamin C is involved in many roles in the body, including the synthesis of collagen, converting dopamine to noradrenalin, aiding absorption of non-haem iron and as a general antioxidant (Skeaff, 2007). Many fruits and vegetables contain vitamin C, with citrus fruits being particularly good sources. Other foods, such as kiwifruit, tomatoes, fruit juices, strawberries, potatoes, kumara also contain vitamin C. Midwives will keep in mind that women who smoke cigarettes will have reduced vitamin C levels, indirectly leading to lowered absorption of iron. Vitamin C intakes for women in New Zealand are adequate, with an estimated only 1.3% of the population having inadequate intakes (Ministry of Health, 2013).

Table 3.2 DRVs, intakes, signs of deficiency and dietary sources and deficiency symptoms of water-soluble vitamins for females in the UK

Micronutrient	DRVs (women 11–50+ years, including pregnancy; Department of Health, 1991)	UK adult intakes (women 19–64 years; Henderson et al., 2003)	Symptoms of deficiency (Groff and Gropper, 2000)	Major dietary sources
Thiamin (Vitamin B1)	11–14 years = 0.7mg/day; 15–50+ years = 0.8mg/day; pregnancy = +0.1mg/day	1.54mg/day	Beri-beri, muscle weakness, anorexia, tachycardia	Cereals and cereal products (many of which are fortified with B group vitamins), meat, whole grains, nuts, wheat germ, yeast, pork, duck, vegetables such as cauliflower and spinach.
Riboflavin (Vitamin B2)	11–50+ years = 1.1mg/day; pregnancy = +0.3mg/day	1.6mg/day	Cheilosis, glossitis, hyperaemia and oedema of oral and pharyngeal mucus membranes	Cereals and cereal products (many of which are fortified with B group vitamins), meat and meat products, milk and dairy products.
Niacin (Vitamin B3)	11–14 years = 12mg/day; 15–18 years = 14mg/day; 19–50 years = 13mg/day; 50+ years = 12mg/day	30.9mg/day	Pellagra, diarrhoea, dermatitis, mental confusion, dementia	Cereals and cereal products (many of which are fortified with B group vitamins), meat, poultry, fish, yeast, peanuts, brans, pulses and wholemeal wheat (Truswell, 2007).
Pantothenic acid	3–7mg/day (safe intake)		Numbness and tingling of periphery, vomiting, fatigue	Widely distributed in foods.
Biotin	10–200µg/day (safe intake)		Anorexia, nausea, glossitis, depression, dermatitis	Kidneys, beans, legumes, peanut butter, breads and other whole-grain foods, dairy products, fish, mushrooms and yeast.
Folic acid	15–50+ years = 200µg/day; pregnancy = +100µg/day	251µg/day	Megaloblastic anaemia, diarrhoea, depression, fatigue, confusion	Cereal, green leafy vegetables such as broccoli, spinach, asparagus, lettuce.
Pyridoxine (Vitamin B6)	11–14 years = 1.0mg/day; 15–50+ years = 1.2mg/day	2.0mg/day	Dermatitis, glossitis, convulsions	Cereals and cereal products (many of which are fortified with B group vitamins), meat and meat products, vegetables.
Cobalamin (Vitamin B12)	11–14 years = 1.2µg/day; 15–50+ years = 1.5 µg /day	4.8µg/day	Megaloblastic anaemia, peripheral neuropathy, glossitis	Meat, fish, poultry, eggs, yogurt, cheese, yeasts, milk and milk products.
Ascorbic acid (Vitamin C)	11–14 years = 35mg/day; 15–50+ years = 40mg/day	81mg/day	Scurvy, loss of appetite, fatigue, impaired wound healing	Citrus fruit, kiwifruit, tomatoes, strawberries, potatoes, kumara.

Iodine

Iodine is a mineral required for thyroid growth and reproductive function. It is very important during pregnancy and lactation, as demands for iodine increase and iodine is required for normal growth and development of the fetus. Good food sources for iodine include seafood, fish, eggs, milk and iodised salt. Fish and freshly cooked seafood are important foods and ideally should be incorporated into a regular weekly dietary intake. Deficiencies in iodine are common, reflecting poor soil content of iodine, and thus poor iodine content of the food supplies in many countries. Deficiencies lead to swelling of the thyroid gland, as seen in goitre, and also can cause miscarriage, stillbirth, intellectual impairment, growth restriction, behavioural problems and; Leung, Pearce and Braverman, 2011). Since 1924, iodine has been added to salt in an attempt to reduce frequent deficiencies in the general population; it has been mandatorily added to bread in New Zealand since 2009. However, even with the compensatory mechanisms of pregnancy, where the body increases its ability to absorb nutrients, these additions are not meeting the increased needs of pregnant and lactating women; hence, in 2010 iodine supplementation was recommended by the New Zealand government for all women (Ministry of Health, 2010).

Iron

Iron is a trace mineral found mostly in haemoglobin in the red blood cells. Iron requirements increase in pregnancy to meet the needs of the growing fetus and to provide for optimal brain growth. However, it should be acknowledged that the body's ability to absorb iron in pregnancy also increases in response to this need. Dietary iron is vitally important for maintaining adequate levels and reducing the risk of iron-deficiency anaemia in pregnancy, which, however, needs to be distinguished from the normal physiological adaptation of haemodilution, which occurs as a normal response to increasing blood volume.

Iron absorption is greatly influenced by inhibitors or promoters. Inhibitors include substances such as coffee, and tannins in tea. Promoters of non-haem iron are vitamin C and meat. Iron can be classified as being either haem or non-haem. Haem iron is found mostly in meat and is protected by the haem molecules, so it is much less influenced by inhibitors, making it more absorbable. Non-haem iron is found in both plant and animal sources and is not as absorbable and is greatly influenced by inhibitors. Absorption can be increased by consuming non-haem iron with vitamin C and/or meat. Iron deficiency and iron-deficiency anaemia are different, with depleted iron stores making the individual deficient; however, anaemia occurs when the haemoglobin itself is deficient. In New Zealand iron supplements should be taken only once iron-deficiency anaemia is diagnosed (Ministry of Health, 2006). Side-effects occur frequently from iron supplementation, as supplements include large doses of iron in the knowledge that it will not all be absorbed. Iron overload and toxicity can occur from supplement overdose and can lead to abdominal pain, vomiting and acidosis.

Calcium

Calcium makes up about 90 per cent of the human skeleton and is needed from our diet for the maintenance of good bones and teeth. Calcium is also required for muscle contraction, nerve conductivity, blood clotting and hormonal release. Intake of calcium is required on a daily basis and food rich in calcium is predominately found in dairy products such as milk, cheese and yogurt and in soy. Calcium can also be found in leafy green vegetables, bread,

Table 3.3 DRVs, intakes, signs of deficiency and dietary sources and deficiency symptoms of minerals for females in the UK

Micronutrient	DRVs (women 11–50+ years, including pregnancy; Department of Health, 1991)	UK adult intakes (women 19–64 years; Henderson et al, 2003)	Symptoms of deficiency (Groff and Gropper, 2000)	Good dietary sources (Groff and Gropper, 2000)
Calcium	11–18 years = 800mg/day 19+ years = 700mg/day lactation = +550mg/day	809mg/day	Poor growth, osteomalacia, osteoporosis	Milk and dairy products, legumes, dried fruit.
Phosphorus	11–18 years = 625mg/day 19+ years = 550mg/day lactation = +440mg/day	1116mg/day	Neuromuscular and skeletal problems, osteomalacia	Milk and dairy products, meat and poultry, nuts, legumes.
Chloride	11+ years = 2500mg/day	3482mg/day	Dehydration and associated conditions	Salts, milk, meat, eggs.
Magnesium	11–14 years = 280mg/day 15–18 years = 300mg/day 19+ years = 290mg/day lactation = +50mg/day	233mg/day	Muscular weakness, tetany, convulsions, growth failure	Nuts, legumes, cereals, chocolate, seafood.
Potassium	11–14 years = 3100mg/day 15+ years = 3500mg/day	2655mg/day	Muscular weakness, arrythmia	Vegetables, fruit, dried fruit.
Sodium	11+ years = 1600mg/day	2303mg/day	Weight loss, poor growth, anorexia	Table salt, meat, dairy products, bread.
Iron	11–49 years = 14.8mg/day 50+ years = 8.7mg/day	11.6mg/day	Anaemia and related problems	Meat and meat products, green leafy vegetables, fortified cereal and cereal products.
Zinc	11–14 years = 9mg/day 14+ years = 7mg/day lactation (0–4mo) = +6mg/day lactation (4mo+) = +2.5mg/day	7.9mg/day	Impaired wound healing, poor growth and development	Oysters, liver, meat and poultry, whole grains.
Copper	11–14 years = 0.8mg/day 15–18 years = 1mg/day 19+ years = 1.2mg/day lactation = +0.3mg/day	1.07mg/day	Anaemia	Liver, whole grains, legumes, meat, fish.
Selenium	11–14 years = 45µg/day 14+ years = 60µg/day lactation = +15µg/day	45µg/day	Cardiac myopathy	Meat, poultry, fish, dairy products.
Iodine	11+ years = 140µg/day	167µg/day	Enlarged thyroid/goitre	Iodised salt, seafoods, liver, eggs.

nuts, seeds, dried fruit and canned fish. Deficiencies can lead to osteomalacia and osteoporosis in adults. Calcium supplementation has been shown in many studies to reduce premature birth, increase birth weight and reduce gestational hypertensive disorders in pregnancy, including pre-eclampsia (Hofmeyr, Lawrie, Atallah and Duley, 2010; Imdad and Bhutta, 2011; Ortega *et al.*, 1999); however the impact of supplementation is greatest in women with calcium deficiencies, highlighting the importance of a calcium-rich diet in pregnancy.

Summary

Understanding the complexities of specific micronutrients and their functions in the body during pregnancy and lactation is important for health professionals, and this is especially so for midwives. Micronutrients do not work in isolation and they form a synergy within the body when consumed in food. Generally, intake through food consumption is preferable to supplementation, and rarely leads to toxicity. However, folic acid and iodine are two supplements available to assist women to meet increased requirements that are not easily gained from the diet. The midwife and other healthcare professionals who are working with women during pregnancy will be further empowered further in their engagement and understanding of mothers-to-be, new mothers and their infants by an understanding of the contribution of micronutrients to health and well-being.

References

Ackermans, M.M., Zhou, H., Carels, C.E., Wagener, F.A. and Von den Hoff, J.W. (2011) Vitamin A and clefting: putative biological mechanisms. *Nutrition Review* 69 (10): 613–624.

Barker, D.J.P. (1994) *Mothers, Babies and Disease in Later Life*. London: BMJ Publishing Group.

Department of Health (1991) *Dietary Reference Values for Food Energy and Nutrients for the United Kingdom*. London: HMSO.

De-Regil, L.M., Palacios, C., Ansary, A., Kulier, R. and Peña-Rosas, J.P. (2012) *Vitamin D supplementation for women during pregnancy: A review*. The Cochrane Collaboration: Wiley Publishers.

Greer, F.R. (2010) Vitamin K the basics: what's new? *Early Human Development*, 86 (Suppl. 1): 43–47.

Groff, J.L. and Gropper, S.S. (2000) *Advanced Nutrition and Human Metabolism*, 3rd edn. London: Thomson Learning.

Harris, A.L. (2011) Vitamin D deficiency and bacterial vaginosis in pregnancy: examining the link. *Nursing and Women's Health*, 5 (5): 423–430.

Harrison, E.H. (2005) Mechanisms of digestion and absorption of dietary vitamin A. *Annual Review of Nutrition*, 25: 87–103.

Hathcock, J.N., Hattan, D.G., Jenkins, M.Y., McDonald, J.P., Sundaresan, P.R. *et al.* (1990) Evaluation of vitamin A toxicity. *American Journal of Clinical Nutrition*, 52 (2): 183–202.

Henderson, L., Gregory, J., Irving, K. and Swan, G. (2003) *The National Diet and Nutrition Survey: Adults aged 19 to 64 years*. Vol. 2. *Energy, Protein, Carbohydrate, Fat and Alcohol Intake*. London: The Stationery Office.

Hofmeyr, G.J., Lawrie, T.A., Atallah, A.N. and Duley, L. (2010) Calcium supplementation during pregnancy for preventing hypertensive disorders and related problems. *Cochrane Database of Systematic Reviews*, (8): CD001059.

Hollis, B.W. and Wagner, C.L. (2004) Assessment of dietary vitamin D requirements during pregnancy and lactation. *American Journal of Clinical Nutrition*, 79: 717–726.

Imdad, I. and Bhutta, Z.A. (2012) Effects of calcium supplementation during pregnancy on maternal, fetal and birth outcomes. *Paediatric and Perinatal Epidemiology*, 26 (Suppl. 1): 138–152.

Kovacs, C.S. (2008) Vitamin D in pregnancy and lactation: maternal, fetal and neonatal outcomes from human and animal studies. *The American Journal of Clinical Nutrition*, 88: 520S–528S.

Leung, A.M., Pearce, E.N. and Braverman, L.E. (2011) Iodine nutrition in pregnancy and lactation. *Endocrinology and Metabolism Clinics of North America*, 40 (4): 765–777. DOI: 10.1016/j.ecl.2011.08.001.

McGuire, S. (2012) WHO guideline: vitamin A supplementation in pregnant women. *American Society of Nutrition Advanced Nutrition*, 3: 215–216, DOI: 10.3945/an.111.001701.

Ministry of Health (2006) *Food and Nutrition Guidelines for Health: Pregnant and Breastfeeding Women: A Background Paper*. Wellington, NZ: Ministry of Health.

Ministry of Health (2011) *A Focus on Nutrition: Key Findings of the 2008/09 New Zealand Adult Nutrition Survey*. Wellington, NZ: Ministry of Health.

Ministry of Health (2013) *Companion Statement on Vitamin D and Sun Exposure in Pregnancy and Infancy in New Zealand*. Wellington, NZ: Ministry of Health.

NICE (National Institute for Health and Care Excellence) (2013) Vitamin D: implementation of existing guidance to prevent deficiency draft scope for consultation 7 January –1 February 2013. *(Online)* Available from: http://guidance.nice.org.uk/PHG/71 [accessed 23 April 2013].

Ortega, R.M., Martinez, R.M., Lopez-Sobaler, A.M., Andres, P. and Quintas, M.E. (1999) Influence of calcium intake on gestational hypertension. *Annals of Nutrition and Metabolism*, 42: 37–46.

Pawlak, R., Parrott, S.J., Raj, S., Cullum-Dugan, S. and Lucus, D. (2013) How prevalent is vitamin B12 deficiency among vegetarians? *Nutrition Reviews*, 71 (2): 110–117.

Poel, Y.H., Hummel, P., Lips, P., Stam, F. and van der Ploeg, T. (2012) Vitamin D and gestational diabetes: a systematic review and meta-analysis. *European Journal of Internal Medicine*, 23 (5): 465–469.

Scientific Advisory Committee on Nutrition (2005) *Review of Dietary Advice on Vitamin A*. London: The Stationery Office.

Shearer, M.J., Fu, X. and Booth, S.L. (2012) Vitamin K nutrition, metabolism, and requirements: current concepts and future research. *American Society of Nutrition Advanced Nutrition*, 3: 182–195. DOI:10.3945/an.111.001800.

Skeaff, M. (2007) Vitamins C and E. In: Mann, J. and Truswell, S.A. (eds), *Essentials of Human Nutrition* (pp. 201–222). New York: Oxford University Press.

Thurnham, D.I. (2007) Vitamin A and carotenoids. In: Mann, J. and Truswell, S.A. (eds), *Essentials of Human Nutrition*. New York: Oxford University Press.

Trusswell, S. (2007) The B vitamins. In Mann, J. and Truswell, S.A. (eds) *Essentials of Human Nutrition*. New York: Oxford University Press.

Tsiaras, W.G. and Weinstock, M.A. (2011) Factors influencing vitamin D status. *ActaDermato Venereologica*, 91 (2): 115–124.

Wagner, C.L., Taylor, S.N., Dawodu, A., Johnson, D.D. and Hollis, B.W. (2012) Vitamin D and its role during pregnancy in attaining optimal health of mother and fetus. *Nutrients*, 4 (3): 208–230.

Whitney, E. and Rolfes, S.R. (2008) *Understanding Nutrition*. (11th ed.). CA: Thomson Wadsworth.

Women's Health Action Trust (2010) Vitamin K. Does My Baby Need It? Information for Parents. *(Online)* Available from: www.womens-health.org.nz [accessed 23 April 2013].

Wong, R.S. and Radhakrishnan, A.K. (2012) Tocotrienol research: past into present. *Nutrition Review*, 70 (9): 483–490.

4

NUTRITIONAL NEEDS FOR LACTATION

Victoria Hall Moran

Pregnancy and breastfeeding are one of the most nutritionally demanding times of a woman's life, when nutritional requirements increase to support fetal, newborn and infant growth and development as well as maternal metabolism and tissue development pertaining to reproduction and breastfeeding (Picciano 2003). In a key strategic document for infant and young child feeding, the World Health Organization (WHO) recognizes the importance of the relation between the nutrition and health of the mother and her child.

> The health and nutritional status of mothers and children are intimately linked. Improved infant and young child feeding begins with ensuring the health and nutritional status of women, in their own right, throughout all stages of life and continues with women as providers for their children and families. Mothers and infants form a biological and social unit; they also share problems of malnutrition and ill-health. Whatever is done to solve these problems concerns both mothers and children together.
>
> (WHO 2003, p. 5)

It is clearly of importance to maintain adequate maternal nutrition whilst breastfeeding, in order to ensure the optimal health of both mother and child.

Breast milk contains energy and nutrients in appropriate amounts for the optimal growth and development of the infant as well as many non-nutrient substances essential for perinatal adaptation to neonatal life. The nutritive requirements of lactation are considerably greater even than those of pregnancy; the milk secreted in four months of lactation requires a level of energy roughly equivalent to the total energy needed for the pregnancy (Picciano 2003).

Despite this increased demand, women are remarkably resilient in their ability to produce breast milk of sufficient quantity and quality to support the growth of their infant, even when the mother is herself deprived of nutrients. In the developing world optimal breastfeeding of infants under two years of age has the potential to prevent 1.4 million deaths in children under five (Black *et al.* 2008). Milk production does, however, have an impact on maternal body composition and nutritional status, and lactating women have an increased requirement for many nutrients (Butte and Hopkinson 1998).

The recommended nutrient intakes for breastfeeding women are based on limited data, less even than are available to inform recommendations for pregnancy. A breastfeeding woman's dietary intake reference values are calculated from data relating to the quantity of milk produced during lactation, its energy and nutrient content and the amount of maternal energy and nutrient reserves. The quantity and nutrient content of milk consumed by the infant who is growing well and maintaining appropriate biochemical indices of nutritional status are often used as proxies to assess maternal nutritional adequacy during lactation (Picciano 2003). Large variations in nutrient recommendations exist across the world. Table 4.1 compares the current micronutrient recommendations in the UK and USA with those of the WHO/FAO. Even within Europe, where physiological requirements of the different populations are very similar, wide disparities exist (Hall Moran *et al.* 2010).

A recent European Commission project (EURRECA 2007–2012) has addressed these disparities, providing tools to help to harmonise the process of setting Dietary Reference Values (DRVs) (www.eurreca.org). DRVs can be used as a basis for reference values in food labelling and for establishing food-based dietary guidelines (FBDG), which translate nutritional recommendations into messages about foods and diet and can guide consumers on what to eat and can help them to make healthy dietary choices.

Nutrient requirements during lactation

Few studies have considered the impact of lactation on the mother's nutritional status. Rather, focus has been placed on the influence of maternal nutritional status on the composition of her breast milk (Hall Moran *et al.* 2010). For many nutrients the mobilization of maternal reserves helps to protect breast milk composition against variations in maternal nutrient intake and status (Langley-Evans 2009). Table 4.2 describes the nutrients in human breast milk that are most likely to be affected by maternal dietary intake.

Energy

The energy requirement of a breastfeeding woman is defined as 'the level of energy intake from food that will balance the energy expenditure needed to maintain a body weight and body composition, a level of physical activity and breast milk production that are consistent with optimal health for the woman and her child' (FAO/WHO/UNU 2004, p. 63). This definition implies that the energy required to produce an appropriate volume of milk must be added to the woman's usual energy requirement and assumes that she resumes her usual level of physical activity soon after giving birth (FAO/WHO/UNU 2004).

The main factors that influence the energy needs of lactating women are breastfeeding duration and the extent of exclusive breastfeeding practices. An exclusively breastfeeding woman has much greater energy and nutrient needs (with the exception of iron, due to the potential protective effect of lactational amenorrhoea) than a woman who is only partially breastfeeding. Dewey (2004) calculated that the average energy costs for milk production for an exclusively breastfeeding woman are 595 kcal/day at 0–2 months postpartum and 670 kcal/day at 3–8 months postpartum. The energy needed to support this would be 440–515 kcal/day, allowing for 500g of fat loss per month. The energy needs are lower for a partially breastfeeding woman, depending on the extent to which non-breast milk foods are consumed by her infant (Dewey 2004). Generally, women who are well nourished and maintain appropriate weight gain throughout pregnancy utilize their body fat reserves to provide a significant proportion of the additional energy needed for lactation.

Studies on the effect of breastfeeding on postpartum weight loss are conflicting. Some studies have identified associations between breastfeeding and postpartum weight loss (Kac *et al.* 2004; Stuebe *et al.* 2010), whilst others have found little or no difference in the rate of weight loss between women who breastfed and those who did not (Sichieri *et al.* 2003;

Table 4.1 UK, US and WHO/FAO micronutrient reference values during lactation

	UK DRV[1] – RNI	US DRI[2-6] – RDA	WHO/FAO[7]
Vitamin A	950 μg RE/d ↑ 350 μg RE/d	1200 μg RE/d (age 14–18y) ↑ 500 μg RE/d 1300 μg RE/d (age 19–50y) ↑ 600 μg RE/d	850 μg RE/d ↑ 350 μg RE/d
Vitamin D	10 μg/d ↑ 10 μg/d	15 μg/d No increment	5 μg/d No increment
Vitamin E	None set	19 mg/d ↑ 4 mg/d	None set
Vitamin K	None set	75 μg/d (age 14–18y) 90 μg/d (age 19–50 y) No increment	55 μg/d No increment
Vitamin C	70 mg/d ↑ 30 mg/d	115 mg/d (age 14–18y) ↑ 50 mg/d 120 mg/d (age 19–50 y) 45 mg/d	70 mg/d ↑ 25 mg/d
Riboflavin	1.6 mg/d ↑ 0.5 mg/d	1.6 mg/d ↑ 0.6 mg/d (age 14–18y) ↑ 0.5 mg/d (age 19–50 y)	1.6 mg/d ↑ 0.5 mg/d
Thiamin	0.4mg/1000 kcal No increment	1.4 mg/d ↑ 0.4 mg/d (age 14–18y) ↑ 0.3 mg/d (age 19–50 y)	1.5 mg/d ↑ 0.4 mg/d
Niacin	8.9 mg/d ↑ 2.3 mg/d	17 mg/d ↑ 3 mg/d	17 mg/d NE ↑ 3 mg/d
Vitamin B6	15 ug/g protein/d No increment	2.0 mg/d ↑ 0.8 mg/d (age 14–18y) ↑ 0.7 mg/d (age 19–50 y)	2.0 mg/d ↑ 0.7 mg/d
Folate	260 μg/d ↑ 60 μg/d	500 μg/d ↑ 100 μg/d	500 μg/d ↑ 100 μg/d
Vitamin B12	2.0 μg/d ↑ 0.5 μg/d	2.8 μg/d ↑ 0.4 μg/d	2.8 μg/d ↑ 0.4 μg/d
Pantothenic acid	None set	7 mg/d (AI) ↑ 2 mg/d	7 mg/d ↑ 2 mug/d

Table 4.1 Continued

	UK DRV¹ – RNI	US DRI²⁻⁶ – RDA	WHO/FAO⁷
Biotin	None set	35 μg/d (AI) ↑10 μg/d (age 14–18y) ↑5 μg/d (age 19–50 y)	35 μg/d ↑5 μg/d
Choline	None set	550 mg/d (AI) ↑150 mg/d(age 14–18y) ↑125 mg/d (age 19–50 y)	None set
Calcium	1350 mg/d (age 15–18y) 1250 mg/d (age 19–50y) ↑550 mg/d	1300 mg/d (age 14–18y) 1000 mg/d (age 19–50y) No increment	750 mg/d No increment (NPNL adolescents 1000 mg/d particularly during the growth spurt)
Iron	14.8 mg/d No increment	10 mg/d (age 14–18y) ↓5 mg/d 9 mg/d (age 19–50) ↓9 mg/d	10–30 mg/d depending on bioavailability of iron (a decrease of around 50% of NPNL values)
Phosphorus	990 mg/d* ↑440 mg/d	1250 mg/d (age 14–18y) 700 mg/d (age 19–50y) No increment	None set
Magnesium	350 mg/d (age 15–18y) 320 mg/d (age 19–50y) ↑50 mg/d	360 mg/d (age 14–18y) 310 mg/d (age 19–30y) 320 mg/d (age 31–50y) No increment	270 mg/d ↑50 mg/d
Zinc	13 mg/d (0–4 months) 9.5 mg/d (4+ months) ↑2.5–6 mg/d	13 mg/d (age 14–18y) 12 mg/d (age 19–50) ↑4 mg/d	Depending on bioavailability of zinc: 5.8–19 mg/d (0–3 months) 5.3–17.5 mg/d (3–6 months) 4.3–14.4 (7–12 months) NPNL adolescents 4.3–14.4 mg/d NPNL women 3.0–9.8 mg/d
Copper	1.3 μg/d (age 15–16y) 1.5 μg/d (age 18–50y) ↑0.3 μg/d	1.3 μg/d ↑0.4 μg/d	None set
Selenium	75 μg/d ↑15 μg/d	70 μg/d ↑15 μg/d	35 μg/d (0–6 months) ↑9 μg/d 42 μg/d (7–12 months) ↑16 μg/d

Iodine	140 µg/d No increment	290 µg/d ↑140 µg/d	200 µg/d ↑50 µg/d
Potassium	3.5 g/d No increment	5.1 g/d (AI) ↑0.4 g/d	None set
Manganese	None set	2.6 mg/d (AI) ↑1.0 mg/d (age 14–18y) ↑0.8 mg/d (age 19–50)	None set
Molybdenum	None set	50 µg/d ↑7 µg/d (age 14–18y) ↑5 µg/d (age 19–50)	None set

Notes: ↑ represents the amount of increase from non-pregnant, non-lactating levels.
↓ represents the amount of decrease from non-pregnant, non-lactating levels.
DRV dietary reference value; RNI reference nutrient intake; DRI dietary reference intakes; RDA recommended daily allowance; RE retinol equivalents; NE niacin equivalents; AI average intake; NPNL non-pregnant, non-lactating.
* RNI for phosphorus set to equal the RNI for calcium in mmol. The increment for pregnancy therefore reflects the increment set for calcium.
1 Committee on Medical Aspects of Food Policy (1991).
2 Institute of Medicine, Food and Nutrition Board (1997).
3 Institute of Medicine, Food and Nutrition Board (1998).
4 Institute of Medicine, Food and Nutrition Board (2000).
5 Institute of Medicine, Food and Nutrition Board (2001).
6 Institute of Medicine, Food and Nutrition Board (2004).
7 WHO/FAO (2004a).

Table 4.2 Nutrients in human breast milk categorised according to whether they are likely to be affected by maternal dietary intake

Nutrients present in breast milk at generally stable concentrations	Nutrients for which material intake is likely to affect breast milk composition
Energy	Monounsaturated fatty acids
Protein	Polyunsaturated fatty acids (LA, ALA, AA, DHA)
Total fat	Trans fatty acids
Saturated fatty acids	Vitamin A (retinol and carotenes)
Carbohydrates (lactose)	Vitamin C
Sodium	Vitamin E
Calcium	Niacin
Magnesium	Thiamin
Phosphors	Riboflavin
Iron	Vitamin B6
Copper	Vitamin B12
Zinc	Folate
Chloride	Pantothenic acid
Manganese	Biotin
Selenium	Iodine
Potassium	
Vitamin D	

Source: SACN (2011).

Onyango *et al.* 2011). In their systematic review of breastfeeding and maternal and infant health outcomes in developed countries, Ip *et al.* (2007) found only seven studies that were of sufficient quality and reported that the effect of breastfeeding in mothers on return to pre-pregnancy weight was negligible (less than 1kg weight change) and the effects of breastfeeding on postpartum weight loss were unclear. The inconsistency within these studies may reflect the degree of accuracy in the measurements of weight change, often inadequate control for numerous covariables including the amount of pregnancy weight gain, and lack of accuracy in the definition of exclusivity and the duration of breastfeeding. However, these studies also consistently revealed that many factors other than breastfeeding had larger effects on weight retention or postpartum weight loss, such as pre-pregnancy weight, age, parity, ethnicity, smoking, exercise and return to work (Ip *et al.* 2007). Thus, Butte and Hopkinson (1998) have suggested that the nutritional aim to ensure optimal maternal well-being should be to ensure balance in the composition of the body over the pregnancy–lactation cycle as a whole.

UK dietary reference values for energy during lactation increase by 330 kcal per day in the first 6 months (SACN 2011), i.e. a daily energy intake of 2270 kcal. Thereafter, the energy intake required to support breastfeeding will be modified by maternal body composition and the breast milk intake of the infant. WHO/FAO recommend an additional 505 kcal/day for well-nourished women with adequate gestational weight gain (see Table 4.1).

Long chained polyunsaturated fatty acids (LCPUFA)

As discussed in Chapter 2, the central nervous system contains high concentrations of n-3 LCPUFAs (omega-3 fatty acids), which are important for infant growth and development.

For the newborn, maternal n-3 LCPUFA intake over the perinatal period has been closely associated with improvement of infant visual and cognitive function. There is also accumulating evidence to support the concept that maternal n-3 LCPUFA intake during gestation and lactation has an impact on the metabolic programming of the infant, which may have long-term implications for later development of metabolic diseases, including obesity, type 2 diabetes, cardiovascular disease (CVD) and hypertension (Innis 2011).

The major n-3 LCPUFA components of breast milk are docosahexaenoic acid (DHA) and alpha linoleic acid (AA). DHA in particular plays a major role in infant neurological development. Research has indicated that the DHA content of breast milk may affect the IQ (Helland et al. 2003) and immune function later in childhood (Prentice and van der Merwe 2011). The transfer of LCPUFA from mother to her fetus/infant during lactation is dependent largely upon maternal status, but genetic influences are also now recognized (Lauritzen and Carlson 2011). Breast milk AA levels tend to be more conserved than DHA, but DHA responds sensitively to dietary DHA and higher levels and have been found in women with diets high in fish intake (Gibson et al. 1997).

Fish and seafood is the only food group that is a significant source of n-3 LCPUFA and, as a whole food, offers a range of nutrients that are frequently under-represented in habitual diets, including iodine, calcium, vitamin D, zinc and iron (Hunt and McManus 2013). Breast milk DHA content is much higher in fish-eating countries as compared with low-income populations, whose supply of PUFA comes mainly from cereals and vegetable oils, some of which have very low α-Linolenic acid (ALA) content (Brenna 2011). Women who do not eat seafood may be advised to increase their DHA intakes whilst breastfeeding by using vegetable oils with higher ALA content (e.g. soybean or rapeseed oil).

Minerals and vitamins

For many minerals, including iron, zinc and copper, the infant is well protected by maternal homeostatic processes, such that moderate deficiency or excessive dietary intake do not significantly alter the levels of these micronutrients in the mother's milk (Domellof et al. 2004). Many minerals are transferred into milk by active transfer rather than by passive diffusion and this process compensates for variations in maternal mineral status.

The concentration of many vitamins in breast milk is dependent upon the vitamin status of the mother, with maternal deficiencies leading to deficiencies in the breastfeeding infant. Vitamins of particular concern in this respect include vitamin A, vitamin D and vitamin B12 (Allen, 2005). Table 4.1 compares the UK, US and WHO/FAO micronutrient reference values for breastfeeding women. Key micronutrients are discussed in further detail below.

Iodine

The iodine concentration of human breast milk varies markedly as a function of the iodine intake of the population. An average consumption of 750ml breast milk per day would provide an intake of iodine of about 60mg/day in Europe and 120mg/day in the United States, which in some areas falls short of the WHO recommendation of 90mg iodine/day from birth (WHO/FAO 2004). For women with marginal iodine status, the demands of lactation can precipitate clinical and biochemical symptoms, including increased thyroid volume, altered thyroid hormone levels and impaired mental function (Dorea 2002; Zimmermann and Delange 2004).

Thyroidal iodine turnover rate is more rapid in infants (Zimmermann 2009), so adequate breast milk iodine levels are particularly important for the neurodevelopment in breastfed infants. A 33 per cent increase in iodine intake is needed to accommodate the changes in maternal thyroid metabolism to support lactation and to supply sufficient iodine for milk to meet the needs for growth and development of the infant (WHO/FAO 2004). The levels recommended to ensure that pregnant and lactating women do not suffer from iodine deficiency post-partum are listed in Table 4.1.

Iodine deficiency affects more than 2.2 billion individuals (38 per cent of the world's population) (ICCIDD 2011) and remains the leading cause of preventable developmental delay worldwide. Although iodine deficiency is certainly much more common in low-income countries it is not confined to them. A study of 737 teenage women from nine areas of the UK found that half had a mild iodine deficiency, while nearly a fifth (18 per cent) had moderate iodine deficiency (Vanderpump et al. 2011). Similar patterns have been seen in Europe, the USA, Australia and New Zealand, where national surveys confirmed the re-emergence of a problem (Zimmermann and Delange 2004; Leung et al. 2011). Other areas, such as Japan, have some of the highest iodine intakes in the world through their consumption of iodine-rich seaweed such as kombu (*Laminaria japonica*). A recent study, combining information from dietary records, food surveys, urine iodine analysis and seaweed iodine content, estimated that the Japanese iodine intake, largely from seaweeds, averages 1,000–3,000μg/day (1–3mg/day) (Zava and Zava 2011). Such excessive iodine ingestion by the mother during pregnancy may lead to hyperthyrotropinemia in their babies (Nishiyama et al. 2004).

It has been suggested that the iodization of salt may be a cost-effective and sustainable solution to the problem. Since 1993 the WHO has conducted a global programme of salt iodization to boost dietary levels and prevent deficiency, but it is currently not compulsory for manufacturers in the UK to add iodine to salt.

Zinc

An adequate supply of zinc is essential for the normal growth and development of the mammary gland function for milk synthesis and secretion. The level of zinc in colostrum is 17 times higher than that in blood, which illustrates the importance of zinc for the growth and development of the newborn infant (Almeida et al. 2008). Zinc concentration of breast milk declines rapidly in the first three months post-partum (Krebs et al. 1995). It has been estimated that about 4–6 per cent of maternal bone mass is lost during six months of full lactation, enabling maternal bone to contribute about 20 per cent of the breast milk zinc over a six-month period (Moser-Veillon 1995).

Although the prevalence of severe zinc deficiency is rare, mild to moderate zinc deficiency is common in lactating women in several regions of the world (Brown et al. 2004). A number of studies of lactating women with marginal zinc status have revealed that homeostatic mechanisms can compensate for low maternal dietary zinc intakes. The proportion of dietary zinc absorbed in such women has been shown to increase by over 70 per cent as compared to non-lactating women or pre-conception values (Sian et al. 2002).

Current WHO recommendations for zinc intake during pregnancy and lactation range from 4.3 to 19mg per day depending upon months post-partum and the bioavailability of zinc from the diet (WHO/FAO 2004). Generally, these dietary recommendations can be met from usual habitual intakes, but intakes can be increased by advising women to integrate more zinc-rich foods into their diets, such as wheat germ, wheat bran, sesame seeds and cheese (Derbyshire 2011).

Calcium

During lactation women typically lose 280–400mg/day of calcium through breast milk (Kovacs 2011). To meet this increased demand the mother must mobilize calcium from her own stores. Physiologic adaptations, such as up-regulation of intestinal calcium absorption and bone resorption, provide much of the calcium in breast milk (Figure 4.1) (Kovacs 2011).

Several investigations of the effect of maternal dietary calcium intake on breast milk calcium levels indicate that the two are independent of each other (Kent *et al.* 2009) and skeletal resorption is not suppressed by increasing the dietary intake of calcium in women (Polatti *et al.* 1999). A randomized control trial of pregnant and lactating women in the Gambia revealed that despite their having low dietary intakes of calcium (300–400mg/day) and low breast milk concentrations, calcium supplements had no significant benefit in terms of breast milk concentration (Jarjou *et al.* 2006). After weaning, the bone density is fully restored over the subsequent six to twelve months (Kovacs and Kronenberg 1997; Polatti *et al.* 1999).

The UK dietary guidelines recommend that breastfeeding women increase their calcium intake to 1250mg/day, an increase of 550mg/day. Women should try to increase their dietary intake of calcium by substituting low-calcium foods (e.g. white bread, low-fat yoghurt, green salad, currants) with calcium-rich alternatives (e.g. granary bread, whole-milk yoghurt, watercress, figs) (Derbyshire 2011). Milk is another important source of calcium and other

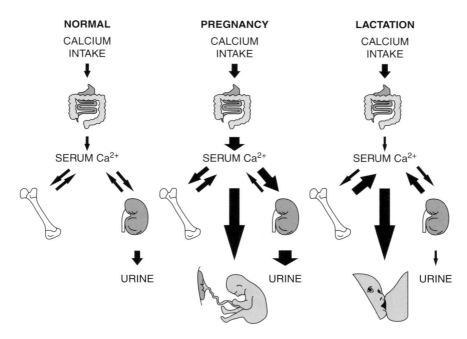

Figure 4.1 Calcium homeostasis in human pregnancy and lactation, contrasted with normal. The thickness of arrows indicates a relative increase or decrease with respect to the normal and non-pregnant state.

Source: Reproduced from Kovacs, C.S. (2011) Calcium and bone metabolism disorders during pregnancy and lactation. *Endocrinology and Metabolism Clinics of North America*, 40(4): 795, with permission.

nutrients. A study in Canada, comparing exclusively breastfeeding mothers who drank milk and those who restricted their milk intake to less than 250ml/day found that drinking milk provided important sources of protein, calcium, thiamin, riboflavin and zinc (Mannion *et al.* 2007).

Vitamin A

Vitamin A is needed for the growth and differentiation of cells and tissues and plays a key role in infant development. Vitamin A deficiency (VAD) is a major public health problem in low-income countries. Globally, it is estimated that 140–250 million children under the age of five years are affected by vitamin A deficiency. These children suffer a dramatically increased risk of death, blindness and illness, especially from measles and diarrhoea. Since breast milk is a natural source of vitamin A, promoting breastfeeding is the best way to protect infants from VAD (WHO, The Micronutrient Initiative 1998). Although high doses of Vitamin A should not be consumed during pregnancy, to avoid teratogenesis, high dose supplementation of post-partum women with vitamin A has been shown to be an effective way of ensuring adequate supplies for the infant through breast milk (Sommer *et al.* 2002) and preventing deficiency. Some caution should be exercised before providing universal high dose vitamin A supplementation, however, as vitamin A (retinol) has been found to have a modulating effect on colostrum vitamin E (alpha-tocopherol) in human breast milk. Generally, vitamin A and beta-carotene are widely available in the diet from foods such as orange and dark, leafy vegetables (Derbyshire 2011).

Vitamin D

Through its action in regulating calcium and phosphate absorption, vitamin D plays a vital role in the growth and development of bones. Babies are particularly at risk of vitamin D deficiency because of their relatively large vitamin D needs, related to the high rate of skeletal growth (WHO/FAO 2004). Vitamin D deficiency in infancy has also been associated with an increased risk of developing type 1 diabetes, respiratory infections, cardiovascular diseases and cancer later in life (Prentice 2008). Whilst our understanding of the ways in which maternal vitamin D levels affect health outcomes in the mother, fetus and breast-fed infant continues to evolve, the precise mechanisms remain unclear (Brannon and Picciano 2011). Vitamin D deficiency has gained a lot of interest in recent years with the resurgence in the prevalence of rickets, particularly among South Asian immigrants to Western Europe (Alfaham *et al.* 1995; Gillie 2004). Reduced UV exposure from sunlight, due to the prevalent use of sunscreen creams, sunlight avoidance or the wearing of traditional Muslim dress can contribute to vitamin D deficiency in pregnant and lactating mothers, which can lead to lowered breast-milk concentrations (Seth *et al.* 2009).

At birth, infants have acquired *in utero* the vitamin D stores that must support them through the first months of life (WHO/FAO 2004). Human breast milk is low in vitamin D, although limited sunlight exposure has been shown to prevent rickets in many breastfed babies. However, breastfed infants who do not receive adequate sunlight exposure or, if necessary, supplementation are at increased risk of developing vitamin D deficiency or rickets (Gartner and Greer 2003).

Vitamin D is not found naturally in many foods (oily fish being an exception), but a growing number of foods are fortified with vitamin D, including milks (cows', soy and rice) and some yogurts, ready-to-eat cereals, margarines and fruit juices (Brannon and Picciano 2011). In the UK, public health guidance has been provided which recommends that pregnant and breastfeeding women should increase their intake of vitamin D to 10µg/day. As there are few dietary sources of vitamin D available to meet this recommended target, vitamin D supplements should be taken. Healthcare professionals are urged to take particular care to ensure that those at greatest risk of vitamin D deficiency, including women who are obese, who have limited skin exposure to sunlight or who are of South Asian, African, Caribbean or Middle Eastern descent, are advised to take vitamin D supplements (NICE 2011).

Allergenic risk

During the last few decades the prevalence of atopy has increased worldwide, particularly in Western countries and amongst children (Beasley *et al.* 1998). Globally, around 7–8 per cent of children develop food allergy, 15–20 per cent acquire atopic eczema and 31–34 per cent develop asthma or recurrent wheezing (Halken 2004). It has been suggested that the observed increase of allergic diseases in populations with a Western lifestyle may, in part, be due to an altered microbial exposure in the gastrointestinal tract (Holt *et al.* 1997). As the efficiency of the gastrointestinal barrier is reduced in the newborn period (Sampson 2004), infants are particularly vulnerable to such exposure. A possible protective role of breastfeeding has been suggested, and differences in intestinal microflora in infants who are breastfed, as compared with formula-fed infants, have been found (Agostoni *et al.* 2004). However, the evidence supporting a protective role for breastfeeding against allergy and asthma is as yet inconclusive (Duncan and Sears 2008; Grimshaw *et al.* 2009).

In August 2009, the UK Department of Health revised its advice about eating peanuts during pregnancy, breastfeeding and early childhood in relation to the risk of developing peanut allergy in childhood (FSA 2009). The change in advice followed a major review of the scientific evidence that revealed that there was no clear association between eating peanuts (or foods containing peanuts) during pregnancy, breastfeeding or early childhood and an increased likelihood of a child's developing a peanut allergy (COT 1998). The new guidelines advise women that they may eat peanuts or foods containing peanuts when they are breastfeeding, unless they are allergic to them or unless their health professional advises them not to.

Factors which may influence the nutritional status of the breastfeeding mother

Veganism and vegetarianism

Vegans, lacto-vegetarian and vegetarian mothers may be at risk of nutrient inadequacy, particularly with regard to vitamin B12 (cobalamin), iron and docosahexaenoic acid (DHA), and consequently their corresponding breast milk nutrient levels may be very low (Specker *et al.* 1990). Additionally, the endogenous metabolism of DHA may be inhibited, due to a high proportion of linoleic versus linolenic acid intake. Studies have shown that infants born to mothers who are vegetarian or vegan may be at risk of cobalamin and iron deficiency (Fadyl and Inoue 2007) and megoblastic anaemia (Erdeve *et al.* 2009).

Case studies have demonstrated severe vitamin B12 deficiency in exclusively breastfed infants of vegetarian and vegan mothers (Weiss *et al.* 2004; Wagnon *et al.* 2005). Infants of vegetarian and vegan mothers may have low vitamin B12 levels at birth if the mother's vitamin B12 intake was suboptimal during pregnancy and her stores are low, and this may be perpetuated if the vitamin B12-deficient mother breastfeeds her infant. There is little information regarding the long-term neurological effects of such deficiencies, but these may include intellectual impairment, severe disturbance of gait and epilepsy (Graham *et al*. 1992).

Vegetarianism is particularly common in adolescent women, with a prevalence of between 8 and 37 per cent (Worsley and Skrzypiec 1998), which may further compound the nutritional challenge of lactation in this particularly vulnerable population. In addition, vegetarian teenagers are also more likely to exhibit health-compromising dietary behaviours such as frequent dieting, binging, purging and laxative use for weight control (Neumark-Sztainer *et al*. 1997; Perry *et al*. 2001) and alcohol use (Greene-Finestone *et al*. 2008). Studies have yet to be conducted on the particular influence of vegetarian diets on the nutritional status of lactating adolescents.

The UK Department of Health recommends that vegan breastfeeding mothers supplement their diet with vitamin D and, if they had been taking B12 supplements during pregnancy, that they continue to do so throughout breastfeeding. Pregnant and lactating women may also be encouraged to incorporate flaxseed oil (cold pressed) into their diets, as this has been shown to significantly improve red blood cell levels of ALA, Eicosapentaenoic acid (EPA) and DHA (Barceló-Coblijn *et al*. 2008), although more research is needed in women of childbearing age.

Adolescence

National nutritional surveys have shown that the highest prevalence of nutritional deficiencies occurs in adolescence (e.g. Gregory *et al*. 2000), and literature reviews have illustrated that poor adolescent nutritional intake and status prevails during pregnancy (Hall Moran 2007a; 2007b) and lactation (Hall Moran *et al*. 2010). The increased nutritional demand to support lactation occurs at a time of rapid growth and development in adolescents, with the attainment of approximately 50 per cent of adult body weight and 15 per cent of final adult height during this period (Rogol *et al*. 2000). Scholl *et al*. (1990; 1993) have demonstrated that adolescents in the US continued to grow in stature and accrue fat mass during pregnancy and early postpartum. In undernourished populations, however, adolescents' linear growth have been shown to cease and lean body mass and per cent body fat to decline during pregnancy and lactation (Rah *et al*. 2008), indicating a depletion of maternal energy and nutrient reserves to meet the demands of both pregnancy and lactation (Rah *et al*. 2010). Clearly, the nutritional demands of pregnancy and lactation seem to have a far greater impact on the nutritional status of under-nourished adolescent mothers, which could augment a cycle of nutritional deprivation in such populations.

Adolescence is a critical time for bone mass acquisition, when bone accretion rates peak during pubertal growth, due to associated hormonal changes. Whilst there is evidence that adolescents experience bone mineral density (BMD) loss during lactation, this effect seems to be transient, with subsequent repletion of BMD once breastfeeding ceases (Bezerra *et al*. 2004). Further, it has been found that adolescents experience less bone resorption associated with lactation, as compared to adults, potentially contributing to protection against excessive bone loss (Bezerra *et al*. 2002). There is also early evidence of a link between vitamin D receptor gene polymorphisms and bone mass in lactating adolescent women, with some genotypes having better bone status than others in a population with habitually low calcium intakes (Bezerra *et al.* 2007).

There is an increased demand for zinc and during the adolescent growth spurt and during lactation. Thus, the lactating adolescent is at particular risk of suboptimal zinc status, with increased requirements to support her own development and maturation as well as her capacity to produce nutritionally adequate milk. Meeting zinc demands during lactation will depend on the dietary supply, bioavailability and the capacity for adaptation of zinc metabolism. Whilst evidence suggests that the biochemical responses of zinc to lactation are similar in adolescents and adults, significant correlations were found between the activity of zinc-dependent enzymes and plasma zinc in adolescents, which may suggest a limiting action of poor maternal zinc status on the metabolic adaptation capacity of this population (Maia *et al.* 2007).

Smoking

The negative influence of maternal smoking on breastfeeding duration has been well described in the literature (Horta *et al.* 2001) and has been shown even after adjusting for socio-economic group and education level (Hopkinson *et al.* 1992). Some studies have suggested that smoking reduces daily milk output by approximately 250–300ml (Vio *et al.* 1991; Hopkinson *et al.* 1992), possibly related to suppressed prolactin production in smokers (Andersen *et al.* 1984; Widström *et al.* 1991). Little is known about the influence of smoking on maternal nutritional status or milk composition, but there is some evidence that smoking is associated with significant reductions in milk fat concentration (Vio *et al.* 1991; Hopkinson *et al.* 1992). The reduction in milk volume and fat content has been given as an explanation for why women who smoke cease to breastfeed earlier than those who do not smoke (Hopkinson *et al.* 1992). However, it is not yet clear whether social and behavioural differences between smokers and non-smokers play a greater role in early cessation of breastfeeding than do physiological factors. In their epidemiological literature review Amir and Donath (2002) claimed that, as women who smoke are less likely to intend to breastfeed and less likely to seek help with breastfeeding problems than non-smoking mothers, it cannot be assumed that the relationship between smoking and breastfeeding duration is a wholly physiological one. Recent qualitative research emphasized the importance of the role of psychosocial factors, reporting that the reasons given by women who ceased to breastfeed earlier related to their perceptions that smoking while breastfeeding constituted a strong risk of harming their baby (Goldade *et al.* 2008).

Alcohol

Studies have shown that alcohol ingestion is associated with decreased oxytocin release, inhibiting the milk ejection reflex in a dose response manner (Anderson 1995; Mennella *et al.* 2005). Alcohol is also passed readily into the milk, with milk concentrations of alcohol closely paralleling maternal blood alcohol concentration at an equal or slightly greater level. A breastfed infant is exposed to only a fraction of the alcohol that the mother ingests, but infants are able to detoxify alcohol at only half the rate of adults in their first weeks of life (Abel 1984). Although the effects of alcohol for the infant vary, depending on the amount of alcohol consumed, even moderate alcohol consumption is associated with reduced milk intake, reduced motor development, impaired sleep patterns and increased risk of hypoglycaemia. It has been suggested that the presence of alcohol in breast milk has the overall effect for the infant of decreasing breast milk consumption by 23 per cent (Mennella and Beauchamp 1991). Although drinking moderate amounts of alcohol does not warrant discontinuation of breastfeeding, mothers who choose to drink while breastfeeding should be aware of the potential effects on their infants (Koren 2002).

Guidelines on alcohol use in the UK remain somewhat vague, with the Royal College of Obstetricians and Gynaecologists advising that one or two units a couple of times a week is 'probably' safe (RCOG 2006). Other countries are less equivocal about their advice and the National Health and Medical Research Council in Australia (2009) recommends that women abstain from drinking alcohol during breastfeeding, rather than drinking small amounts.

Obesity

Obese women are less likely to breastfeed their babies than women who are not obese, causing some public health concern due to the rising prevalence of obesity in women of reproductive age and the association between formula feeding and greater risk of obesity in children (Arenz et al. 2004). A systematic review that assessed the association between maternal obesity and infant feeding intention, initiation and duration found that obese women plan to breastfeed for a shorter period than do normal-weight women and are less likely to initiate breastfeeding (Amir and Donath 2007). The reasons for this have not yet been fully explained, but depressive symptoms, perceived stress and anxiety do not appear to explain the association (Mehta et al. 2011). Evidence from systematic reviews suggests that obese women have significantly delayed lactogenesis and lower milk transfer, as compared to women who are not obese (Amir and Donath 2007; Turcksin et al. 2012). Furthermore, fewer obese women perceived that their milk supply was adequate, as compared with non-obese women, suggesting that there may be a physiological influence (Turcksin et al. 2012). As more obese women have been shown to cite 'insufficient milk' as a reason to cease breastfeeding (24 per cent vs 13 per cent), there are clear implications for the duration of breastfeeding in obese women (Guelinckx et al. 2011). There is a clear and urgent need for further qualitative studies to further explore obese women's behaviour and infant feeding decisions in relation to these factors. As obese women are less likely to initiate or continue breastfeeding than non-obese women, health professionals should be aware that obese women may need additional support with breastfeeding. Midwifery management of obesity-related lactation issues should begin with education about optimal prenatal weight gain and regular weight assessment to avoid excessive gain (Jevitt et al. 2007).

Birth spacing and the recuperative interval

There is a large nutritional demand associated with closely spaced consecutive births, particularly when lactation overlaps with pregnancy (King 2003). The duration and intensity of lactation influences the ability of the mother to replenish her nutrient reserves during the interval between pregnancies (Dewey and Cohen 2007). Pregnancies with short 'recuperative intervals' (defined as the amount of time that the woman was not lactating prior to the next conception) are particularly vulnerable to nutrient depletion. A recent systematic review concluded that current evidence is conflicting and further studies are needed to understand the role that breastfeeding (and its intensity) plays in the relationship between birth spacing and infant and child mortality (Conde-Agudelo et al. 2012).

Socio-economic and cultural perspectives

There is a range of deeply embedded cultural practices that will influence what the mother selects to eat during lactation. For example, Hispanic cultures, Chinese and some South Asian groups adhere to a set of implicit rules around 'hot' and 'cold' foods (Davis 2001; Wambach and Riordan 2010). This does not relate to temperature but, rather, to a set of foods that are considered to affect the body in particular ways. The practice of giving herbs and galactogogues (foods thought to enhance the quality and/or quantity of milk) to the mother is a widespread cultural practice which varies from community to community. Ramadan fasting has been found to be associated with a reduction in the micronutrient (zinc, magnesium and potassium), but not macronutrient, content of breast milk, although infant growth does not appear to be affected, largely because the energy requirements of the infant are still met (Rakicioğlu *et al.* 2006). There is some evidence that fasting may alter the infant-feeding behaviour of mothers who fast. A study of 129 mothers of infants aged six months or younger on their attitudes to and perceptions of fasting while breastfeeding during Ramadan found that 22 per cent of mothers believed that fasting caused a decrease in the volume of their breast milk and 23 per cent thought that they should increase the amount of solid supplements that the infant received during fasting (Ertem *et al.* 2001). Such practices need further exploration in order to assess their implications for maternal and child nutrition and health.

Socio-economic considerations at both macro and micro levels influence the dietary intake of women; for example, mothers living in conditions of poverty may have little opportunity to obtain foods known to be important during pregnancy and lactation (Stapleton and Keenan 2009). Poor nutritional status in pregnancy and the postpartum period may exert its effect throughout the life course and can be transmitted across generations, which, if left unchecked, may lead to an inter-generational cycle of nutritional deprivation.

Conclusion

Recent research is providing new knowledge on the nutrient requirements of breastfeeding women. Given the wide variation in breastfeeding practices across the world, making nutritional recommendations for lactating women is challenging. It is crucial to first examine the cultural practices within and across populations and to assess their relevance before making recommendations. We need to avoid assumptions that providing the 'correct' information on nutritional requirements during lactation will lead women to make the 'right choices' in terms of their own nutrition and the patterns and practices of breastfeeding. This consumerist concept of decision making (knowledge in, behaviour out) is based on an illusion of linearity and it ignores the complexities of decision making. In reality, decisions will be made based on macro-level (structural) factors such as socio-economic and political contexts, gender relationships and food availability, along with micro-level factors such as local cultural practices, norms, lifestyles, attitudes and beliefs (Pelto 1987; Bilson and Dykes 2009).

References

Abel, E.L. (1984) *Pharmacology of alcohol relating to pregnancy and lactation.* Buffalo, NY: Plenum Press: 29–45.

Agostoni, C., Axelsson, I., Goulet, O., Koletzko, B., Michaelsen, K.F. *et al.* (2004) Prebiotic oligosaccharides in dietetic products for infants: a commentary by the ESPGHAN Committee on Nutrition. *Journal of Pediatric Gastroenterology and Nutrition* 39: 465–473.

Alfaham, M., Woodhead, S., Pask, G. and Davies, D. (1995) Vitamin D deficiency: a concern in pregnant Asian women. *British Journal of Nutrition* 73 (6): 881–887.

Allen, L.H. (2005) Multiple micronutrients in pregnancy and lactation: an overview. *American Journal of Clinical Nutrition* 81: 1206S–1212S.

Almeida, A.A., Lopes, C.M., Silva, A.M. and Barrado, E. (2008) Trace elements in human milk: correlation with blood levels, inter-element correlations and changes in concentration during the first month of lactation. *Journal of Trace Elements in Medicine & Biology* 22: 196–205.

Amir, L.H. and Donath, S.M. (2002) Does maternal smoking have a negative physiological effect on breastfeeding? The epidemiological evidence. *Birth* 29, 112–123.

Amir, L. and Donath, S. (2007) A systematic review of maternal obesity and breastfeeding intention, initiation and duration. *BMC Pregnancy Childbirth* 7: 9.

Andersen, A.N., Rønn, B., Tjønneland, A., Djursing, H. and Schiøler, V. (1984) Low maternal but normal fetal prolactin levels in cigarette smoking pregnant women. *Acta Obstetricia et Gynecologica Scandinavica* 63 (3): 237–239.

Anderson, P.O. (1995) Alcohol and breastfeeding. *Journal of Human Lactation* 11 (4): 321–323.

Arenz, S., Rückerl, R., Koletzko, B. and Von Kries, R. (2004) Breast-feeding and childhood obesity: a systematic review. *International Journal of Obesity* 28 (10): 1247–1256.

Barceló-Coblijn, G., Murphy, E.J., Othman, R., Moghadasian, M.H., Kashour, T. and Friel, J.K. (2008) Flaxseed oil and fish-oil capsule consumption alters human red blood cell n-3 fatty acid composition: a multiple-dosing trial comparing 2 sources of n-3 fatty acid. *American Journal of Clinical Nutrition* 88 (3): 801–809.

Beasley, R., Keil, U., von Mutius, E. *et al.* (1998) Worldwide variation in prevalence of symptoms of asthma, allergic rhinoconjunctivitis, and atopic eczema: ISAAC. *The Lancet*, 351: 1225–1232.

Bezerra, F.F., Laboissiere, F.P., King, J.C. and Donangelo, C.M. (2002) Pregnancy and lactation affect markers of calcium and bone metabolism differently in adolescent and adult women with low calcium intakes. *Journal of Nutrition* 132: 2183–2187.

Bezerra, F.F., Mendonca, L.M.C., Lobato, E.C., O'Brien, K.O. and Donangelo, C.M. (2004) Bone mass is recovered from lactation to postweaning in adolescent mothers with low calcium intakes. *American Journal of Clinical Nutrition* 80: 1322–1326.

Bezerra, F.F., Cabello, G.M.K., Mendonca, L.M.C. and Donangelo, C.M. (2007) Bone mass and breast milk calcium are associated with vitamin D receptor gene polymorphisms in adolescent mothers. *Journal of Nutrition* 138: 277–281.

Bilson, A. and Dykes, F. (2009) A bio-cultural basis for protecting, promoting and supporting breastfeeding. In Dykes, F. and Hall Moran, V. (eds) *Infant and young child nutrition: challenges to implementing a global strategy*. Oxford: Wiley-Blackwell.

Black, R.E., Allan, L.H., Bhutta, Z.A., Caulfield, L.E., De Onis, M. *et al.* (2008) Maternal and child undernutrition: global and regional exposures and health consequences. *The Lancet* 371 (9608): 243–260, doi: 10.1016/S0140-6736(07)61690-0.

Brannon, P.M. and Picciano, M.F. (2011) Vitamin D in pregnancy and lactation in humans. *Annual Review of Nutrition* 31: 89–115.

Brenna, J.T. (2011) Animal studies of the functional consequences of suboptimal polyunsaturated fatty acid status during pregnancy, lactation and early post-natal life. *Maternal and Child Nutrition* 7: 59–79.

Brown, K.H., Rivera, J.A., Bhutta, Z., Gibson, R.S., King, J.C. *et al.* (2004) International Zinc Nutrition Consultative Group (IZiNCG) technical document# 1. Assessment of the risk of zinc deficiency in populations and options for its control. *Food and Nutrition Bulletin* 25 (1) Suppl. 2: S99.

Butte, N.F. and Hopkinson, J.M. (1998) Body composition changes during lactation are highly variable among women. *Journal of Nutrition* 128: 381S–385S.

Committee on Medical Aspects of Food Policy (COMA) (1991) *Dietary Reference Values for food energy and nutrients for the United Kingdom*. London: The Stationery Office.

Conde-Agudelo, A., Rosas-Bermudez, A., Castaño, F. and Norton, M.H. (2012) Effects of birth spacing on maternal, perinatal, infant, and child health: a systematic review of causal mechanisms. *Studies in Family Planning* 43 (2): 93–114.

COT (2008) *Committee on Toxicity of Chemicals in Food, Consumer Products and the Environment.* Statement on the review of the 1998 COT recommendations on peanut avoidance. [Available at: http://cot.food.gov.uk/cotstatements/cotstatementsyrs/cotstatements2008/cot200807peanut].

Davis, R.E. (2001) The postpartum experience for Southeast Asian women in the United States. *Maternal and Child Nursing* 26 (4): 208–213.

Derbyshire, E. (2011) *Nutrition in the childbearing years.* Oxford: Wiley-Blackwell.

Dewey, K.G. (2004) Impact of breastfeeding on maternal nutritional status. *Advances in Experimental Medicine & Biology* 554: 91–100.

Dewey, K.G. and Cohen, R.J. (2007) Does birth spacing affect maternal or child nutritional status? A systematic literature review. *Maternal & Child Nutrition* 3: 151–173.

Domellof, M., Lonnerdal, B., Dewey, K.G., Cohen, R.J. and Hernell, O. (2004) Iron, zinc, and copper concentrations in breast milk are independent of maternal mineral status. *American Journal of Clinical Nutrition* 79: 111–115.

Dorea, J.G. (2002) Iodine nutrition and breast feeding. *Journal of Trace Elements in Medicine & Biology* 16: 207–220.

Duncan, J.M. and Sears, M.R. (2008) Breastfeeding and allergies: time for a change in paradigm? *Current Opinion in Allergy and Clinical Immunology* 8 (5): 398.

Erdeve, O., Arsan, S., Atasay, B., Ileri, T. and Uysal, Z. (2009) A breast-fed newborn with megaloblastic anemia: treated with the vitamin B12 supplementation of the mother. *Journal of Pediatric Hematology/Oncology* 31 (10): 763–765.

Ertem, I. O., Ulukol, B. and Gulnar, S. B. (2001). Attitudes and practices of breastfeeding mothers regarding fasting in Ramadan. *Child: Care, Health and Development* 27 (6), 545–554.

EURRECA (EURopean micronutrient RECommendations Aligned), www.eurreca.org.

Fadyl, H. and Inoue, S. (2007) Combined B12 and iron deficiency in a child breast-fed by a vegetarian mother. *Journal of Pediatric Hematology/Oncology* 29 (1): 74.

FAO/WHO/UNU (2004) *Human energy requirements.* Report of a Joint FAO/WHO/UNU Expert Consultation. Rome, 17–24 October 2001.

FSA (2009) Peanuts during pregnancy, breastfeeding and early childhood. www.food.gov.uk/policy-advice/allergyintol/peanutspregnancy#.UTXPzndtYXU [accessed 5 May 2012].

Gartner, L.M. and Greer, F.R. (2003) Prevention of rickets and vitamin D deficiency: new guidelines for vitamin D intake. *Pediatrics* 111 (4): 908–910.

Gibson, R.A., Neumann, M.A. and Makrides, M. (1997) Effect of increasing breast milk docosahexaenoic acid (DHA) on plasma and erythrocyte phospholipid fatty acids and neural indices of exclusively breast fed infants. *European Journal of Clinical Nutrition* 51: 578–584.

Gillie, O. (2004) *Sunlight robbery.* Health Research Forum Occasional Reports, No. 1, p. 20. www.healthresearchforum.org.uk.

Goldade, K., Nichter, M., Nichter, M., Adrian, S., Tesler, L. *et al.* (2008) Breastfeeding and smoking among low-income women: results of a longitudinal qualitative study. *Birth* 35: 230–240.

Graham, S.M., Arvela, O.M. and Wise, G.A. (1992) Long-term neurologic consequences of nutritional vitamin B12 deficiency in infants. *Journal of Pediatrics*, 121: 710–714.

Greene-Finestone, L.S., Campbell, M.K., Evers, S.E. and Gutmanis, I.E. (2008) Attitudes and health behaviours of young adolescent omnivores and vegetarians: a school-based study. *Appetite* 51: 104–110.

Gregory, J., Lowe, S., Bates, C., Prentice, A., Jackson, L. *et al.* (2000) *Report of the Diet and Nutrition Survey. Volume 1, National diet and nutrition survey: young people aged 4 to 18 years.* London: The Stationery Office.

Grimshaw, K.E., Allen, K., Edwards, C.A., Beyer, K., Belay, A. *et al.* (2009) Infant feeding and allergy prevention: a review of current knowledge and recommendations. A EuroPrevall state of the art paper. *Allergy* 64: 1407–1416.

Guelinckx, I., Devlieger, R., Bogaerts, A., Pauwels, S. and Vansant, G. (2011) The effect of pre-pregnancy BMI on intention, initiation and duration of breast-feeding. *Public Health Nutrition* 15: 840–848.

Halken, S. (2004) Prevention of allergic disease in childhood: clinical and epidemiological aspects of primary and secondary allergy prevention. *Pediatric Allergy and Immunology* 15 Suppl 16: 4–5.

Hall Moran, V. (2007a) A systematic review of dietary assessments of pregnant adolescents in industrialised countries. *British Journal of Nutrition* 97: 411–425.

Hall Moran, V. (2007b) Nutritional status in pregnant adolescents: a systematic review of biochemical markers. *Maternal & Child Nutrition* 3: 74–93.

Hall Moran, V., Lowe, N., Berti, C., Cetin, I., Hermoso, M. *et al.* (2010) Nutritional requirements during lactation. Towards European alignment of reference values: the EURRECA network. *Maternal & Child Nutrition* 6: 39–54.

Helland, I.B., Smith, L., Saarem, K., Saugstad, O.D. and Drevon, C.A. (2003) Maternal supplementation with very-long-chain n-3 fatty acids during pregnancy and lactation augments children's IQ at 4 years of age. *Pediatrics*, 111 (1): e39–e44.

Holt, P.G., Sly, P.D. and Björkstén, B. (1997) Atopic versus infectious diseases in childhood: a question of balance? *Pediatric Allergy and Immunology* 8: 53–8.

Hopkinson, J.M., Schanler, R.J., Fraley, J.K. and Garza, C. (1992) Milk production by mothers of premature infants: influence of cigarette smoking. *Pediatrics* 90: 934–938.

Horta, B.L., Kramer, M.S. and Platt, R.W. (2001) Maternal smoking and the risk of early weaning: a meta-analysis. *American Journal of Public Health* 91: 304–307.

Hunt, W. and McManus, A. (2013) Seafood and omega 3s for maternal and child mental health. In: Hall Moran, V. (ed.) *Maternal and infant nutrition and nurture: controversies and challenges*, 2nd edn. London: Quay Books.

ICCIDD (International Council for the Control of Iodine Deficiency Disorders) (2011), www.iccidd.org [accessed 31 August 2011].

Innis, S.M. (2011) Metabolic programming of long-term outcomes due to fatty acid nutrition in early life. *Maternal & Child Nutrition* 7 (Suppl. 2), 112–123.

Institute of Medicine, Food and Nutrition Board (1997) *Dietary Reference Intakes for calcium, phosphorus, magnesium, vitamin D and fluoride.* Washington DC: National Academy Press.

Institute of Medicine, Food and Nutrition Board (1998) *Dietary Reference Intakes for thiamin, riboflavin, niacin, vitamin B6, folate, vitamin B12, pantothenic acid, biotin, and chlorine.* Washington DC: National Academy Press.

Institute of Medicine, Food and Nutrition Board (2000) *Dietary Reference Intakes for vitamin C, vitamin E, selenium, and carotenoids.* Washington DC: National Academy Press.

Institute of Medicine, Food and Nutrition Board (2001) Dietary Reference Intakes for vitamin A, vitamin K, *arsenic, boron, chromium, copper, iodine, iron, manganese, molybdenum, nickel, silicon, vanadium, and zinc.* Washington DC: National Academy Press.

Institute of Medicine, Food and Nutrition Board (2004) *Dietary Reference Intakes for water, potassium, sodium, chloride, and sulphate.* Washington DC: National Academy Press.

Ip, S., Chung, M., Raman, G., Chew, P., Magula, N. *et al.* (2007) Breastfeeding and maternal and infant health outcomes in developed countries. *Evidence Report/Technology Assessment* 153.

Jarjou, L.M., Prentice, A., Sawo, Y., Laskey, M.A., Bennett, J. *et al.* (2006) Randomized, placebo-controlled, calcium supplementation study in pregnant Gambian women: effects on breast-milk calcium concentrations and infant birth weight, growth, and bone mineral accretion in the first year of life. *American Journal of Clinical Nutrition* 83 (3): 657–666.

Jevitt, C., Hernandez, I. and Groër, M. (2007) Lactation complicated by overweight and obesity: supporting the mother and newborn. *Journal of Midwifery & Women's Health* 52 (6): 606–613.

Kac, G., Benicio, M.H.A., Velasquez-Melendez, G., Valente, J.G. and Struchiner, C.J. (2004) Breastfeeding and postpartum weight retention in a cohort of Brazilian women. *American Journal Clinical Nutrition* 79: 487–93.

NUTRITIONAL NEEDS FOR LACTATION

Kent, J.C., Arthur, P.G., Mitoulas, L.R. and Hartmann, P.E. (2009) Why calcium in breastmilk is independent of maternal dietary calcium and vitamin D. *Breastfeeding Review: Professional Publication of the Nursing Mothers' Association of Australia* 17 (2): 5.

King, J.C. (2003) The risk of maternal nutritional depletion and poor outcomes increases in early or closely spaced pregnancies. *Journal of Nutrition* 133 (5): 1732S–1736S.

Koren, G. (2002) Drinking alcohol while breastfeeding. Will it harm my baby? *Canadian Family Physician* 48 (1): 39–41.

Kovacs, C.S. (2011) Calcium and bone metabolism disorders during pregnancy and lactation. *Endocrinology and Metabolism Clinics of North America* 40 (4): 795.

Kovacs, C.S. and Kronenberg, H.M. (1997) Maternal–fetal calcium and bone metabolism during pregnancy, puerperium and lactation. *Endocrine Reviews* 18: 832–872.

Krebs, N.F., Reidinger, C.J., Hartley, S., Robertson, A.D. and Hambidge, K.M. (1995) Zinc supplementation during lactation: effects on maternal status and milk zinc concentrations. *American Journal of Clinical Nutrition* 61, 1030–1036.

Langley-Evans, S. (2009) *Nutrition: a lifespan approach*. Chichester: Wiley-Blackwell.

Lauritzen, L., and Carlson, S.E. (2011) Maternal fatty acid status during pregnancy and lactation and relation to newborn and infant status. *Maternal & Child Nutrition* 7: 41–58.

Leung, A.M., Pearce, E.N. and Braverman, L.E. (2011) Iodine nutrition in pregnancy and lactation. *Endocrinology and Metabolism Clinics of North America* 40: 765.

Maia, P.A., Figueiredo, R.C.B., Anastácio, A.S., Porto da Silveira, C.L. and Donangelo, C.M. (2007) Zinc and copper metabolism in pregnancy and lactation of adolescent women. *Nutrition* 23: 248–253.

Mannion, C.A., Gray-Donald, K., Johnson-Down, L. and Koski, K.G. (2007) Lactating women restricting milk are low on select nutrients. *Journal of the American College of Nutrition* 26 (2): 149–155.

Mehta, U.J., Siega-Riz, A.M., Herring, A.H., Adair, L.S. and Bentley, M.E. (2011) Pregravid body mass index, psychological factors during pregnancy and breastfeeding duration: is there a link? *Maternal & Child Nutrition* 8 (4): 423–433.

Mennella, J.A. and Beauchamp, G.K. (1991) The transfer of alcohol to human milk. Effects on flavor and the infant's behavior. *New England Journal of Medicine* 325: 981–985.

Mennella, J.A., Pepino, M.Y. and Teff, K.L. (2005) Acute alcohol consumption disrupts the hormonal milieu of lactating women. *Journal of Clinical Endocrinology & Metabolism*, 90 (4): 1979–1985.

Moser-Veillon, P.B. (1995) Zinc needs and homeostasis during lactation. *Analyst* 120: 895–897.

National Health and Medical Research Council, Australia (2009) Australian Alcohol Guidelines to Reduce Health Risks from Drinking Alcohol, www.nhmrc.gov.au/media/releases/2009/new-alcohol-guidelines-say-reduce-drinking-reduce-risk.

Neumark-Sztainer, D., Story, M., Resnick, M.D. and Blum, R.W. (1997) Adolescent vegetarians, a behavioural profile of a school-based population in Minnesota. *Archives of Pediatrics and Adolescent Medicine* 151: 833–838.

NICE (2011) Guidance for midwives, health visitors, pharmacists and other primary care services to improve the nutrition of pregnant and breastfeeding mothers and children in low income households. *Public Heath Guidance*. London: Department of Health.

Nishiyama, S., Mikeda, T., Okada, T., Nakamura, K. and Kotani, T. (2004) Transient hypothyroidism or persistent hyperthyrotropinemia in neonates born to mothers with excessive iodine intake. *Thyroid* 14 (12): 1077–1083.

Onyango, A.W., Nommsen-Rivers, L., Siyam, A., Borghi, E., Onis, M. *et al.* (2011) Post-partum weight change patterns in the WHO Multicentre Growth Reference Study. *Maternal and Child Nutrition* 7: 228–240.

Pelto, G. (1987) Cultural issues in maternal and child health and nutrition. *Social Science and Medicine* 25 (6): 553–559.

Perry, C.L., McGuire, M.T., Neumark-Sztainer, D. and Story, M. (2001) Characteristics of vegetarian adolescents in a multiethnic urban population. *Journal Adolescent Health* 29: 406–416.

Picciano, M.F. (2003) Pregnancy and lactation: physiological adjustments, nutritional requirements and the role of dietary supplements. *Journal of Nutrition* 133: 1997S–2002S.

Polatti, F., Capuzzo, E., Viazzo, F. *et al.* (1999) Bone mineral changes during and after lactation, *Obstetrics & Gynecology* 94 (1): 52–56.

Prentice, A. (2008) Vitamin D deficiency: a global perspective. *Nutrition Reviews* 66 (s2): S153–S164.

Prentice, A.M. and van der Merwe, L. (2011) Impact of fatty acid status on immune function of children in low-income countries, *Maternal & Child Nutrition* 7: 89–98.

Rah, J.H., Christian, P., Shamim, A.A., Arju, U.T., Labrique, A.B. and Rashid, M. (2008) Pregnancy and lactation hinder growth and nutritional status of adolescent girls in rural Bangladesh. *Journal of Nutrition* 138: 1505–1511.

Rah, J.H., Shamim, A.A., Arju, U.T., Labrique, A.B., Klemm, R.D. *et al.* (2010) Difference in ponderal growth and body composition among pregnant vs. never-pregnant adolescents varies by birth outcomes. *Maternal & Child Nutrition* 6 (1): 27–37.

Rakicioğlu, N., Samur, G., Topçu, A. and Topçu, A.A. (2006) The effect of Ramadan on maternal nutrition and composition of breast milk. *Pediatrics International* 48 (3): 278–283.

RCOG (2006) Alcohol and pregnancy: information for you. www.rcog.org.uk/files/rcog-corp/Alcohol%20and%20Pregnancy.pdf [accessed 18 March 2013].

Rogol, A.D., Clark, P.A. and Roemmich, J.N. (2000) Growth and pubertal development in children and adolescents: effects of diet and physical activity, *American Journal of Clinical Nutrition* 72: 521S–528S.

SACN (2011) Paper for discussion: Dietary reference values for lactating women. SACN, London. www.sacn.gov.uk/pdfs/sacn_dietary_reference_values_for_energy.pdf.

Sampson, H.A. (2004) Update on food allergy. *Journal of Allergy and Clinical Immunology* 113: 805–819.

Scholl, T.O., Hediger, M.L. and Ances, I.G. (1990) Maternal growth during pregnancy and decreased infant birth weight. *American Journal of Clinical Nutrition* 51: 790–793.

Scholl, T.O., Hediger, M.L., Cronk, C.E. and Schall, J.I. (1993) Maternal growth during pregnancy and lactation. *Hormone Research* 39 (Suppl. 3): 59–67.

Seth, A., Marwaha, R.K., Singla, B., Aneja, S., Mehrotra, P. *et al.* (2009) Vitamin D nutritional status of exclusively breast fed infants and their mothers. *Journal of Pediatric Endocrinology* 22: 241–246.

Sian, L., Krebs, N.F., Westcott, J.E., Fengliang, L., Tong, L. *et al.* (2002) Zinc homeostasis during lactation in a population with a low zinc intake. *American Journal of Clinical Nutrition* 75: 99–103.

Sichieri, R., Field, A.E., Rich-Edwards, J. and Willett, W.C. (2003) Prospective assessment of exclusive breastfeeding in relation to weight change in women. *International Journal of Obesity and Related Metabolic Disorders* 27: 15–20.

Sommer, A., Davidson, F.R. and Annecy, A. (2002) Assessment and control of vitamin A deficiency: the Annecy Accords. *Journal of Nutrition* 132: Suppl. 2850S.

Specker, B.L., Black, A., Allen, L. and Morrow, F. (1990) Vitamin B12 low milk concentrations are related to low serum, concentrations in vegetarian women and to methylmalonic aciduria in their infants. *American Journal of Clinical Nutrition* 52: 1073–1076.

Stapleton, H. and Keenan, J. (2009) Bodies in the making: reflections on women's consumption practices in pregnancy. In: Dykes, F. and Hall Moran, V. (eds) *Infant and young child nutrition: challenges to implementing a global strategy*. Oxford: Wiley-Blackwell.

Stuebe, A.M., Kleinman, K., Gillman, M.W., Rifas-Shiman, S.L., Gunderson, E.P. and Rich-Edwards, J. (2010) Duration of lactation and maternal metabolism at 3 years postpartum. *Journal of Women's Health* 19: 941–950.

Turcksin, R., Bel, S., Galjaard, S. and Devlieger, R. (2012) Maternal obesity and breastfeeding intention, initiation, intensity and duration: a systematic review. *Maternal & Child Nutrition*, DOI: 10.1111/j.1740-8709.2012.00439.x.

Vanderpump, M.P.J., Lazarus, J.H., Smyth, P.P. *et al.* (2011) On behalf of the British Thyroid Association UK Iodine Survey Group. Iodine status in UK schoolgirls: a cross-sectional survey. *Lancet*, 377: 2007–2012.

Vio, F., Salazar, G. and Infante, C. (1991) Smoking during pregnancy and lactation and its effects on breast-milk volume. *American Journal of Clinical Nutrition* 54: 1011–1016.

Wagnon, J., Cagnard, B., Bridoux-Henno, L., Tourtelier, Y., Grall, J.Y. and Dabadie, A. (2005) Breast-feeding and vegan diet. *Journal de Gynecologie, Obstetrique et Biologie de la Reproduction* 34: 610–2.

Wambach, K. and Riordan, J. (2010) The cultural context of breastfeeding. In: Riordan, J. and Wambach, K., *Breastfeeding and human lactation*. London: Jones and Bartlett Publishers.

Weiss, R., Fogelman, Y. and Bennett, M. (2004) Severe vitamin B12 deficiency in an infant associated with a maternal deficiency and strict vegetarian diet, *Journal of Pediatric Hematology & Oncology* 26: 270–1.

WHO (2003) *Global strategy for infant and young child feeding*. Geneva: WHO.

WHO, The Micronutrient Initiative (1998) *Safe vitamin A dosage during pregnancy and lactation. Recommendations and report of a consultation*. Geneva: WHO.

WHO/FAO (Food and Agriculture Organization of the United Nations) (2004) *Vitamin and mineral requirements in human nutrition*, 2nd edn. Geneva: WHO/FAO.

WHO/FAO (2004a) *Joint WHO/FAO expert consultation on human vitamin and mineral requirements*. Geneva: WHO/FAO.

Widström, M., Werner, S., Matthiesen, A.S., Svensson, K. and Uvnaas Moberg, K. (1991) Somatostatin levels in plasma in nonsmoking and smoking breast-feeding women. *Acta Paediatrica* 80 (1): 13–21.

Worsley, A. and Skrzypiec, G. (1998) Teenage vegetarianism: prevalence, social and cognitive contexts. *Appetite* 30: 151–170.

Zava, T.T. and Zava, D.T. (2011) Assessment of Japanese iodine intake based on seaweed consumption in Japan: a literature-based analysis. *Thyroid Research* 4 (14): 1–7.

Zimmermann, M.B. (2009) Iodine deficiency, *Endocrine Reviews* 30 (4): 376–408.

Zimmermann, M. and Delange, F. (2004) Iodine supplementation of pregnant women in Europe: a review and recommendations. *European Journal of Clinical Nutrition* 58: 979–984.

Part II

CONTEXT AND CULTURAL ISSUES

5

NOURISHMENT

A sociological exploration of food, culture and identity

Rea Daellenbach

Introduction

British celebrity chef Jamie Oliver has a mission. As he explained in his TED Prize Wish talk, 'I have a wish for everyone to help create a strong, sustainable movement to educate every child about food, inspire families to cook again and empower people everywhere to fight obesity' (Oliver 2010). Through his television series, cookbooks, Ministry of Food community initiatives and the school dinner programme, he is trying to change the way food is produced, prepared and consumed. He promotes cooking food from fresh ingredients, with enticing and varied menus. He has taken on politicians and the food industry and has inspired an enthusiastic following, but also numerous critics.

In the Christmas 2012 issue of the *British Medical Journal* (*BMJ*), another voice was added to Oliver's critics. Howard, Adams and White (2012) published research results casting doubt over whether home-cooked recipes are healthier than supermarket convenience foods in the United Kingdom. They randomly selected 100 recipes from cookbooks by the television chefs Jamie Oliver, Nigella Lawson and Hugh Fearnley-Whittingstall and compared these with 100 'ready meals' from UK supermarkets. They found that, on average, the ready meals contained less fat and saturated fat and more fibre than those made from the recipes. On this basis, they conclude that the TV chefs' 'recipes seem to be less healthy than the ready meals' (Howard, Adams and White 2012: 4).

The controversy about the relative health benefits of the chefs' recipes and supermarket ready meals is embedded in a larger global debate about food. The participants in this debate include transnational and government public health agencies, vast numbers of non-governmental organisations such as national heart foundations, nutritionists, dieticians and medical associations, social movement groups, as well as the food industry, food sector interest groups and dieting and health food enterprises. All these are competing for the hearts, minds and stomachs of the world's population. As a consequence, we are constantly bombarded with conflicting messages about what we should and should not eat.

Midwives are caught up in the web of promoting dietary messages well. They are expected to provide nutritional assessment and advice to women during pregnancy and for breastfeeding. This has intensified in recent years amidst growing concerns about adverse neonatal and maternal outcomes associated with food-borne pathogens, obesity and alcohol consumption. Also, there is growing recognition that nutritional status and exposure to environmental toxins during pregnancy have lifelong effects for babies as well as for mothers. But how can midwives make sense of the plethora of contradictory advice while providing individualised advice to women that is respectful of their cultural beliefs and the personal circumstances that determine their food choices? On the one hand, pregnancy and caring for a new baby can offer an ideal opportunity to make positive lifestyle changes. Often, however, the women who would most benefit from information about good nutrition are the least interested or able to take it up (Crozier, Robinson, Borland, Godfrey, Cooper and Inkskip 2009; Wennberg, Lundqvist, Högberg, Sandström and Hamberg, in press).

This chapter presents a sociological account of some of the current debates around people's food consumption. It rests on the premise that eating and drinking, like birth, is both a biological and a cultural reality (see Chapter 1). Drawing on insights from archaeology and food psychology about the genetic human predispositions related to food consumption, the chapter begins by examining the links between humans' biological food needs and culture. Then it asks: what are the salient aspects of culture that shape our current beliefs about food? A question that is particularly relevant for midwifery is: what are the cultural values and expectations that shape women's relationship with food? These questions are addressed through tracing the effects of industrialisation on women's roles within the household and the tensions and contradictions that these produce for women in the new millennium.

The term 'culture' refers to the way of life of a particular group of people based on shared language, values and expected forms of behaviour. Culture is not simply a kind of programming. Rather, a culture can be thought of as a specific 'menu' of options, and this explains, for example, why siblings often make dissimilar lifestyle or dietary choices. At the same time, choices that are not on the menu of options are unthinkable or not accepted as valid by others within the cultural milieu.

Food is an essential part of each human being's daily life, even in contexts where food is not available or a person is focused on avoiding eating. Eating is not just about satisfying bodily needs. Anthropologist Claude Lévi-Strauss is often quoted as saying that 'food is good for thinking'. He argued that, for humans, food is laden with symbolic meanings that define social cohesion and social boundaries (Darnton 2002). The food 'we' eat smells and tastes good, the food eaten by 'others' is less appetising and sometimes even disgusting. Thus, eating fulfils a critical social function, enabling people to construct and accomplish self-identity and a sense of belonging to a cultural group.

Our genetic inheritance

The public health campaigns aimed at promoting healthy food choices are based on the assumption that people need nutritional advice because they do not naturally prefer foods that are good for them. In a hypothetical world in which unhealthy food choices were not available, would we not naturally seek out well-balanced healthy diets, choosing foods that contained the micronutrients we needed and avoiding those that were detrimental to our health? This proposition was given widespread credibility through a study done by paediatrician Clara Davis in the 1930s. She conducted an experiment with infants (six to eleven months old at the beginning of the study) in an orphanage where at meal times each child was presented with a wide range of nutritious foods (such as cereals, fruits, vegetables, meat, eggs and milk) that they could choose from (Logue 2004). Caregivers would give the children any food they pointed to without in any way trying to influence their choices. She found that while some children would binge on one particular food for a time, overall each child ended up with a well-balanced diet. She concluded that young children instinctively know what they need to eat, a theory that she called the 'wisdom of the body' (Strauss 2006).

Davis's ideas are appealing, and certainly had an impact on the medical advice subsequently given to parents about infant feeding. However, there was a problem with her experiment. Children had to point to the food they wanted and then a nurse would feed it to them. This social interaction meant that the children had to develop a range of complex cognitive and social skills, and to learn not just that food could relieve hunger and the tastes of different foods, but also that pointing would elicit specific caregiver responses. The children will have also learned to read the inadvertent and unconscious cues from caregivers while negotiating their food intake (Logue 2004). Thus, the results do not necessarily support the theory that humans innately know what to eat if cultural influences are stripped away. They may instead point to how food preferences are learned and become embodied in social contexts.

Food psychologists Roizin and his team argue that the lack of knowing instinctively what to eat is part of our genetic inheritance as omnivores:

> Many animals are born knowing what to eat, and they instinctively seek out the visual image, scent, or taste of a particular food (for instance, koala bears eat only the leaves of a few species of eucalyptus trees). Human beings, however, must learn what to eat. Like rats, pigs, herring gulls and cockroaches, we are omnivores. The omnivorous strategy has the advantages of flexibility and freedom of dependence on any one food source. But omnivores face the attendant risk of consuming toxins or a nutritionally unbalanced diet. These two opposing facts create the 'omnivore's dilemma'.
>
> (Haidt, Roizin, McCauley and Imada 1997: 108–109)

As in rats and cockroaches, the innate flexibility and adaptability of food preferences has enabled humans to extend their range of habitation to virtually any terrain on this planet and to withstand massive environmental changes. However, unlike rats and cockroaches, humans have evolved complex pro-social feeding strategies to deal with the omnivore's dilemma. What most definitively separates humans from the rest of the natural world is the use of cooking for food preparation (Jones 2007). Cooking is a universal human activity. All societies have means of cooking some of the food they consume. Even the Inuit peoples of the Arctic Circle, who traditionally ate a lot of their food raw, did cook some, using seal and whale fat as fuel.

Bioarchaeologist Jones (2007) argues that the development of food cooking transformed not only food but also the human species. He suggests that early human gatherers and hunters may have consumed a lot of food where they found it. Cooking food, however, required more social cooperation and organisation. Cooking brought people together around the fire to plan, prepare and eat a meal. The fire also provided warmth, and protection from predators. Around the fire, people shared food, space, time and stories of their experiences, and thus developed the 'essence of conviviality that defines humanity' (Jones 2007: 2). Food sharing was also involved in social decisions such as who not to share food with and how to prioritise who would be fed first in situations when food was scarce. Following the work of anthropologist Lévi-Strauss, Jones suggests that the use of fire to cook food was an important resource in the development of culture and civilisation (Jones 2007).

Cooking food has had a massive effect on our genetic inheritance (Jones 2007). Thermal processing transforms raw food by breaking down many toxins and fibres found in the food and increasing the available calories. In making foods more nutritious and easier to digest, cooking can be described as a form of external digestion. The shift from dependence on raw food to consumption of some cooked food reduced the high energy demands of the digestive system. This enabled the expansion of the size of the human brain, particularly the neocortex, which in turn increased intelligence and the ability to create and manage increasing complexity in social relationships (Jones 2007).

For humans, physiology and culture are intertwined in their relation to food consumption. Humans do not instinctively know what to eat and instead rely on cultural knowledge to tell them what is good for them. This does not mean that individuals cannot work out for themselves how different foods affect them, but this is learned through critical reflection on bodily sensations and memory, mediated through cultural schemas that categorise food.

More recent thinking about genetic determinants of food preferences suggests that humans do have universal preferences for sweet and salty tastes and the sensation of fats. Fetuses *in utero* swallow more amniotic fluid when it contains more glucose, and babies also demonstrate a preference for sweetness. The preference for the taste of salt develops at about four months of age. The appreciation of umami (yummy) tastes develops in the second year of life (Lanfer 2012). It is not clear whether there is a universal human preference for umami tastes. However, some health food advocates see attention to this taste as a potentially effective way of encouraging people to eat a greater range of healthy foods. As well as meat and fish, umami foods include soy bean products, tomatoes, mushrooms, seaweed, yeast extract and roasted nuts, seeds and vegetables.

The innate human taste preferences are excellent evolutionary adaptations in the context of food insecurity. This has been the reality for most humans until only very recently and continues to be an issue for 870,000,000 people worldwide (Food and Agriculture Organization 2012). However, when food is plentiful, the predisposition to prefer foods that are sweet and have a high fat content becomes a harmful adaptation, as is evidenced by the 1.4 billion of the world's adults who are overweight and at increased risk of developing diabetes, heart disease and certain cancers (World Health Organization 2012).

The omnivore's dilemma has resulted in humans, as a species, having a deep ambivalence about food. We need to eat a wide range of different foods so as to ensure that our micronutrient needs are met, and at the same time to be averse to flavours and sensations that might be indicative of harmful constituents. Food psychologists suggest that people tend to fall at either one end or the other of a scale between being sensation seeking or neophobic (Haidt, Roizin, McCauley and Imada 1997; Logue 2004). This is determined to some extent by genetic diversity. However, it is also influenced by epigenetic mechanisms. Research by Shim, Kim and Mathai (2011) found that children who were exclusively breastfed for the first six months after birth had significantly reduced rates of rejection of vegetables, fruits, meat and fish, as compared to those who were not (odds ratio 0.19, 95, % confidence interval 0.06.–0.69). They propose that this could be due to breast milk containing the flavours of the foods eaten by the mother. Rappoport (2003) also suggests that another factor could be that the quality-controlled consistency of infant formula does not prime a baby to learn to like novel flavours. Children develop likings for different foods through repeated exposure and observing adults or other children eating foods (Lanfer 2012). This makes sense for an omnivore who has developed a reliance on shared food preparation and consumption. The next section explores the current contexts for the organising of meals within the household and charts how this developed over time.

Families and the industrialisation of food in the twentieth century

Women, particularly mothers in households with dependent children, tend to bear the primary responsibility for decisions around what foods are bought and how they are prepared

(De Vault 2008; Walter 2009). Organising the food for the family is more than just work. It is laden with ideological meanings and social expectations. As Lupton explains, 'One major concern that is constantly linked with food is that of love, particularly maternal love, romantic love and wifely concern about the well-being of one's husband' (Lupton 1996: 37). Trying to ensure that family members' bodily and emotional nutritional needs are met has become symbolic of a woman's love for her partner and children and her status as a 'good mother'. This configuration of practices and meanings emerged with the rise of industrialisation towards the end of the 1800s (Aronson 1980; Thomas 1995).

Industrialisation had different effects for different classes within industrialising nations. However, for most, the household no longer functioned as a unit of production in which both the care of the family and economic work were combined (Aronson 1980). For the urban middle classes, as business enterprises had to expand in order to compete, the production of goods and services was no longer an affair that involved all members of the family. As a result, middle-class women found a new vocation in the roles of housekeeper, wife and mother (Skocpol 1992: 323).

Industrialisation also resulted in substantial numbers of people living in poverty in cities throughout Europe and the North America and Australasia (Klaus 1993). Changes in techniques of agricultural production and landownership led to masses of people migrating to urban centres in search of paid employment. As many as two million people left Ireland during the 'potato famine' of 1845–55 (Kiple 2007). However, the wages for men, women and children working in the cities were so low that many could barely afford the necessities of life. In addition, the length of the working day was such that people had little time or energy for household labour (Thomas 1995). Many of the working class lived in overcrowded and unsanitary housing. Some did not even have access to cooking facilities, and those that were available were often inefficient and had to be shared with the other tenants of the building. Infant and child mortality rates among the poor were very high and many people suffered from chronic ill-health, due to malnutrition (Klaus 1993).

In the last decades of the 1800s, a number of social movements arose that began to view urban poverty as a social problem, not just a private trouble. The most important of these in effecting changes to women's roles and responsibility within society was the emerging women's movement, made up of a large number of women's organisations around the world. The diversity of the social and political agendas of different women's groups is too complex to do justice to it here. However, women's suffrage was an important political goal for many. This was based on a concept of 'maternal citizenship', asserting that mothers were just as important as soldiers for protecting the security and prosperity of the nation, and thus they should be entitled to the right to vote (Skocpol 1992).

Many women reformers were influenced by a belief that women are naturally more pious and nurturing than men, referred to as the cult of 'True Womanhood' (Skocpol 1992). Based on Christian principles and middle-class ideals, supporters of True Womanhood argued that society could be improved from within, by mothers' tender and unselfish care for the physical and moral health of their children and husbands. They believed that women also had a natural 'caretaking and nurturing role . . . outside the home . . . to succor the poor and educate the wayward' (Skocpol 1992: 324). Women's organisation members visited women living in poverty and sought to educate them about them about nutrition, hygiene and childcare (Aronson 1980). They also lobbied governments to introduce labour and welfare reforms so that working-class women would also be able to afford to adopt the 'universal' function of women as wives, homemakers and mothers (Skocpol 1992).

It is probable that, prior to industrialisation, the responsibility for food preparation, cleaning and childcare fell primarily on women. However, in extended households that were comprised of several generations and non-family members such as workers and servants, these tasks were assigned according to the needs and skills within each household (Kiple 2007) and not necessarily only a mother's responsibility. Thomas (1995) notes that many working-class women aspired to the new Victorian ideal of motherhood. The ideological and economic reforms that resulted from the turn-of-the-century political activism enabled more women to take up this role. This brought about significant improvements in health.

Even though nature (or God) had created women to be mothers, they were increasingly seen as needing all sorts of expert advice to help them fulfil this role. Cookbooks and housekeeping manuals became immensely popular in this era (Rappoport 2003). For example, Queen Victoria's chef, Francatelli (perhaps the first celebrity chef), produced a cookbook for working-class families in 1852. It included recipes for vegetable soups, potatoes and cheap cuts of meat as well as 'a pudding made of small birds' that the boys might have caught (Francatelli 1852). In recognition that some working-class families did not own the necessary cookware, Francatelli began with a list of what was needed and advised readers to 'strive to lay by a little of your weekly wages to purchase these things, that your families may be well fed, and your homes made comfortable' (Francatelli 1852: 1). Books such as Francatelli's were published in many countries around the world. In a study of Bengali domestic manuals that were written as an indigenous response to the imported British books, Walsh quotes advice asserting that cooking is a 'beautiful and important ingredient of family life' that should not be left to hired cooks who would not give it the required 'attention and devotion', nor 'enjoy the same pleasure' as a wife has in cooking for her family (Walsh 2005: 191).

Many cookbooks had a dual purpose. As well as offering recipes to promote domestic felicity, they provided the opportunity for business enterprises to advertise their new products and inform women about how to use them. Francatelli's cookbook included advertisements for new refined grains, food additives, drinks and patent medicines. Some business enterprises produced their own cookbooks, such as the *Edmonds Sure to Rise Cookery Book* in New Zealand. Initially written in 1908 to promote the company's line of baking products, it expanded to include all meals and became the definitive guide to New Zealand cooking for several generations (Ministry for Culture and Heritage, 2012).

Doctors also found a new role as advisors to mothers. Armed with insights from the emerging nutrition sciences and new substances produced by the food processing industry (for example, infant formulas), doctors increasingly began to instruct women about the nutritional needs of their families and the best way to raise healthy children (Apple 1997; Aronson 1980). Apple refers to this as the growth of scientific motherhood. In Britain, a number of other European countries and New Zealand, one effect of this was the registration of midwives, with the aim of ensuring that poor and working-class women had access to maternity services. The new, registered midwives also were expected to be 'health missionaries' and to inform women about hygiene, diet, infant feeding and family healthcare (Marland 1997). While mothers have perhaps been the health workers within the family for much longer, this now became a moral imperative and an expected responsibility under the guidance of health professionals (Apple 1997).

Families and food in the new millennium

The ideal of women's place in the home was fraught with contradictions. Women were supposed to be contributing to the well-being of the nation, whilst at the same time being marginalised in public and political arenas. They were expected to cater for their families without having control over the resources to do this. This included control over the safety and healthiness of the food on the market. Also, after the Second World War, women were expected meet the needs of each family member as an individual, with their own individual needs coming last. These contradictions came to a head with the second wave of feminism in the 1970s and 1980s. At the same time, economic changes required a larger workforce and made it more difficult for families to live on one income. Consequently, most mothers are now in paid employment and there are new ideas about gender equality. How has this affected family food consumption?

In 2006, the Health Sponsorship Council of New Zealand commissioned a qualitative study into the eating patterns of New Zealand families (TNS New Zealand 2007). Over one hundred families participated in focus groups, family/whānau (Maori extended family) interviews and individual interviews. Care was taken to ensure that participants were representative of the diversity of ethnic and socio-economic groups in New Zealand. The findings from this study provide insight into the issues facing families in relation to food consumption today.

The research in New Zealand found that mothers were generally the ones who were responsible for planning, purchasing and preparing the families' meals, even if they were in paid employment (TNS New Zealand 2007). Some participants in the study described cooking family meals as pleasurable and satisfying. These families were more likely to have shared meals around a table. However, most identified it as a chore for which they often did not have the time and energy at the end of the working day or after looking after young children all day. Thus, they were more likely to eat convenience foods, including takeaway fast foods, and to leave out vegetables. Convenience foods were perceived by some participants as being more filling and better value for money than home-cooked meals with vegetables (TNS New Zealand 2007).

Many participants also reported that family meals were marked by emotional conflict over getting children to eat healthy foods, e.g. vegetables (TNS New Zealand 2007). The researchers identified that 'partner drag' – partners who did not eat healthy foods – contributed to this. Some families found that eating in front of the television reduced this tension, though without necessarily improving children's diets. Others gave up trying, in the interests of harmony, as '[h]aving to deal with conflict that could arise from insisting on healthy eating was seen as something that would eat into time – already a scarce commodity' (TNS New Zealand 2007: 128).

Struggling to get children eat healthy foods is not a new problem for families. It was one of the main issues for which mothers sought medical advice in the era of scientific motherhood (Apple 1997). Medical advice in the early 1900s tended to advocate authoritarian measures to make children eat the foods doctors had identified as healthy. Davis's research in the 1930s was so influential because it advocated a more child-led approach (Strauss 2006). Both approaches to encouraging children to eat healthy foods focus on intra-familial dynamics, particularly on mothers' responsibility to ensure that children have a healthy diet. And mothers can choose between an authoritarian approach, which can create conflict, or a more facilitative approach that requires organisation, perseverance and time. However, in the new millennium powerful forces outside the family can also have profound effects on children's food choices.

Many parents and children in the TNS NZ study talked about kinds of foods that children particularly wanted to eat. The report notes that '[c]hildren frequently asked their parents to buy specific foods they had seen advertised on television (or had seen in other children's lunchboxes)' (TNS NZ 2007: 8) and '[w]hen having takeaways the children may have got to choose what type of takeaways they had. They could also influence the decision to get takeaways' (TNS NZ 2007: 143). These children had food preferences that were clearly shaped by food industry advertising.

A report produced by the Rudd Center (Harris, Weinberg, Schwartz, Ross, Ostroffa, and Brownell 2010) used data on the actual hours of television watched and found that for the year 2008, on average, an American child (aged 2–17) watched 4484 food advertisements. A quarter of these were for fast foods, while the next two categories, breakfast cereals and prepared meals combined, contributed another quarter. Other categories included soft drinks, candy and snacks. By comparison, children saw on average only twenty advertisements for fruits and vegetables over the entire year. Thus, children's education about food, outside of what they might get at home, comes primarily from the processed food industry promoting foods that are high in sugar, salt and fat. It is interesting to note that food companies are aware of the potentially addictive nature of the overconsumption of the sugary and high-fat foods they produce (Schor and Ford 2007). This was revealed in the evidence gained from the legal proceedings against tobacco companies in the United States, as tobacco companies had bought out major food companies in order to diversify away from cigarettes.

Schor and Ford (2007) argue that the power of food advertising aimed at children lies in the way that 'branded (i.e. junk) food comes to occupy an increasingly central position in children's sense of identity, their relationships to other children and adults and the construction of meaning and value that structure their lives' (Schor and Ford 2007: 16). This is set within a social context of increasing individualisation in which children are pushed to develop their own future identity in order to be able to have a 'life of one's own'. Identity, rather from being inherited through birth, as it was in the past and still is in many communities around the world, has become a personal project (Beck and Beck-Gernsheim 2002). Advertising aimed at children taps into this in various ways. Some promise future success. Others offer identification with a brand, e.g. 'Weetbix Kid' in New Zealand (Weetbix is a popular breakfast cereal), or an identity position as a child (not adult) through the use of childish fantasy images (Schor and Ford 2007). Even if children resist messages about particular brands, they may still assimilate the message that food is a significant personal identity choice.

As concerted food advertising aimed at children took off in the 1990s and has continued into the new millennium, the children first exposed to this are now adults and having children of their own. How has their orientation to food been shaped by this experience? Younger generations are now likely to have quite different diets to their parents and grandparents. This is true whether they live in the United States, Italy, Japan or India (Rappoport 2003). The evidence from New Zealand shows that millennials (born 1980 onwards) eat fewer vegetables and fruits and eat significantly more fast food than do older generations (University of Otago 2011). Millennials have also grown up with public health messages about nutrition and social movement activism related to food consumption, and thus there is also a high degree of variability in diets within this generation (McPhail, Chapman and Beagan 2011). While many eat more processed and fast foods, others choose a greater range of vegetables, organic and locally grown foods, or become vegetarian or vegan. The new cultural imperative is to construct your own diet. Eating is increasingly becoming a way of feeding our identities as individuals and an important way to express our sense of self-worth as entitled and moral agents (Lupton 1996).

The new millennium is marked globally by the growing diversity of foods and cuisines on offer and also by the diverse and multiple cultural and nutritional meanings attached to each food ingredient. Salecl (2010) argues that choice related to food is laden with anxiety, as choosing invariably leads to questions as to whether this is really the best choice and what other people will think about this choice. People's food choices are obviously determined first by the material constraints of what foods are available on the market and what they can afford to buy. However, even with the same material conditions, people differ in the foods they choose to purchase and consume.

Rappoport (2003) suggests that the link between food choices and identity can be analysed through three competing food ideologies: hedonism, nutritionism and ethical/spiritual orientations. These ideologies do not determine what people eat, but why they make the food choices that they do. These three ideologies provide justificatory frameworks for decision making in relation to food, and people often use several at once. While these ideologies are expressed through individuals' orientations to food, they are embedded in the globalised economics of the food industry and the politics of health and cultural diversity.

Hedonist justifications for food choices include satiating hunger, comfort and enjoyment. Taste, flavour and the sensations of food are important. The aesthetics of food can be important also, although what counts as aesthetically pleasing is highly variable. For some, this might be the advertised brands of processed foods, while for others it is gourmet meals (Rappoport 2003). Selecting foods primarily on the basis of convenience might also be counted under a hedonist approach, as it confers benefits in terms of reducing the time required for meal planning and preparation.

Bordo (2003) argues that capitalism places women (and increasingly men) in a double bind. They are exhorted to indulge desires, to buy and consume food with the promise of happiness (the hedonist ideology). At the same time they are expected to strive for self-control and self-improvement to achieve the slender body that is so highly valued in the employment market and for attracting a partner. Preoccupation with this double bind is ever present in the lives of many women as they oscillate between overeating for emotional comfort and restrictive dieting in an attempt to shed the extra calories they have consumed.

Rappoport (2003) refers to the second important ideology of food consumption in modern societies as 'nutritionism'. This refers to a raft of different theories about what constitute healthy foods (see also Pollan 2006), including the advice from dieticians, nutritionists and doctors as well as the recommendations put forward by various health food specialists and dieting programmes. What these have in common is the conviction that health should be the primary determinant of food choices through identifying the risks associated with 'bad' foods and the benefits of 'good' foods, although there is little consensus about what these might be. The focus is on changing individuals' eating behaviours, based on a moralist discourse that we are each individually responsible for our health (Lupton 1996). Without radically changing the market-driven food industry, it not clear how effective this strategy can be. Research on eating patterns suggests that many people try to accommodate both hedonist and nutritionist food ideologies and consume food that they know to be unhealthy and then feel guilty about it (see for example McPhail, Chapman and Beagan 2011). The TNS New Zealand (2012) food survey found that many people were confused by the different and conflicting dietary health messages. Some of the respondents reported being resistant to these messages, not trusting nutrition experts, while others did not bother trying to understand them at all.

Hedonism and nutritionism are both internally focused ideologies – 'I eat what I eat for my own happiness or health'. Religious and ethical concerns that can determine people's food choices are externally oriented as expressions of wider cultural, social and ethical concerns.

67

These include Halal, Kosher or Hindu food rules, vegetarianism prompted by the motivation not to be complicit in causing the suffering and killing of animals, or eating only seasonal and locally produced foods as a commitment to planetary and community sustainability. Making family eating choices to pass on a cultural heritage or family values, such as the shared meal as a focus for quality family time, could also be considered as an externally oriented ideology. The TNS NZ survey found that some Maori New Zealanders placed high value on the ethical principle of manākitanga, or sharing and hospitality in relation to food. This ideology is based on the precept that what we eat connects us to larger social questions and relationships.

Identification with a peer group has been found to be a significant external orientation for youth. The 13- to 16-year-old participants in a study conducted in the North of England linked food brand choices to identity and were able to articulate a clear hierarchy of 'best' and 'wrong brands' (Stead, McDermott, MacKintosh and Adamson 2011). Food has invariably functioned in this way in culture; food choices signal identity and belonging to a particular peer group within the social milieu.

These different food ideologies highlight the complexity of diets in our times and it can easily seem too complicated for midwives. However, in avoiding talk of nutrition, women's and babies' health and well-being may be neglected, with possible long-term implications. The recognition that these food ideologies determine people's food choices can enable midwives to provide individualised care. It prompts midwives to ask more than just what food women eat, but also to ask what is important for them in deciding what to eat.

Over the past 150 years, the responsibility for food choices in families has rested primarily on women, but there is nothing intrinsically gendered about this. Midwives might be able to find opportunities during appointments and in classes to encourage partners and other significant people in women's lives to consider healthy eating as a very real way of supporting the woman and her baby. Through the sharing of food preparation and eating together, healthy eating can become a shared family responsibility with potential benefits to health and family well-being.

Conclusion

Humans have sought to resolve the omnivore's dilemma by collective strategies of food collection, preparation and eating. Through cooking food, humans have evolved the brain capacity to construct elaborate cultural schemas that determine what, how and even to some extent why they eat. Thus, humans learn what to eat as members of families and communities. Unfortunately, in today's world, many learn to eat from the food industry, with devastating health consequences, while at the same time they are seen as being morally culpable for these consequences. As the introductory paragraphs of this chapter indicate, the omnivore's dilemma is again the subject of intense public attention and private anxieties (Pollan 2006).

Midwives can make a significant contribution to a culture of healthy eating through talking to women and their families about food and nutrition. In recognising that we are what we eat, in surprising and complex ways, midwives can play their part in inspiring and empowering people to eat delicious and healthy foods and help to create strong, sustainable families.

References

Apple, R. (1997) 'Constructing Mothers, Scientific Motherhood in the Nineteenth and Twentieth Centuries', in R. Apple and J. Golden (eds) *Mothers and Motherhood: Readings in American History*, Columbus, OH: Ohio State University Press.

Aronson, N. (1980) 'Working Up an Appetite', in J. Kaplan (ed.) *A Woman's Conflict: The Special Relationship between Women and Food*, Englewood Cliffs, NJ: Prentice-Hall.

Beck, U. and Beck-Gernsheim, E. (2002) *Individualization*, London: Sage Publications.

Bordo, S. (2003) *Unbearable Weight, Feminism, Western Culture and the Body*, 10th edn, Berkeley, CA: University of California Press.

Crozier, S., Robinson, S., Borland, S., Godfrey, K., Cooper, C. and Inkskip, H. (2009) 'Do Women Change Their Food Habits during Pregnancy? Findings from the Southampton Women's Study', *Paediatric Perinatal Epidemiology*, 23 (5) 446–453. Online. Available www.ncbi.nlm.nih.gov/pmc/articles/PMC3091015/pdf/ukmss-35209.pdf (accessed 13 October 2012).

Darnton, R. (2002) 'Sex for Thought', in K. Phillips and B. Reay, B. (eds) *Sexualities in History: A Reader*, London: Routledge.

De Vault, M. (2008) 'Conflict and Deference', in C. Counihan and P. Van Esterik (eds) *Food and Culture: A Reader*, 2nd edn, New York, NY: Routledge.

Food and Agriculture Organization (2012) *The State of Food Insecurity in the World*, Rome: Food and Agriculture Organization of the United Nations. Online. Available www.fao.org/publications/sofi/en/ (accessed 3 December 2012).

Francatelli, C. E. (1852, 1977) *Plain Cookery Book for the Working Classes*, London: Scholar Press. Online. Available www.gutenberg.org/files/22114/22114-h/22114-h.htm (accessed 3 February 2013).

Haidt, J., Roizin, P., McCauley, C. and Imada, S. (1997) 'Body, Psyche, and Culture: The Relationship between Disgust and Morality', *Psychology and Developing Studies*, 9 (1) 107–131.

Harris, J., Weinberg, M., Schwartz, M., Ross, C., Ostroffa, J. and Brownell, K. (2010) *Rudd Report, Trends in Television Food Advertising*, Englewood, CN: Yale University. Online. Available www.yaleruddcenter.org/resources/upload/docs/what/reports/RuddReport_TVFoodAdvertising_5.12.pdf (accessed 6 February 2013).

Howard, S., Adams, J. and White, M. (2012) 'Nutritional Content of Supermarket Ready Meals and Recipes by Television Chefs in the United Kingdom: Cross Sectional Study', *British Medical Journal*, 345, e7607: 1–10. Online. Available www.bmj.com/content/345/bmj.e7607 (accessed 20 December 2012).

Jones, M. (2007) *Feast: Why Humans Share Food*, New York, NY: Oxford University Press.

Kiple, K. (2007) *A Movable Feast, Ten Millennia of Food Globalization*, New York, NY: Cambridge University Press.

Klaus, A. (1993) *Every Child a Lion: The Origins of Maternal and Infant Health Policies in the United States and France, 1890–1920*, Ithaca, NY: Cornell University Press.

Lanfer, A. (2012) 'Taste Preferences, Diet and Overweight in European Children, An Epidemiological Perspective', PhD Dissertation, University of Bremen. Online. Available http://elib.suub.uni-bremen.de/edocs/00102773-1.pdf (accessed 2 November 2012).

Logue, A. (2004) *The Psychology of Eating and Drinking*, 3rd edn, New York, NY: Brunner-Routledge.

Lupton, D. (1996) *Food, the Body and the Self*, London: Sage Publications.

Marland, H. (1997) 'The Midwife as Health Missionary', in H. Marland and A.M. Rafferty (eds) *Midwives, Society and Childbirth: Debates and Controversies in the Modern Period*, London: Routledge.

McPhail, D., Chapman, G. and Beagan, B. (2011) ''Too Much of That Stuff Can't Be Good': Canadian Teens, Morality, and Fast Food Consumption', *Social Science & Medicine*, 73, 301–307. Accessed from ScienceDirect Database.

Ministry for Culture and Heritage (2012) 'Edmonds Cookery Book', *New Zealand History Online*. Available from www.nzhistory.net.nz/media/photo/edmonds-cookbook (accessed 3 February 2013).

Oliver, J. (February, 2010) *TED Prize Wish: Teach Every Child about Food*. Video Online. Available www.ted.com/talks/jamie_oliver.html (accessed 2 November 2012).

Pollan, M. (2006) *The Omnivore's Dilemma: A Natural History of Four Meals*, New York, NY: Penguin Press.

Rappoport, L. (2003) *How We Eat: Appetite, Culture and the Psychology of Food*, Toronto: ECW Press.

Salecl, R. (2010) *Choice*, London: Profile Books.

Schor, J. and Ford, M. (2007) 'From Tastes Great to Cool: Children's Food Marketing and the Rise of the Symbolic', *Journal of Law, Medicine & Ethics*, 35 (1) 10–21. Available from ProQuest database.

Shim, J.E., Kim, J. and Mathai, R. (2011) 'Association of Infant Feeding Practices and Picky Eating Behaviours of Preschool Children', *Journal of the American Dietetic Association*, 111 (9) 1363–1368. Accessed from Science Direct Database.

Skocpol, T. (1992) *Protecting Soldiers and Mothers: The Political Origins of Social Policy in the United States*, Cambridge, MA: First Harvard University Press.

Stead, M., McDermott, L., MacKintosh, A.M. and Adamson, A. (2011) 'Why Healthy Eating Is Bad for Young People's Health: Identity, Belonging and Food', *Social Science & Medicine*, 72 (2011) 1131–1139. Accessed from Science Database.

Strauss, S. (2006) 'Clara M. Davis and the Wisdom of letting Children Choose Their Own Food?' *Canadian Medical Association Journal*, 175 (10) 1199–1201. Available from ProQuest database.

Thomas, C. (1995) 'Domestic Labour and Health: Bringing It All Back Home', *Sociology of Health and Illness* 17 (30) 328–352.

TNS New Zealand (2007) *Healthy Eating in New Zealand Families/Whānau*, Health Sponsorship Council. Online. Available http://archive.hsc.org.nz/researchpublications.html (accessed 25 October 2012).

University of Otago and Ministry of Health (2011) *A Focus on Nutrition: Key Findings of the 2008/09 New Zealand Adult Nutrition Survey*, Wellington: Ministry of Health. Online. Available www.health.govt.nz/publication/focus-nutrition-key-findings-2008-09-nz-adult-nutrition-survey (accessed 25 October 2012).

Walsh, J. (2005) *How To Be the Domestic Goddess of Your Home, An Anthology of Bengali Domestic Manuals*, New Delhi: Yoda Press.

Walter, L. (2009) Slow Food. Available www.uwgb.edu/cfcc/Provisions/SlowFood%26HomeCooking.pdf (accessed 5 February 2013).

Wennberg, A., Lundqvist, A.H., Högberg, U., Sandström, H. and Hamberg, K. (in press) 'Women's Experiences of Dietary Advice and Dietary Changes in Pregnancy', *Midwifery*, in press. Available from ScienceDirect Database.

World Health Organization (March, 2013) Obesity and Overweight, Fact sheet no. 311. Available www.who.int/mediacentre/factsheets/fs311/en/ (accessed 11 August 2013)

6

CARING FOR WOMEN WITH EATING DISORDERS

From conception to birth and beyond

Lydia Jade Turner

> She [midwife] treated me like I was about the 100th person she'd seen that day
> . . . I was terrified the baby was dead or handicapped. That was all I was thinking
> about. I was still vomiting and I felt terrible about that . . . She didn't look at me,
> she was just asking me all these questions like: 'Are you going to breastfeed or
> bottle feed?'
>
> (Stapleton 2007: 45)

Eating disorders affect a significant proportion of women during their childbearing experience. A recent Australian study found that approximately 7.5 per cent of women meet the clinical criteria for diagnosis, whilst a quarter were very concerned about their shape and weight (Edwards 2013). Perhaps this should not come as a surprise, given that more than 913,000 people in Australia suffered from eating disorders in 2012 (Deloitte Access Economics 2012). However, this may be a conservative estimate, taking into account the fact that the National Eating Disorders Collaboration reports that approximately one in twenty Australians has an eating disorder (National Eating Disorders Collaboration) and that eating disorders have increased two-fold over the five-year period between 2007 and 2012 (National Eating Disorders Collaboration).

The etiology of eating disorders is complex and multifactorial. Some evidence suggests a genetic predisposition for anorexia nervosa and bulimia nervosa (Collier *et al*. 1999); however, the chance of developing an eating disorder is influenced by psychological and social factors. Bulimia nervosa in particular has been linked to trauma, including childhood sexual abuse, although not everyone with this illness has been abused. Psychological factors including perfectionism, obsessive-compulsiveness, core low self-esteem, negative emotionality, neuroticism, harm avoidance, and traits associated with avoidant personality disorder have been identified as increasing vulnerability to the development of eating disorders (Belasco 2008).

In terms of sociocultural influence, evidence shows that the internalisation of the Western beauty ideal of thinness is a significant factor (Bordo 2013). Spread through a range of mediums, exposure to images glorifying thinness significantly contribute to risky and harmful weight-loss behaviours (Turner and Tankard Reist 2012). In fact dieting, which is often embarked on in a bid to achieve thinness, is the most common pathway into the development of an eating disorder. As will be seen in Chapters 12 and 13, a culture that pathologises and holds prejudicial attitudes against those deemed fat is likely to play a role, as many diet in a bid to escape discrimination. While some embark on a diet in good faith that they are improving their health, for many women this will lead to the development of an eating disorder or other dysfunctional eating pattern (Eating Disorders Association of New Zealand).

Eating disorders may strike at any time during a woman's life, with the typical first onset occurring during adolescence (Micali 2010). Many women will conceive without having recovered or had their symptoms go into remission (Easter *et al.* 2011). For those whose symptoms have remitted, pregnancy can be a vulnerable time for relapse (Micali *et al.* 2006). For other women, pregnancy may lead to the onset of an eating disorder. In vulnerable women, the hormonal changes that take place during pregnancy may increase feelings of instability and despair (Vandenberg and Baker-Townsend 2012). For those who have not developed effective coping strategies, pregnancy may act as a trigger for the development of an eating disorder (Little and Lowkes 2000; Harris 2010; Broussard 2012; Vandenberg and Baker-Townsend 2012; Zauderer 2012; Tierney *et al.* 2013).

Left undetected and unaddressed, eating disorders can lead to serious medical and psychological consequences for both the mother and her baby (Table 6.1).

The perinatal mortality rate of babies born to mothers with eating disorders increases significantly, with one North American study finding women with anorexia nervosa to have six times the national average risk for perinatal mortality (Little and Lowkes 2000). Eating disorders are typically cloaked in shame and secrecy and it is not common for women to volunteer information about their eating difficulties to health professionals in discussions about conception or from the antenatal to postpartum period (Franko and Walton 1993). It is therefore vital that tools enabling health professionals to recognise that a woman may have an eating disorder, or for the woman to self-identify, are made available. Such tools would facilitate women being offered help earlier rather than later during their pregnancy. This chapter will therefore explore how we can identify and care for women affected by eating disorders from conception to postpartum.

Diagnosing an eating disorder

The *Diagnostic Statistical Manual of Mental Disorders* (DSM-IV-TR) is published by the American Psychiatric Association (2000) and provides standard criteria for the diagnosis of mental illnesses. Clinicians, researchers, pharmaceutical companies, health insurance companies, and policy makers use it globally. The DSM-IV-TR criteria for eating disorders include three main categories: anorexia nervosa (Box 6.1), bulimia nervosa, and eating disorders not otherwise specified (EDNOS) (Box 6.2), although a fourth category of Binge Eating Disorder has been proposed for the DSM-V (Box 6.3).

Table 6.1 Potential consequences of disordered eating on mother and infant

Antenatal	Intrapartum	Postnatal
Miscarriage	Low Apgar scores	Cleft lip and palate
Stillbirth	Preterm birth	Small for gestational age
Breech presentation	Caesarean section	Large for gestational age
Hypertension	Forceps-assisted birth	Infection
Antepartum haemorrhage		Postpartum haemorrhage

Box 6.1 **The DSM-IV-TR criteria for eating disorders**

Anorexia Nervosa

A. Refusal to maintain body weight at or above a minimally normal weight for age and height (e.g. weight loss leading to maintenance of body weight less than 85 per cent of that expected; or failure to make expected weight gain during period of growth, leading to body weight less than 85 per cent of that expected).

B. Intense fear of gaining weight or becoming fat, even though underweight. [Please note: clarification with regard to 'fear of weight gain' was discussed under the proposed changes for DSM-V. A significant minority of individuals with the syndrome explicitly deny such fear. Therefore, the addition of a clause to focus on behaviour was recommended.]

C. Disturbance in the way in which one's body weight or shape is experienced, undue influence of body weight or shape on self-evaluation, or denial of the seriousness of the current low body weight.

D. In post menarche females, amenorrhea i.e. the absence of at least three consecutive menstrual cycles. (A woman is considered to have amenorrhea if her periods occur only following hormone, e.g. oestrogen, administration.)

Specify type:
Restricting Type: during the current episode of Anorexia Nervosa, the person has not regularly engaged in binge eating or purging behaviour (i.e. self-induced vomiting or the misuse of laxatives, diuretics or enemas).
Binge-Eating/Purging Type: during the current episode of Anorexia Nervosa, the person has regularly engaged in binge eating or purging behaviour (i.e. self-induced vomiting or the misuse of laxatives, diuretics or enemas).

Source: American Psychiatric Association (2000)

Eating Disorders Not Otherwise Specified (EDNOS) is one of the lesser-known eating disorders, although the majority of those with eating disorders fall into this category (American Psychiatric Association, 2000). It is important to recognise that all eating disorders are serious, regardless of the size of the person. Whilst anorexia nervosa typically leads to rapid weight loss and underweight presentation, people with bulimia nervosa (Box 6.4) typically present in their healthy weight range according to Body Mass Index (BMI) or higher (American Psychiatric Association, 2000). In fact, a recent study in Australia found one in five 'obese' Australian women now suffers from symptoms of eating disorders (Darby (née Star), Hay, Mond, Quirk, Buettner and Kennedy 2009).

Eating disorders are recognized under the DSM-IV-TR as genuine psychiatric illnesses (American Psychiatric Association, 2000), and Australia's national eating disorders charity The Butterfly Foundation reports eating disorders as having the highest mortality rate out of any other psychiatric illness. According to the Paying the Price Report (Deloitte Access Economics 2012), the annual death rate for eating disorder sufferers is higher than the 2011 death toll on Australia's roads (Deloitte Access Economics 2012). Many die from suicide or

---

Box 6.2 Eating Disorder Not Otherwise Specified

The Eating Disorder Not Otherwise Specified category is for disorders of eating that do not meet the criteria for any specific eating disorder. Examples include:

1. For women all of the criteria for Anorexia Nervosa are met except that the woman has regular menses.
2. All of the criteria for Anorexia Nervosa are met except that, despite significant weight loss, the individual's current weight is in the normal range.
3. All of the criteria for Bulimia Nervosa are met except that the binge eating and inappropriate compensatory mechanisms occur at a frequency of less than twice a week or for a duration of less than 3 months.
4. The regular use of inappropriate compensatory behaviour by an individual of normal body weight after eating small amounts of food (e.g., self-induced vomiting after the consumption of two cookies).
5. Repeatedly chewing and spitting out, but not swallowing, large amounts of food.
6. Binge-eating disorder: recurrent episodes of binge eating in the absence of the regular use of inappropriate compensatory behaviours characteristic of Bulimia Nervosa (see Appendix B in DSM-IV-TR for suggested research criteria).

Box 6.3 The proposed clinical criteria for Binge Eating Disorder

The proposed changes for the DSM-V included a new category of eating disorder:

A. Recurrent episodes of binge eating. An episode of binge eating is characterized by both of the following:

1. Eating in a discrete period of time (for example, within any 2-hour period), an amount of food that is definitely larger than most people would eat in a similar period of time under similar circumstances
2. A sense of lack of control over eating during the episode (for example, a feeling that one cannot stop eating or control what or how much one is eating)

B. The binge-eating episodes are associated with three (or more) of the following:

1. eating much more rapidly than normal
2. eating until feeling uncomfortably full
3. eating large amounts of food when not feeling physically hungry
4. eating alone because of feeling embarrassed by how much one is eating
5. feeling disgusted with oneself, depressed, or very guilty afterwards

C. Marked distress regarding binge eating is present
D. The binge eating occurs, on average, at least once a week for three months
E. The binge eating is not associated with the recurrent use of inappropriate compensatory behaviour (for example, purging) and does not occur exclusively during the course of Bulimia Nervosa or Anorexia Nervosa.

Source: American Psychiatric Association (2000)

Box 6.4 Bulimia nervosa

A. Recurrent episodes of binge eating. An episode of binge eating is characterized by both of the following:

1. Eating, in a discrete period of time (e.g. within any two-hour period), an amount of food that is definitely larger than most people would eat during a similar period of time and under similar circumstances
2. A sense of lack of control over eating during the episode (e.g. a feeling that one cannot stop eating or control what or how much one is eating)

B. Recurrent inappropriate compensatory behaviour in order to prevent weight gain, such as self-induced vomiting; misuse of laxatives, diuretics, enemas or other medications; fasting or excessive exercise.

C. The binge eating and inappropriate compensatory behaviours both occur, on average, at least twice a week for 3 months.

D. Self-evaluation is unduly influenced by body shape and weight.

E. The disturbance does not occur exclusively during episodes of Anorexia Nervosa.

Specify type:
Purging Type: during the current episode of Bulimia Nervosa, the person has regularly engaged in self-induced vomiting or the misuse of laxatives, diuretics, or enemas
Non Purging Type: during the current episode of Bulimia Nervosa, the person has used other inappropriate compensatory behaviours, such as fasting or excessive exercise but has not regularly engaged in self-induced vomiting or the misuse of laxatives, diuretics or enemas.

---

medical complications resulting from the disorder (Treasure *et al.* 2007). Depression and anxiety are also common co-morbid illnesses that also require screening and treatment (American Psychiatric Association 2000; Knopf *et al.* 2013).

Unfortunately, health professionals working with women with eating disorders are not free from prejudice. All healthcare professionals are advised to take a compassionate approach, as laying blame on the woman either explicitly or implicitly is unlikely to lead to improved outcomes. Sufferers of eating disorders often use their disorder as a way of regulating their emotions (Safer *et al.* 2009; Knopf *et al.* 2013), so feeling judged or criticised is likely to lead to the sufferer clinging more tightly to their disorder.

It is important that all health professionals examine their own biases prior to working with individuals or groups of people who have eating disorders. Sufferers often feel shame and demonstrate secrecy, and they are fearful of being judged. It is especially important therefore that health professionals foster trust in a pregnant woman who presents with anorexia nervosa, bulimia or one of the other, unspecified eating disorders. This will enable the woman to feel safe enough to disclose her disorder and the difficulties that arise from it (Little and Lowkes 2000).

Conception and eating disorders

Eating disorders affect approximately 5 to 10 per cent of women of childbearing age (Micali 2010). Given that the average age of onset is during adolescence, it is not surprising that many women with eating disorders will experience fertility problems (Easter *et al*. 2011). Two small studies have indicated that approximately one in ten women presenting at a fertility clinic will have a current eating disorder (Steward *et al*. 1990; Thommen *et al*. 1995) and many will experience absent or irregular menstrual cycles. However, many will be able to conceive using assisted reproductive technology in spite of having a low body weight or not having recovered from their specific condition (Micali 2010).

Women with anorexia nervosa – whether past or current – are more likely to suffer amenorrhoea, as compared to those with bulimia nervosa or other eating disorders (Easter *et al*. 2011). This may be because those with bulimia nervosa typically present within the healthy weight range or higher within the parameters of the BMI scale. Anorexia nervosa, in particular, can wreak havoc on the endocrine system, leading to under-functioning of the hypothalamo-pituitary-gonadal axis. This is because plasma concentrations of luteinising hormone (LH) and follicle-stimulating hormone (FSH) including oestrogens are lower than normal (Micali 2010). FSH and LH act synergistically in reproduction (Micali 2010). Bulimia nervosa in particular has been associated with polycystic ovaries and other follicular abnormalities – the reasons why being poorly understood (Zerbe 2007).

Irregular menstrual cycles also lead many women to believe that they are infertile, subsequently leading to unwanted pregnancies. Unwanted pregnancies increase the risk of unstable emotion and despair (Vandenberg and Baker-Townsend 2012), potentially exacerbating an existing eating disorder and increasing the likelihood of negatively impacting on pre- and postpartum mother–baby attachment. It is therefore essential for health professionals to inform women with irregular periods that, while they may experience increased fertility problems, they are not necessarily infertile. Health professionals may wish to encourage women with eating disorders to use contraception and delay pregnancy until their eating disorder symptoms have reduced, and to refer them to an eating disorder specialist for treatment.

Many women with binge eating disorder present as 'overweight' or 'obese', according to their BMI. In recent years, complications associated with 'obesity' such as large-for-gestational-age babies (LGA) and caesarean birth have led some doctors who are not screening for eating disorder to advise 'obese' women to lose weight during their first trimester. Advice to diet is ill advised at any time during pregnancy because of poor outcomes for the woman and baby (Broussard 2012).

Concerns about weight, instead of the promotion of overall health (see Chapter 13), are linked to dietary restraint. Typically, the body 'fights' against weight loss, as dietary restriction produces hormonal responses in the body, so that appetite-stimulating hormones increase while appetite-suppressing hormones reduce, along with metabolic changes (Sumithran *et al*. 2011). It is common for binge eating to occur in response to restriction – the very behaviour that health professionals want to reduce. This may explain why women with binge eating disorder who show greater worry about weight gain during pregnancy are likely to gain more weight in pregnancy, as compared to those with anorexia or bulimia nervosa (Harris 2010). Advising women to diet during pregnancy could therefore be considered dangerous practice, and likely to backfire.

The potential lifelong consequences for the mother and fetus, coupled with evidence that eating disorders usually go undetected by healthcare providers, mean that it is crucial that measures are put in place to detect, assess, and assist women with eating disorders so as to treat them as early as possible during pregnancy (Jacobi *et al*. 2004). As already discussed above, women are not generally willing to volunteer information about their eating difficulties, due to feelings of shame and secrecy. One study found that 93.3 per cent of participants presenting with eating disorder symptoms did not report eating disorders during pregnancy (Broussard 2012). Therefore any discussion initiated by midwives and other health practitioners should be non-judgemental and compassionate (see Chapter 8) and parallel to other conversations that midwives have with women about other difficult areas in their lives (e.g. domestic abuse). Eating issues need to be treated in a similarly sensitive manner as are HIV status and drug use.

Women with eating disorders are often overly afraid of giving up their eating disorder behaviours, due to a fear of being unable to cope with feelings of distress or being out of control around food. Intense fear of gaining weight, along with rigid thinking patterns, is typically present in women with eating disorders (Jacobi *et al*. 2004). They may not be ready to trust the possibility that alternative coping and distress tolerance strategies will work as effectively as the dysfunctional patterns they have developed to help them to survive emotionally. Many will also struggle with depression, anxiety, self-harm, or substance abuse/dependency (Jacobi *et al*. 2004). Previous trauma, such as child sexual abuse, is also higher amongst those presenting with eating disorders – although not everyone with an eating disorder has been abused (Varcarolis 1998).

One qualitative study found that women with a history of eating disorders prior to pregnancy were not asked once about their eating disorder or eating habits throughout their entire pregnancy (Harris 2010). Thus, ignoring the issue can lead women into thinking that their eating difficulties are not of interest. Identifying such women before conception would be ideal, because they may well consider delaying pregnancy and seeking advice and/or treatment before becoming pregnant. This might then facilitate the restoration of nutritional status, eating disorder remission or significant reduction in the symptoms. When women present with infertility, exploring the possibility of an eating disorder is therefore recommended.

A number of tools that can help to identify eating disorders exist for those who match the clinical criteria according to the DSM-IV-TR. These include the Eating Attitudes Test (EAT) for anorexia nervosa, or the Bulimia Investigatory Test Edinburgh (BITE) for those presenting with bulimia nervosa (Harris 2010). The SCOFF[1] questionnaire is another tool, which consists of five questions designed to detect the possibility of an eating disorder (Morgan *et al*. 2000; Harris 2010). As most women with eating disorders do not meet the strict clinical criteria for either anorexia or bulimia nervosa, subclinical eating disorders which still carry serious and potentially lifelong consequences may go undetected.

By routinely including caring questions in on-going assessments (see Chapter 8), health professionals may be able to tease out the more subtle subclinical eating disorders; for example, by asking questions such as 'How do you feel about your weight?' 'Do you spend a lot of time worrying about your appearance or thinking you are fat?' 'Are you engaging in weight control efforts now', Do friends or family members tell you that you over-exercise or don't eat enough?' or asking questions about reproductive history such as absence of menses over a period of three months (Zerbe 2007). More specific questions could include asking about highest and lowest weight and asking specific questions about compensatory behaviours such as laxative abuse or purging (Harris 2010). For a woman diagnosed with an eating disorder, it would be useful to consider possible co-morbid behaviours, because eating disorders are often used to regulate emotion and other behaviours that serve a similar function. These may include self-harm, compulsive over-exercising, and substance abuse, including smoking and alcohol use. One study found that 14 to 37 per cent of mothers matching the clinical criteria for eating disorders reported smoking, as compared to 9 per cent of those who did not (Harris 2010).

Levels of self-harm are particularly high in women with eating disorders. Between 25 and 45 per cent of individuals with eating disorders engage in self-harm, as compared to less than 1 per cent of the general US population (Harris 2010). It is not uncommon for self-harm to occur alongside substance abuse, including alcohol, and sometimes these co-morbid behaviours increase as the eating disorder subsides because they are viewed as 'safer' alternative coping strategies. Therefore, asking questions specifically about self-harm and other co-morbid behaviours is essential (Harris 2010).

'Diabulimia' is another eating disorder that was identified in 2007 (Harris 2010). Diabulimia occurs when a person with Type 1 diabetes intentionally abstains from injecting insulin, in an effort to lose weight. Without the injected insulin, the person's energy intake is drastically reduced. There is no available evidence yet to demonstrate how diabulimia affects pregnant women or birth outcomes. However, diabulimia in a non-pregnant woman can result in diabetic ketoacidosis, long-term vascular disease and peripheral nerve damage, and increases the risk of death from diabetes three-fold (Harris 2010). It is hypothesised that birth outcomes would be similar to those in pregnant women whose diabetes is poorly managed (Harris 2010). These would include birth defects, pre-eclampsia, stillbirth, neonatal morbidity, and macrosomia. Therefore it would be prudent to refer any woman with Type 1 diabetes in pregnancy who is suffering from diabulimia to the diabetic specialist team, and also to make a referral to specialist help such as a psychologist.

For those who are not as severely affected, psychoeducation about eating disorders and basic nutrition may be particularly useful. Education about the ineffectiveness of laxatives in weight loss, or how bulimia nervosa is considered a failed form of dieting because it typically does not lead to noticeable weight loss, may be enough to increase motivation in some women to loosen their grip on the eating disorder behaviours and actively engage with treatment. Regardless, if a midwife has any suspicion of any level of eating disorder, then referral to an eating disorder specialist is warranted.

Pregnancy

The study of the progression of eating disorder behaviours during pregnancy has resulted in mixed findings. Retrospective studies have found that eating disorder symptoms reduce significantly during pregnancy – although they do not entirely disappear – but return to pre-pregnancy levels during the postpartum period. Other studies have demonstrated that eating disorder symptoms can worsen during the course of pregnancy and continue to do so into the postpartum period (Pui-yee Lai *et al*. 2006). These findings suggest that awareness on the part of the professional by appropriate screening and monitoring from the point of conception through to the postpartum period is warranted. One of the more noticeable early warning signs may be a lack of weight gain over two consecutive visits during the second trimester (Harris 2010). Further investigation through sensitive questioning may elicit more evidence. Midwives and other health professionals need to regularly 'check in' during pregnancy, asking questions that may assist in detecting the presence of an eating disorder.

In a study involving 12,254 women, the researchers found that participants who experienced a recent episode of an eating disorder were found to be more likely to engage in dieting for weight loss, laxative abuse, self-induced vomiting, and to exercise more as compared to other groups during pregnancy. They also reported that eating-disordered thoughts and concerns about their weight and shape were more prevalent among these women than in control groups throughout pregnancy (Micali *et al*. 2006). Specifically, approximately 25 per cent of the participants maintained purging behaviour, while about 10 per cent continued to diet for weight loss at 32 weeks, in addition to expressing high levels of concern about weight gain during the third trimester. Women with a recent episode of eating disorder had the highest rates of dieting as well as the highest levels of concern about weight gain and shape. Intervention techniques by an eating disorder specialist may assist by targeting negative thought patterns, with the aim of increasing awareness and reducing them (Micali *et al.* 2006).

The same study also found that women who were classified as 'obese' were more likely to experience a desire to lose weight, to diet for weight loss during pregnancy, and to experience dissatisfaction in response to weight gain, as compared to women in a control group who were of normal weight. However, the researchers found that the women had very low levels of compensatory behaviour, such as vomiting to reduce caloric absorption or abusing laxatives. Shape and weight concerns decreased significantly during pregnancy, as compared to pre-pregnancy. This may indicate that the concerns of larger women for the well-being of their baby are of greater significance than concerns about their weight and shape.

Another study has suggested that anorexia nervosa, in particular, increases the risk of low birth-weight babies (Micali 2008) and that the risk of miscarriage increases two- to three-fold in women with active bulimia nervosa (Micali 2008). Limited research is available on the risks associated with binge eating disorder, as it is a relatively new area of study. However, another study found that women with binge eating disorder gave birth to a greater number of babies considered to be LGA (Bulik *et al.* 2009).

Treatments or interventions for women with eating disorders may include addressing cognitive distortions, providing support, and referring to an eating disorder specialist (Table 6.2). Helping to differentiate between different types of hunger, including physical, emotional, and sensory is also beneficial. Health professionals may wish to describe emotional hunger as being typically experienced as 'neck up,' in contrast to physical hunger, which is typically experienced as 'neck down.' Helping to develop alternative and safe coping strategies, addressing family members' feelings of guilt, and reducing prejudice towards the illness should also be included in intervention strategies.

Studies have shown that the stronger the emotional attachment a woman has to her baby in the antenatal period, the more likely her diet and eating patterns are to be healthy and protective (Pui-yee Lai *et al.* 2006). In addition, these studies have also found that the stronger the emotional attachment, the more positive the adjustment from pregnancy to the postpartum period will be (Pui-yee Lai *et al.* 2006). Therefore, midwives and others health professionals need to promote mother and baby attachment wherever possible, with the aim of helping the woman to engage with her baby (Harris 2010). The support of the partner during pregnancy has also been shown to increase the likelihood of positive outcome (Harris 2010).

There is evidence to show that a significant number of women with bulimia nervosa have been subjected to experiences of domestic violence, childhood trauma, sexual abuse, or rape (Zerbe 2007). Women with bulimia nervosa are also more inclined to experience difficulties with impulse control that are not limited to food intake or purging. These may include substance abuse, self-harm, and unsafe sexual practices. Treatment may therefore include appropriate trauma interventions and support, in addition to encouragement to adopt healthy behaviours around food and weight management.

Unfortunately, the pressure for women to be vigilant about their weight, to diet, and to count calories continues unabated, and weight loss programmes in recent years have begun to target pregnant women. For example, in Australia The Biggest Loser's head trainer, Michelle Bridges, launched a twelve-week 'body transformation' programme targeted at

Table 6.2 Interventions for women with eating disorders

Suggested action	How this may be achieved
Referral to an eating disorder specialist	Contact your national eating disorders referral service: *Australia*: The Butterfly Foundation, http://thebutterflyfoundation.org.au/ Centre for Eating and Dieting Disorders (CEDD), www.cedd.org.au/ *New Zealand*: Eating Difficulties Education Network (EDEN), www.eden.org.nz/ *UK*: beat UK, www.b-eat.co.uk *USA*: National Eating Disorders Association (NEDA), http://nationaleatingdisorders.org Canada: National Eating Disorder Information Centre, www.nedic.ca/index.shtml
Help to differentiate between different types of hunger, including physical, emotional, and sensory	www.tcme.org/documents/ADifferentTypesofHungerHandout.pdf
Help to develop alternative and safe coping strategies	Seeing an eating disorder specialist or other mental health practitioner will be necessary in order to develop these.
Address family members' feelings of guilt	Reassure the woman and family that eating disorders have a complex etiology and are likely to be the result of a complex interaction between genetic and cultural factors.
Reduce prejudice towards the illness	Include posters or brochures in the waiting room or midwife's office that invite conversation and provide information about eating disorders; ask non-confronting questions about the patient's eating, e.g. 'Some women find pregnancy really affects their eating – what changes have you experienced?' Observe any non-verbal bodily communication that may suggest body shame.

pregnant women, advising them to eat no more than 1700 calories per day (Bridges 2012). Dieting during pregnancy is not advisable, as adequate weight gain is necessary to ensure the healthy development of the baby (McKevith 2002). Celebrity magazines and tabloid newspapers such as the *Daily Mail* continue the harmful practice of monitoring and surveillance of the pregnant bodies of celebrities (Hill and Kent-Smith 2013), comparing pre- and post-pregnancy weight loss and size of baby bumps, and relentlessly fat-shaming. Some women may over-exercise or attempt to lose weight during breastfeeding, in a bid to return to their pre-pregnancy shape and weight. However, dieting during breastfeeding is not advisable because more nutrients and energy are necessary at this stage, as compared to during pregnancy (Amorim Adegboye, Linne and Lourenco 2007).

Some evidence suggests that women who engage in moderate to intense levels of exercise may negatively affect fetal development and put their baby at risk of being born at a lower birth weight (McKevith 2002). For women who exercise, the UK's National Childcare Trust advises women to check their pulse and to slow down if it exceeds 140 beats per minute (McKevith 2002). However, other evidence suggests that moderate exercise does not increase the risk of poor fetal outcomes.

Postpartum

While the causes of eating disorders are complex, a bio-psycho-social model based on increasing evidence suggests that eating disorders are caused by an interaction involving genetic, psychological, and social factors. Genetic factors have been identified for both anorexia nervosa and bulimia nervosa (Sullivan *et al.* 1998; Torgersen *et al.* 2008). Psychological factors include difficulties resulting from a parent's eating disorder and co-morbid illnesses. Social factors include internalisation of a thin ideal and cultural shunning of those who do not conform to thinness (Davies and Wardle 1994). Children of women who have a history of or a current eating disorder are at increased risk of developing eating disorders themselves (Little and Lowkes 2000).

There is some evidence now to suggest that eating disorders return shortly after birth, and that in some cases they return to pre-pregnancy levels (Lacey and Smith 1987; Steward *et al.* 1990; Morgan *et al.* 1999; Crow *et al.* 2004, 2008). Concerns about weight gain, eating, and body shape during this time can have detrimental effects on the woman's baby, for several reasons. These include the mother underestimating her baby's nutritional needs, attempts to make the baby thinner, and modelling eating disordered behaviour (Zerbe 2007). As one woman states in Little and Lowkes (2000: 304):

> My husband and I started having marital problems, and we were in marital counselling, and one day I just broke down and started crying and said I just can't do this anymore. Because my daughter started to display running to the bathroom to throw up. She started that at 18 months. She would sit and eat and eat and eat until she literally would throw up, because she had seen me doing it . . . I would sit and watch her, and she would just eat until she threw up. You see at the time I was completely out of control with my own bingeing and purging and M would watch me. She would come into the bathroom and pat my back saying 'Mama sick, poor Mama.' And then when she started to do it, I would sit on the bathroom floor and cradle her and soothe her. Finally I went for treatment and I started to get my own symptoms under control and then I stopped letting her stuff herself and she would get so angry and cry and cry. I think I put some of my guilt and anger at myself on to her. I wanted her to stop and I suddenly stopped letting her have so much food. It was a hard time. She's still got some problems with it and she's three now.
>
> (Little and Lowkes 2000: 304)

And another:

> No, I never did it in front of the kids. It was my little secret and I didn't want them to know . . . Well maybe once, my son saw me purge when he was a baby, and I told him I was sick. I think an effect of my eating disorder is dinnertime. He's one not to sit and eat. I felt my pressure on him when he didn't eat and I immediately got upset. I felt a lot of guilt about that. He wouldn't touch his food. I fed him. This started at age two. But if he didn't want to eat I'd get ugly . . . I'd yell at him . . . something I don't want to remember.
>
> (Little and Lowkes 2000: 304)

Problems identified in mothers with eating disorders include disturbed perceptions of their baby's weight and hunger, difficulties with feeding their baby, difficulties with their own eating, and exposing their baby to these symptoms. In children common problems include food refusal and fussiness, anxiety, mimicking vomiting and overeating behaviour, underweight, and growth delays (Little and Lowkes 2000).

Some studies have demonstrated that mothers with eating disorders are also more likely to experience difficulties with breastfeeding, which may lead to them resorting to breast milk substitute (Little and Lowkes 2000). However, other studies have shown the opposite. A prospective study of over 12,050 women in the United Kingdom found that women with a history of anorexia or bulimia nervosa were more likely to breastfeed, as compared to women with or without psychiatric illnesses, and that women with bulimia nervosa were more likely to breastfeed throughout the baby's first year (Harris 2010). Education about the benefits of breastfeeding will be helpful, regardless.

Additional attention to a woman's eating behaviours is advisable during the postnatal period, as this is the time when eating disorder symptoms are likely to return. With the rise of the 'yummy mummy' phenomenon (Donnelly 2008) and scaremongering about 'obesity', women with a history of eating disorders may feel pressure from relatives, their local doctor, the media, and various industries to lose weight and get back quickly to their pre-baby weight. High antenatal BMI has also been associated with postnatal disordered eating (BMI>30). If health professionals do not ask about their eating habits, they may feel too ashamed to raise the difficulties they are experiencing themselves.

Assessment tools and eating disorder inventories can be used, in addition to appropriate and sensitive questioning. Engendering a relationship where the woman feels safe to express her feelings, and validating her worries whilst increasing her confidence in her ability to look after herself and her baby, may increase motivation and willingness to try to overcome an eating disorder. Helping to identify triggers and using imagery, metaphor, and language to communicate may help her in doing the above. Above all, referring the woman to an eating disorder specialist is crucial. As another woman quoted in Little and Lowkes (2000: 305) stated:

> I think if they suspect something they should ask, and even if they don't get an answer they were looking for because deep down they know it is true, they need to probe a little bit more. I had morning sickness, but I think I was glad I did, so I could not gain the weight . . . probably if I didn't have morning sickness, I still would have been [purging].

Our current culture values thinness, and women are bombarded with thin body images in advertising, film, and television. Just as obesity has become a global issue, so too has an obsession with thinness and an increase in eating disorders. As such, it can be expected that midwives will repeatedly be assisting women affected by eating disorders or other unusual eating behaviours over the course of their professional careers. Having appropriate education and tools to detect, assess, and assist pregnant and postnatal women with eating disorders will play a vital role in restoring the health of these women and their babies throughout each stage of the childbearing experience. Creating a non-judgemental, supportive and compassionate environment that welcomes discussions about eating concerns, and facilitating referral to eating disorder specialists where necessary, will assist in each woman's journey towards the management of symptoms and eventual restoration of health.

Note

1 SCOFF is an acronym for the following questions:

Do you make yourself *S*ick because you feel uncomfortably full?
Do you worry you have lost *C*ontrol over how much you eat?
Have you recently lost more than *O*ne stone in a 3 month period?
Do you believe yourself to be *F*at when others say you are too thin?
Would you say that *F*ood dominates your life?

References

American Psychiatric Association (2000) *Diagnostic and statistical manual of mental disorders* (4th edn). DOI: 10.1176/appi.books.9780890423349.

Amorim Adegboye, A.R., Linne, Y.M. and Lourenco, P.M.C. (2007) Diet or exercise, or both, for weight reduction in women after childbirth, *Cochrane Database of Systematic Reviews* 3.

Belasco, W. (2008) *Food, the key concepts*, New York: Berg.

Bordo, S. (2013) Not just 'a white girl's thing': the changing face of food and body image problems. In: C. Counihan P. and Van Esterik (eds) *Food and culture: a reader* (3rd edn), London: Routledge.

Bridges, M. (2012) *Pregnancy program*. Online. Available at: www.12wbt.com/programs/pregnancy/ (accessed 29 May 2013).

Broussard, B. (2012) Psychological and behavioural traits associated with eating disorders and pregnancy: a pilot study, *Journal of Midwifery & Women's Health*, 57: 61–66. DOI: 10.1111/j.1542-2011.2011.00089x.

Bulik, C., Von, H., Siega-Riz, A., Torgersen, L., Lie, K. *et al.* (2009) Birth outcomes in women with eating disorders in the Norwegian mother and child cohort study (MoBa), *International Journal of Eating Disorders*, 42: 9–18.

Collier, P.A., Sham, P.C., Arranz, M.J., Xun, H. and Treasure, J. (1999) Understanding the genetic predisposition to anorexia nervosa, *European Eating Disorders Review*, 72: 96–102.

Crow, S., Keel, P., Thuras, P. and Mitchell, J. (2004) Bulimia symptoms and other risk behaviors during pregnancy in women with bulimia nervosa, *International Journal of Eating Disorders*, 36: 220–223.

Crow, S., Agras, W., Crosby, R., Halmi, K. and Mitchell, J. (2008) Eating disorder symptoms in pregnancy: a prospective study, *International Journal of Eating Disorders*, 41: 277–279.

Darby (née Star), A., Hay, P., Mond, J., Quirk, F., Buettner, P. and Kennedy, L. (2009). The prevalence of co-morbid obesity and eating disorder behaviours 1995–2005, *International Journal of Eating Disorders*, 42: 104–108.

Davies, K. and Wardle, J. (1994) Body image and dieting in pregnancy, *Journal of Psychosomatic Research*, 38 (8): 787–799.

Deloitte Access Economics (2012) 'Paying the Price' report, the economic and social impact of eating disorders in Australia, http://thebutterflyfoundation.org.au/wp-content/uploads/2012/12/Butterfly_Report.pdf.

Donnelly, L. (2008) 'Yummy mummies' make mothers depressed. *Telegraph*. Online. Available at: www.telegraph.co.uk/news/uknews/1580472/Yummy-mummies-make-mothers-depressed.html (accessed 29 May 2013).

Easter, A., Treasure, J. and Micali, N. (2011) Fertility and prenatal attitudes towards pregnancy in women with eating disorders: results from the Avon Longitudinal Study of Parents and Children, *International Journal of Obstetrics & Gynaecology*, 118: 1491–1498.

Eating Disorders Association of New Zealand, www.ed.org.nz/index.asp?pageID=2145862940.

Edwards, K. (2013) 'Fat shaming Kim Kardashian.' *Daily Life*. Available at: www.dailylife.com.au/news-and-views/dl-opinion/fat-shaming-kim-kardashian-20130328-2gwnd.html (accessed 1 April 2013).

Franko, D. and Walton, B. (1993) Pregnancy and eating disorders: a review and clinical implications, *International Journal of Eating Disorders*, 13 (1): 41–48.

Harris, A. (2010) Practical advice for caring for women with eating disorders during the perinatal period, *Journal of Midwifery & Women's Health*, 55: 579–586, DOI: 10.1016/j.jmwh.210.07.008.

Hill, E. and Kent-Smith, E. (2013) It's Kate v Kim . . . The bump off! One's an English duchess. The other is Hollywood royalty. And when it comes to maternity wear, they really ARE oceans apart. *Mail Online*. Available at: www.dailymail.co.uk/femail/article-2305066/Kate-Middleton-v-Kim-Kadashian-baby-bump-Duchess-Cambridges-maternity-style-oceans-apart.html (accessed 29 May 2013).

Jacobi, C., Abascal, L. and Taylor, C. (2004) Screening for eating disorders and high-risk behaviour: caution, *International Journal of Eating Disorders*, 36: 280–295.

Knopf, C., Von Holle, A., Zerwas, S., Torgersen, L., Tambs, K. *et al.* (2013) Course and predictors of maternal eating disorders in the postpartum period, *International Journal of Eating Disorders*, 46 (4): 355–368. DOI: 10.1002/eat.22088.

Lacey, J. and Smith, G. (1987) Bulimia nervosa, the impact of pregnancy on mother and baby, *British Journal of Psychiatry*, 150: 777–781.

Little, L. and Lowkes, E. (2000) Critical issues in the care of pregnant women with eating disorders and the impact on their children, *Journal of Midwifery & Women's Health*, 45 (4): 299–307.

McKevith, B. (2002) *Nutrition Bulletin*, British Nutrition Foundation, 27: 161–163.

Micali, N. (2008) Eating disorders and pregnancy, *Psychiatry*, 7 (4): 191–193.

Micali, N. (2010) Management of eating disorders during pregnancy, *Progress in Neurology and Psychiatry*, 14 (2): 24–26.

Micali, N., Treasure, J. and Simonoff, E. (2006) Eating disorder symptoms in pregnancy: a longitudinal study of women with recent and past eating disorders and obesity, *Journal of Psychosomatic Research*, 63: 297–303.

Morgan, J., Lacey, J. and Sedgwick, P. (1999) Impact of pregnancy on bulimia nervosa, *British Journal of Psychiatry*, 174: 135–140.

Morgan, J., Reid, F. and Lacey, J. (2000) The SCOFF questionnaire: a new screening tool for eating disorders, *The Western Journal of Medicine*, 172: 164–165.

National Eating Disorders Collaboration, www.nedc.com.au/for-the-media.

Pui-yee Lai, B., So-kum Tang, C. and Kwok-lai Tse, W. (2006) A longitudinal study investigating disordered eating during the transition to motherhood among Chinese women in Hong Kong, *International Journal of Eating Disorders*, 39: 303–311.

Safer, D., Telch, C. and Chen, E. (2009) *Dialectical Behavior Therapy for binge eating and bulimia*, New York: The Guilford Press.

Stapleton, H. (2007) *'I'm not pregnant, I'm fat.' The experiences of some eating disordered childbearing women and mothers*, Report, School of Nursing and Midwifery, University of Sheffield GRiP (Getting Research into Practice).

Steward, D., Robinson, E., Goldbloom, D. and Wright, C. (1990) Infertility and eating disorders, *American Journal of Obstetric Gynaecology*, 163: 1196–1199.

Sullivan, P., Bulik, C. and Kendler, K. (1998) Genetic epidemiology of binging and vomiting, *British Journal of Psychiatry*, 173: 75–79.

Sumithran, P., Prendergast, L., Delbridge, E., Purcell, K., Shulkes, A. *et al.* (2011) Long-term persistence of hormonal adaptations to weight loss, *New England Journal of Medicine*, 365: 1597–1604.

Thommen, M., Vallach, L. and Kiencke, S. (1995) Prevalence of eating disorders in a Swiss family planning clinic, *Eating disorders*, 3: 324–331.

Tierney, S., McGlone, C. and Furber, C. (2013) What can qualitative studies tell us about the experiences of women who are pregnant that have an eating disorder? *Midwifery*, 29 (5): 542–549. http://dx.doi.org/10.1016/j.midw.2012.04.013.

Torgersen, L., Von Holle, A., Reichborn-Kjennerud, T., Knopf, C., Hamer, R. *et al.* (2008) Nausea and vomiting of pregnancy in women with bulimia nervosa and eating disorders not otherwise specified, *International Journal of Eating Disorders*, 41: 722–727.

Treasure, J., Smith, G. and Crane, A. (2007) *Skills-based learning for caring for a loved one with an eating disorder: the new Maudsley method*, New York: Routledge.

Turner, L.J. and Tankard Reist, M.T. (2012) Teen magazine blows its cover in search of impossible perfection, *Sydney Morning Herald*, July, www.smh.com.au/opinion/society-and-culture/teen-magazine-blows-its-cover-in-search-of-impossible-perfection-20120710–21tq0.html.

Vandenberg, K. and Baker-Townsend, J. (2012) 25 pounds and counting: binge-eating disorder during pregnancy, *Journal of Obstetric, Gynecologic, & Neonatal Nursing*, 41: S188. DOI: 10.1111/j.1552-6909.2012.01363.x.

Varcarolis, E. (1998) *Fundamentals of psychiatric mental health nursing*, Philadelphia: W.B. Saunders.

Zauderer, C. (2012) Eating disorders and pregnancy: supporting the anorexic or bulimic expectant mother, *Journal of Obstetric, Gynecologic, & Neonatal Nursing*, 41: S177–S178. DOI: 10.1111/j.1552-6909.2012.01363.x.

Zerbe, K. (2007) Eating disorders in the 21st century: identification, management, and prevention in obstetrics and gynecology, *Best Practice & Research Clinical Obstetrics and Gynaecology*, 21 (2): 331–343, DOI: 10.1016/j.bpobgyn.2006.12.001.

7

VEGETARIAN AND VEGAN
PREGNANCY

Emma Derbyshire

Introduction

Vegetarianism and veganism are becoming increasingly popular dietary choices. Although many vegetarian and vegan women are able to provide themselves with a healthy and nutritious diet preconception, once pregnant they may need to reconsider some aspects of their diet to accommodate the changing needs for both their own needs and that of their baby. This chapter sets out to explain which nutrients are most likely to be lacking from vegetarians' diets and describes how to achieve a balanced diet, as, for many, their intake may be lacking in certain nutrients. In particular, protein, long chain (LC) n-3 polyunsaturated (PUFA) fatty acids, vitamin B12, vitamin D, calcium, iron, zinc and iodine intakes tend to be lower amongst vegetarians and vegans. These dietary deficiencies can have health implications for mother and baby if the woman is not fully aware of the changing needs of her body at this time. The importance of communicating this information to appropriate health practitioners and organisations is also discussed. Midwives can play a key role in ensuring that women are aware of the latest nutrition guidelines, although these are not always the same for every woman and can depend on the individual's health at the time. The use of supplements and fortified foods is also an important conversation point for vegetarians and vegans in pregnancy, when there are extensive physiological changes which may need to be met with suitable dietary changes.

A vegetarian diet is generally defined as one consisting mostly of plant foods including fruit, legumes, nuts, seeds and grains, although some vegetarians choose to eat eggs and dairy foods (Marsh *et al.* 2009). However, it is a somewhat nebulous term and there are many different forms of 'vegetarian' diets and some even include certain types of meat. Individuals who include such sources generally fall under the umbrella of 'demi-' or 'semi-vegetarians'. For example, women including fish or chicken in their diets may also be respectively referred to as 'pesco-' or 'pollo-vegetarian' (pesco-/pollo-vegetarians eat some meats but exclude others). In vegan diets, individuals exclude all red meat, poultry, fish, dairy and other foods of animal origin from their food (Timko *et al.* 2012). In macrobiotic diets grains are eaten as a main staple food and the diet is supplemented with legumes, vegetables and fruits, seeds and nuts (although to a lesser extent). Refined foods and most animal products are typically avoided in macrobiotic diets (Penney and Miller 2008). A summary of the different classifications is provided in Table 7.1.

Women may choose to be vegetarian, or vegan, for a host of different reasons. For example, because of religious or ethical beliefs, due to concerns over animal welfare or for a range of health benefits (Marsh *et al.* 2009). Younger women have greater a tendency to be motivated for moral and environmental reasons, while middle-aged adults tend to turn to vegetar-

Table 7.1 Different types of vegetarian diet

Diet type	Description
Demi (semi) vegetarian	Occasionally includes meat/poultry/fish.
Fruitarian	Typically comprised of fresh and dried fruits, nuts, seeds and a few vegetables.
Lacto-ovo-vegetarian	Excludes meat produce but includes dairy and eggs.
Lacto-vegetarian	Excludes meat produce and eggs but includes dairy produce.
Macrobiotic	Generally excludes meat and refined produce. Grains are mainly eaten, supplemented with legumes, vegetables and fruits, seeds and nuts (to a lesser extent).
Ovo-vegetarian	Excludes meat and dairy produce but includes eggs.
Pesco-vegetarian	Excludes meat produce but includes fish (and possibly other seafood).
Pollo-vegetarian	Excludes meat produce but includes chicken.
Vegan	Avoids all foods of animal origin.

Source: Adapted from Philips (2005).

ian diets for their health benefits (Pribis *et al.* 2010). For example, there is good evidence that vegetarian diets reduce coronary heart disease and the risk of type 2 diabetes (McEvoy *et al.* 2012) and help to maintain body weight without compromising the nutrient density of diets (Farmer *et al.* 2011). In some cases there is evidence that women may use vegetarianism as a vehicle to manage their weight, which may manifest in eating disorders. For example, in one study 52 per cent of women with a history of an eating disorder had been vegetarian, as compared with 12 per cent in non-vegetarian controls (Bardone-Cone *et al.* 2012).

Turning to recent trends, a more sustainable diet which places less reliance on foods of animal origin has also become of increasing interest (Schösler *et al.* 2012). Scientists have calculated that a non-vegetarian diet (beef consumption especially) requires 2.9 times more water, 2.5 times more primary energy, 13 times more fertiliser and 1.4 times more pesticides than a vegetarian diet (Marlow *et al.* 2009). A Norwegian study investigating the eating habits of pregnant women found that women seem to be becoming more health conscious, reporting frequent consumption of organically produced foods and following dietary trends that are more in line with public advice for healthy and sustainable diets (Torjusen *et al.* 2012). This trend to a more sustainable diet is discussed further in Chapter 9.

Presently, in the United Kingdom around 3 per cent of adults are vegetarian, which, in the present population of 61.4 million, amounts to over 1.8 million individuals (Vegetarian Society 2012a). As discussed in the introduction to this chapter, vegetarians may make this lifestyle choice for many different reasons, including the potential health benefits (Hoek 2004). From information contained in nutritional epidemiological studies it is now well recognised that vegetarian diets are associated with a range of health benefits, including a lower body mass index, lower serum total and low-density lipoprotein cholesterol levels, lower blood pressure and reduced risk of diabetes, cancer, stroke and heart disease (Craig 2010). These potential health benefits are mainly attributed to the fact that vegetarian diets tend to be lower in saturated fat and cholesterol and higher in dietary fibre and health-promoting phytochemicals, due to the frequent consumption of fruits, vegetables, whole grains, legumes, nuts and soy products, which are associated with a lower risk for developing degenerative diseases (Craig 2010).

This chapter sets out to explain how vegetarian/vegan women can ensure that they are eating a healthy, balanced diet and how midwives and other health professionals can support them to do so. Recommendations will be given on how diets can be adapted to prevent those nutritional deficiencies that are more commonly associated with vegetarianism/veganism, with a focus on the nutrients that are important for pregnancy.

Diet quality of vegetarians/vegans

The diet quality of vegetarian and vegan adults has been well studied. However, whether women make any further changes to their diets once they are pregnant is a question that is largely unanswered. Research carried out on non-pregnant vegetarians shows that women generally have a healthy lifestyle but their diets have a tendency to be low in protein, fat and saturated fat (Cade *et al.* 2004) and lacking in thiamine, folate and vitamin B6 (Bedford and Barr 2005). One of the largest studies carried out to date is the German Vegan Study. Findings from this work showed that 40 per cent of the young women (<50 years) were iron deficient (Waldmann *et al.* 2004) and strict vegans had inadequate vitamin B6 concentrations, despite having adequate dietary intakes (Waldmann *et al.* 2006). In the UK, figures from the National Diet and Nutrition Survey indicate that a smaller proportion of girls aged 11–18 years (5.6 per cent) and women aged 19–64 years (3.3 per cent) were iron deficient (Bates *et al.* 2012). Nutritional shortfalls have also been reported in the European Prospective Investigation into Cancer (EPIC) Study (the UK Oxford branch), with vegans reporting some of the lowest intakes of retinol, vitamin B12, vitamin D, calcium and zinc (Davey *et al.* 2003). A summary of the overall nutritional adequacy of vegetarian/vegan diets is included in Figure 7.1.

Focus on protein

Protein is needed in pregnancy for the growth of the developing child, formation of new red blood cells and circulating proteins (Derbyshire 2011a). During pregnancy it is advised that women should aim to eat around 51g protein daily (DH 1991). For vegetarian/vegan mothers this could be obtained from foods such as pulses, seeds, soy products (such as tofu, textured soy protein and milk), cereals, free-range eggs and dairy foods, consumed on a regular basis. Other examples of protein-rich foods suitable for vegetarian/vegan mothers are provided in Table 7.2 and dietary guidelines are presented in Table 7.3.

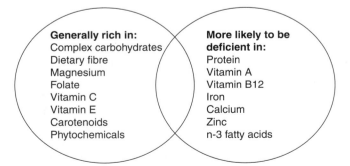

Figure 7.1 Nutritional adequacy of vegetarian diets

Source: Adapted from Leitzmann (2005).

Table 7.2 Dietary Reference Values for vegetarian mothers during pregnancy

Macronutrients	Recommended daily intake
Energy (kcals)	2140
Protein (g/day)	51
Carbohydrate (% energy intake)	47
Total fat (% energy intake)	33
Saturated fat (% energy intake)	No more than 10
Omega-3	200mg DHA (Koletzko *et al.* 2007)
Micronutrients	
Vitamin A (µg)	950
Vitamin C (mg)	50
Vitamin D (µg)	10
Folate (µg)	300
Thiamine (mg)	0.9
Riboflavin (mg)	1.4
Niacin (mg)	13–14
Vitamin B6 (µg)	1.2
Vitamin B12(µg)	1.5
Calcium (mg)	700–800
Iodine (µg)	140
Iron (mg)	14.8
Magnesium (mg)	270
Selenium (µg)	60
Zinc (mg)	7.0
Sodium (g)	1.6

Source: DH (1991).
Key: DHA = docosahexaenoic acid.

Table 7.3 Food sources of key nutrients for vegetarians/vegans (excluding dairy)

Nutrient	Food sources
Protein	Chickpeas, baked beans, tofu, boiled lentils, muesli, hard cheese, hummus.
n-3 fatty acids	Linseed (or flaxseed), soybean oil, rapeseed oil, tofu, walnuts.
Vitamin A (retinol equivalents)	Milk, eggs, yogurt, green leafy vegetables, yellow/orange vegetables or fruits
Vitamin B2 (riboflavin)	Fortified breakfast cereal, milk, yogurt, cheese, eggs, fortified soya drink, almonds.
Vitamin B12	Fortified breakfast cereal, yeast extract (e.g. Marmite), fortified soya drink, eggs, milk.
Vitamin D	Fortified breakfast cereal, fortified soya drink, all margarines, other fortified fat spreads, eggs, milk.
Calcium	Fortified soya drink, sesame seeds, white/brown bread, fortified fruit juice, dried figs, broccoli, green leafy vegetables (except spinach), molasses, milk, cheese, yogurt, beans and pulses, tofu, soya mince.
Zinc	Tofu, legumes (e.g. baked beans, chick peas, lentils), peas, nuts and seeds (e.g. cashew nuts, sunflower seeds), whole grain cereals and wholemeal bread, milk, eggs, cheese, yogurt.
Iron	Fortified breakfast cereal, wholemeal bread, dried fruit (e.g. apricots, prunes, raisins), green leafy vegetables, beans and pulses, molasses, nuts and seeds (almonds, pumpkin seeds, sesame seeds), tofu.
Selenium	Brazil nuts, sunflower seeds, molasses, wholemeal bread.
Iodine	Iodised salt, seaweed, milk.

Source: FSA (2006).

EMMA DERBYSHIRE

Focus on vitamin B12

Vitamin B12 (cobalamin) deficiency is common in vegetarians, mainly due to their limited dietary intake of animal foods (O'Leary and Samman 2010). Vitamin B12 is essential for DNA synthesis and cellular energy production and is central to fetal and child development. Pregnant women who are vegetarian or vegan often have an increased risk of B12 deficiency, which is thought to impact negatively on fetal cognitive, motor and growth outcomes (Pepper and Black 2011).

Most recently, alongside folate deficiency, low maternal vitamin B12 status is thought to be a risk factor for the development of neural tube defects (NTDs; when the baby's spinal cord does not close properly) (Wang *et al.* 2012). In regions where foods have been fortified with folic acid, low vitamin B12 status has been associated with three times the risk of NTDs (Ray *et al.* 2007). However, there is much debate about folic acid fortification, with scientists reporting that this may exacerbate the biochemical and clinical status of vitamin B12 deficiency and recommending that food fortification policies including folic acid should also include vitamin B12 (Selhun and Paul 2011).

Recent evidence has also linked vitamin B12 deficiency in pregnancy to higher levels of maternal adiposity and increased risk of insulin resistance and gestational diabetes, particularly amongst South Asian Indians (Krishnaveni *et al.* 2009). As vegetarian diets tend not to include meat and fish, and vegan diets are generally devoid of milk and eggs, eating fortified cereals could be an important dietary source of vitamin B12 for individuals following such diets (Watanabe 2007). Further studies are now needed to determine the pathways of cobalamin influence on fetal development, as well as strategies to prevent B12 deficiency in pregnant women.

Focus on iron

One of the main functions of iron is to support the formation of haemoglobin. In pregnancy what may be considered as mild anaemia may simply be a physiological state of pregnancy, as a result of the normal haemodilution that takes place in pregnancy (Stables and Rankin 2006). Anaemia in pregnancy is generally defined as haemoglobin levels less than 110g/l, but this is a somewhat simplistic assessment and, wherever possible, a more comprehensive use of biochemical indicators of iron status, including serum ferritin (SF) and serum transferrin receptor (sTfR), should be used to assess the iron status of a woman. Iron deficiency anaemia has been reported to affect as many as 56 million women globally, although this largely depends on the region in which the woman is living (rates are generally higher in low-income countries), the stage of pregnancy (anaemia is more common in the third trimester) and whether the woman is having her first or second child (Goonewardene *et al.* 2012).

Iron deficiency in pregnancy has been associated with unfavourable pregnancy outcomes, including preterm deliveries and reduced infant birth weight, length and iron stores (Daily and Wylie 2008). A cohort study investigating the iron intakes of 1274 pregnant women aged 18–45 years assessed diet quality using 24-hour recalls in each of the three trimesters of pregnancy. Eighty per cent of women had dietary iron intakes below the UK Reference Nutrient Intake of 14.8 mg/day. Interestingly, in this study vegetarians were less likely to have low iron intakes (possibly because they were more likely to be taking supplements in the first two trimesters). Total iron intake (but not from foods alone) was associated with higher birth weight centiles; a relationship that was also stronger in women with the highest vitamin C intakes (Alwan *et al.* 2011). This study is one of the largest conducted to date and emphasises the importance of iron supplementation in pregnancy for vegetarians and its possible benefits in terms of improving birth weights.

Focus on calcium

For most women, dairy products provide a substantial number of important nutrients, including calcium, potassium and magnesium. Diets where these food groups are restricted, e.g. in the case of vegans, can mean that these nutrients are under-consumed (Weaver 2009). Consequently, vegans need to ensure that they get enough calcium from alternative food products. For example, fortified soya milk provides 98mg per 100g eaten, and calcium-set tofu 510mg, sesame seeds 670mg and tahini paste 680mg calcium per 100g (NHS 2012; FSA 2006).

Women with higher calcium intakes in pregnancy are also more likely to have a higher bone density and so are their babies (Prentice 2011). A recent review of randomised controlled trials showed that calcium supplementation may help to protect against pre-eclampsia in pregnancy (Buppasiri et al. 2011). However, when interpreting the findings from these studies it is also important to consider that dairy foods also contain other components, e.g. amino acids and conjugated linoleic acids, which may also have their own separate health benefits (Weaver 2009).

Focus on n-3 fatty acids

Omega-3 fatty acids are polyunsaturated fatty acids (PUFAs) that play a key role in fetal and retina and brain development during pregnancy. These can be classified into omega-3 (alpha-linolenic acid; ALA) and omega-6 (linoleic acid). The health benefits of omega-3 are thought to come from the omega-3 fatty acids docosahexaenoic acid (DHA) and eicosapentaenoic acid (EPA), which the body makes from the parent essential fatty acid alpha-linolenic acid. For vegetarians, marine algae are an important direct source of DHA and EPA (oily fish derive their DHA and EPA from marine algae) which can be found in some supplement brands. ALA (which may be converted to EPA and DHA) is found in flaxseed and also in walnuts and hempseed. One tablespoon of flaxseed oil (14g) is thought to provide around 7.2g of omega-3 (Vegetarian Society 2012). It has been recommended by Koletzko et al. (2007) that pregnant and lactating women should aim to achieve dietary intakes of least 200mg DHA/day, as intakes of the DHA precursor ALA are thought to be less effective in promoting DHA deposition in the fetal brain, when compared with preformed DHA or fatty acids from oily fish.

Looking at omega-3 intakes, one Austrian observational study comprised of 98 adult vegetarians, vegans, omnivores and semi-omnivores measured omega-3 intake and status using foods recalls and gas chromatography, respectively. Researchers found that vegetarian diets had an average n-6:n-3 ratio of 10:1, a risk factor for omega-3 tissue decline, and recommended that this be corrected through dietary or supplementation strategies (Kornsteiner 2010). Similarly, other researchers have found that vegan diets are devoid of DHA, with those including dairy produce and eggs providing only about 0.02g/day and, again, they recommend that supplementation with small amounts of preformed DHA (as low as 200mg) could help to increase the proportion of DHA in blood lipids in vegetarians and vegans (Sanders 2009).

An earlier study of 24 South Asian vegetarian and 24 white omnivore non-pregnant premenopausal women from North London showed that intakes of linoleic acid (18: 2n-6) and the ratio of linoleic to ALA (18: 3n-3) were higher in the vegetarian women, while EPA and DHA were absent from their diets. Vegetarians also gave birth to babies with less DHA in their plasma and cord artery phospholipids (Reddy *et al.* 1994).

Focus on iodine

Iodine is an essential component of thyroid hormones and is also needed for the development of the fetal brain (Pemberton *et al.* 2005). The American National Health and Nutrition Examination Survey found that dairy foods were a particularly important source of iodine in pregnancy, and that vegetarian and vegan women's iodine status was borderline sufficient (Perrine *et al.* 2010). Given these findings, further studies are now also needed specifically in pregnant vegans, whose diets are more likely to be lacking in iodine (because dairy products are not typically eaten).

A cross-sectional study has also investigated the iodine status and thyroid function of vegetarians and vegans. Scientists found that the urinary iodine concentration of vegans was significantly lower than that of vegetarians (78.5µg/l versus 147.0µg/l), with the authors concluding that vegan women of childbearing age should ideally supplement with 150µg iodine daily (Leung *et al.* 2011).

Focus on vitamin D

According to Kaludjerovic and Vieth (2010), vitamin D deficiency may be present in 40 to 80 per cent of all pregnant women. Vitamin D deficiency has been linked to adverse pregnancy outcomes, including pre-eclampsia, gestational diabetes, low birth weight, preterm labour, caesarean delivery and infectious diseases, although results are conflicting (Urrutia and Thorp 2012). Year-round vitamin D deficiency has been found to be particularly prevalent amongst vegetarian UK South Asian women, due to the combined effects of vegetarianism and limited sun exposure (Darling *et al.* 2012).

As foods derived from animal sources generally have the highest vitamin D content per gram, vegetarians who limit their intakes of these foods and vegans may be at greatest risk of vitamin D deficiency. This was investigated using data from the Adventist Health Study, where the vitamin D status of vegetarians was compared between different ethnic groups. Results showed that vitamin D levels were not linked to a vegetarian diet; however, factors including vitamin D supplementation, degree of skin pigmentation and amount and intensity of sun exposure were found to have a greater influence on vitamin D status (Chan *et al.* 2009). Further studies, particularly in pregnant populations, are now needed to reconfirm these findings.

Health in pregnancy and beyond

In terms of potential health benefits there is some evidence that a vegetarian diet could help to prevent excessive weight gain in pregnancy. Findings from the American Project Viva Cohort Study found that women who were vegetarian in their first trimester of pregnancy were less likely to gain excess weight in pregnancy (Stuebe *et al.* 2009). It is possible, however, that these women had a generally healthier lifestyle overall, e.g. may have also been more active.

Some studies also link a vegetarian diet in pregnancy to less favourable health outcomes in the baby. For example, the Indian Pune Maternal Nutrition Study found that children born to mothers who were more likely to eat calcium-rich foods during pregnancy, e.g. milk, milk products, pulses, non-vegetarian foods, green leafy vegetables and fruit, had a higher total and spine bone mineral content and bone mineral density, measured using dual X-ray absorptiometry, six years after birth (Ganpule *et al.* 2006). Equally, findings from the Avon Longitudinal Study of Pregnancy and Childhood Study (ALSPAC) found that women who were vegetarian in pregnancy were more likely to give birth to boys with hypospadias (a birth defect where the urethra is not correctly placed). Researchers proposed that this may be because vegetarians have greater exposure to phytoestrogens, when compared with omnivores, which may affect the development of the male reproductive system *in utero* (North and Golding 2000).

Only a few studies have compared the outcome of pregnancy between lacto-ovo vegetarians, fish eaters and meat eaters. In a UK study no differences were observed between the three study groups in length of gestation, birth weight, birth length or head circumference (Drake *et al.* 1998). Earlier work by Sanders (1995), in contrast, reported lower birth weights of infants born to white women following vegan diets, and also of infants born to Caucasian women eating macrobiotic diets, as compared with the general population. In a study comprised of Hindu vegetarian women living in the UK, duration of pregnancy was, on average, four to five days shorter, onset of labour was earlier and emergency Caesarean section was more prevalent, than in white, non-vegetarians (Reddy *et al.* 1994).

Tailoring the diet

In general, pregnant vegetarians may wish to follow the same advice as meat eaters with respect to food safety issues and good nutrition. They should avoid excess vitamin A, unpasteurised cheeses such as brie or camembert and eating raw or uncooked eggs. Some types of fish, such as marlin, swordfish and tuna, may contain mercury, which could damage the developing nervous system of an unborn infant, should be avoided and no more than two weekly portions of fish should be consumed (including one portion of oily fish) (SACN/CoT 2004). As with non-vegetarians, high intakes of saturated fat and salt should be carefully avoided and alcohol, ideally, should not be consumed in pregnancy.

Vegetarian/vegan diets should be varied but well balanced. When optimal nutrient intakes are achieved vegetarian diets may be beneficial to both maternal and infant health (Craig and Mangels 2009). Pregnant vegetarians/vegans should be encouraged to eat a wide variety of foods, in amounts needed for good health. It must be emphasised that no single food contains all of the nutrients that the body needs for good health. Visual models such as traffic-light systems, the pyramid system and the Eatwell plate can be useful in helping to depict and communicate healthy eating messages (Derbyshire 2011b). For example, a non-vegetarian balanced diet generally includes plenty of potatoes, bread, rice, pasta and starchy foods, plenty of fruit and vegetables, some milk and dairy foods, some meat, fish, eggs, beans and other non-dairy sources of protein and should include just small amounts of food and drinks high in fat and/or sugar (NHS 2012). Obviously meat, fish, eggs and dairy are not eaten by traditional vegetarians/vegans, so appropriate substitution is needed. Foods such as quinoa, lentils, tofu and tempeh (made from fermented soybeans) are good alternative sources of protein, but may still be lacking in micronutrients, e.g. iron and vitamin B12.

Midwives and nutrition professionals can play a key role in informing vegetarians and vegans about food sources that provide adequate levels of protein, omega-3 fatty acids and micronutrients, explaining how the daily diet may be modified to meet nutritional needs (Table 7.2). Women should be referred to nutrition services when further guidance is required or necessary. For example, as mentioned earlier in the chapter, some women may choose to become vegetarian or vegan as a vehicle to promote weight control, which could mean that their diets are not as balanced or as healthy as they might be. Women should be guided in terms of how deficiencies of certain nutrients may affect their own and their baby's health.

On a final note, the use of supplements and fortified foods may help to top up daily nutrient intakes and shield against deficiencies (Craig 2010). This is particularly important in pregnancy, when the extensive physiological changes that take place need to be met with an adequate diet.

Conclusions

It may be possible for vegetarians and vegans to get the key nutrients they need from their diets. However, it is important that women do not fall into eating monotonous diets that may limit the range of nutrients they are getting (McEvoy *et al.* 2012). Diets should be as varied as possible, including a range of different foods groups, i.e. protein, dairy substitute and fresh fruits and vegetables, and supplements where appropriate. For example, women may benefit from taking a specially formulated pregnancy supplement containing the essential nutrients needed during this important time. In particular, these should contain vitamin D, B12 and appropriate omega-3 fatty acids.

Key messages

- Pregnant vegetarians/vegans should aim to ensure that their diets are as balanced and varied as possible.
- Pregnant vegetarians/vegans should follow the same advice as meat-eaters with regard to food safety issues in pregnancy.
- Alternative sources of protein should be included in the diet, e.g. quinoa, lentils, tofu and tempeh, although these may not provide the same levels of micronutrients.
- During pregnancy it is important to include omega-3 fatty acids in the diet, e.g. from flaxseed and flaxseed oil, olive oil, canola (rapeseed) oil and avocado, which are all good sources.
- It is also useful to incorporate fortified foods within the daily diet, e.g. cereals or bedtime drinks.
- Pregnant vegetarians/vegans may benefit from taking prenatal/pregnancy supplements that include vitamins D and B12, in addition to the other nutrients important for health in pregnancy.

References

Alwan, N.A., Greenwood, D.C., Simpson, N.A., McArdle, H.J., Godfrey, K.M. *et al.* (2011) 'Dietary iron intake during early pregnancy and birth outcomes in a cohort of British women', *Human Reproduction*, 26 (4): 911–9.

Bardone-Cone, A.M., Fitzsimmons-Craft, E.E., Harney, M.B., Maldonado, C.R., Lawson, M.A. *et al.* (2012) 'The inter-relationships between vegetarianism and eating disorders among females', *Journal of the Academy of Nutrition & Dietetics*, 112 (8): 1247–52.

Bates, B., Lennox, A., Prentice, A., Bates, C. and Swan, G. (2012) *National Diet and Nutrition Survey Headline Results from Years 1, 2 and 3 (combined) of the Rolling Programme (2008/2009–2010/11)*. London: Food Standards Agency/Department of Health.

Bedford, J.L. and Barr, S.I. (2005) 'Diets and selected lifestyle practices of self-defined adult vegetarians from a population-based sample suggest they are more "health conscious"', *International Journal of Behaviour, Nutrition & Physical Activity*, 2 (1): 4.

Buppasiri, P., Lumbiganon, P., Thinkhamrop, J., Ngamjarus, C. and Laopaiboon, M. (2011) 'Calcium supplementation (other than for preventing or treating hypertension) for improving pregnancy and infant outcomes', *Cochrane Database of Systematic Reviews*, 10: CD007079.

Cade, J.E., Burley, V.J., Greenwood, D.C and UK Women's Cohort Study Steering Group (2004) 'The UK Women's Cohort Study: comparison of vegetarians, fish-eaters and meat-eaters', *Public Health Nutrition*, 7 (7): 871–8.

Chan, J., Jaceldo-Siegl, K. and Fraser, G.E. (2009) 'Serum 25-hydroxyvitamin D status of vegetarians, partial vegetarians, and nonvegetarians: the Adventist Health Study-2', *American Journal of Clinical Nutrition*, 89 (5): 1686S–1692S.

Craig, W.J. (2009) 'Health effects of vegan diets', *American Journal of Clinical Nutrition*, 89 (5): 1627S–1633S.

Craig, W.J. (2010) 'Nutrition concerns and health effects of vegetarian diets', *Nutrition in Clinical Practice*, 25 (6): 613–20.

Craig, W.J. and Mangels, A.R. (2009) 'Position of the American Dietetic Association: vegetarian diets', *Journal of the American Dietetic Association*, 109 (7): 1266–82.

Daily, J.P. and Wylie, B.J. (2008) 'Iron deficiency during pregnancy: blessing or curse?' *Journal of Infectious Diseases*, 98 (2): 157–8.

Darling, A.L., Hart, K.H., Macdonald, H.M., Horton, K., Kang'ombe, A.R. *et al.* (2012) 'Vitamin D deficiency in UK South Asian Women of childbearing age: a comparative longitudinal investigation with UK Caucasian women', *Osteoporosis International*. [Epub ahead of print].

Davey, G.K., Spencer, E.A., Appleby, P.N., Allen, N.E., Knox, K.H. *et al.* (2003) 'EPIC-Oxford: lifestyle characteristics and nutrient intakes in a cohort of 33 883 meat-eaters and 31 546 non meat-eaters in the UK', *Public Health Nutrition*, 6 (3): 259–69.

Derbyshire, E.J. (2011a) 'Macronutrients in pregnancy'. In: *Nutrition in the Childbearing Years*. London: Wiley-Blackwell, pp. 100–25.

Derbyshire, E.J. (2011b) 'Preparing the body for pregnancy'. In: *Nutrition in the Childbearing Years*. London: Wiley-Blackwell, pp. 25–49.

DH (Department of Health) (1991) *Dietary Reference Values for Food Energy and Nutrients for the United Kingdom. Report of the Panel on Dietary Reference Values of the Committee on Medical Aspects of Food Policy*. London: Her Majesty's Stationery Office.

Drake, R., Reddy, S. and Davies, G. (1998) 'Nutrient intake during pregnancy and pregnancy outcome of lacto-ovo-vegetarians, fish-eaters and non-vegetarians', *Vegetarian Nutrition: an International Journal*, 2: 45–50.

Farmer, B., Larson, B.T., Fulgoni, V.L., Rainville, A.J. and Liepa, G.U. (2011) 'A vegetarian dietary pattern as a nutrient-dense approach to weight management: an analysis of the national health and nutrition examination survey 1999–2004', *Journal of the American Dietetic Association*, 111 (6): 819.

FSA (Food Standards Agency) (2006) *McCance and Widdowson's The Composition of Foods*. 6th edn. Cambridge: Royal Society of Chemistry.

Ganpule, A., Yajnik, C.S., Fall, C.H., Rao, S., Fisher, D.J. *et al.* (2006) 'Bone mass in Indian children – relationships to maternal nutritional status and diet during pregnancy: the Pune Maternal Nutrition Study', *Journal of Clinical Endocrinology & Metabolism*, 91 (8): 2994–3001.

Goonewardene, M., Shehata, M. and Hamad, A. (2012) 'Anaemia in pregnancy', *Best Practice & Research Clinical Obstetrics & Gynaecology*, 26 (1): 3–24.

Hoek, A.C., Luning, P.A., Stafleu, A. and de Graaf, C. (2004) 'Food-related lifestyle and health attitudes of Dutch vegetarians, non-vegetarian consumers of meat substitutes, and meat consumers', *Appetite* 42 (3): 265–72.

Kaludjerovic, J. and Vieth, R. (2010) 'Relationship between vitamin D during perinatal development and health', *Journal of Midwifery and Women's Health*, 55 (6): 550–60.

Koletzko, B., Cetin, I., Brenna, J.T., Perinatal Lipid Intake Working Group, Child Health Foundation *et al.* (2007) 'Dietary fat intakes for pregnant and lactating women', *British Journal of Nutrition*, 98 (5): 873–7.

Kornsteiner, M., Singer, I. and Elmadfa, I. (2008) 'Very low n-3 long-chain polyunsaturated fatty acid status in Austrian vegetarians and vegans', *Annals of Nutrition & Metabolism*, 52 (1): 37–47.

Krishnaveni, G.V., Hill, J.C., Veena, S.R., Bhat, D.S., Wills, A.K. *et al.* (2009) 'Low plasma vitamin B12 in pregnancy is associated with gestational "diabesity" and later diabetes', *Diabetologia*, 52 (11): 2350–8.

Leitzmann, C. (2005) 'Vegetarian diets: what are the advantages?' *Forum of Nutrition*, 57: 147–56.

Leung, A.M., Lamar, A., He, X., Braverman, L.E. and Pearce, E.N. (2011) 'Iodine status and thyroid function of Boston-area vegetarians and vegans', *Journal of Clinical Endocrinology & Metabolism*, 96 (8): E1303–7.

Marlow, H.J., Hayes, W.K., Soret, S., Carter, R.L., Schwab, E.R. *et al.* (2009) 'Diet and the environment: does what you eat matter?' *American Journal of Clinical Nutrition*, 89 (5): 1699S–1703S.

Marsh, K., Zeuschner, C., Saunders, A. and Reid, M. (2009) 'Meeting nutritional needs on a vegetarian diet', *Australian Family Physician*, 38 (8): 600–2.

McEvoy, C.T., Temple, N. and Woodside, J.V. (2012) 'Vegetarian diets, low-meat diets and health: a review', *Public Health Nutrition*, 3: 1–8.

NHS (National Health Service) NHS Choices: The Eatwell Plate. Available HTTP: www.nhs.uk/Livewell/Goodfood/Pages/eatwell-plate.aspx (accessed 12 August 2012).

North, K. and Golding, J. (2000) 'A maternal vegetarian diet in pregnancy is associated with hypospadias. The ALSPAC Study Team. Avon Longitudinal Study of Pregnancy and Childhood', *British Journal of Urology International*, 85 (1): 107–13.

O'Leary, F. and Samman, S. (2010) 'Vitamin B12 in health and disease', *Nutrients*, 2 (3): 299–316.

Pemberton, H.N., Franklyn, J.A. and Kilby, M.D. (2005) 'Thyroid hormones and fetal brain development', *Minerva Ginecologica*, 57 (4): 367–78.

Penney, D.S. and Miller, K.G. (2008) 'Nutritional counselling for vegetarians during pregnancy and lactation', *Journal of Midwifery and Women's Health*, 53 (1), 37–44.

Pepper, M.R. and Black, M.M. (2011) 'B12 in fetal development', *Seminars in Cell and Developmental Biology*, 22 (6): 619–23.

Perrine, C.G., Herrick, K., Serdula, M.K. and Sullivan, K.M. (2010) 'Some subgroups of reproductive age women in the United States may be at risk for iodine deficiency', *Journal of Nutrition*, 140 (8): 1489–94.

Philips, F. (2005) 'Vegetarian nutrition', *Nutrition Bulletin*, 30: 132–67.

Prentice, A. (2011) 'Milk intake, calcium and vitamin D in pregnancy and lactation: effects on maternal, fetal and infant bone in low- and high-income countries', *Nestlé Nutrition Workshop Series: Pediatric Program*, 67: 1–15.

Pribis, P., Pencak, R.C. and Grajales, T. (2010) 'Beliefs and attitudes toward vegetarian lifestyle across generations', *Nutrients*, 2 (5): 523–31.

Ray, J.G., Wyatt, P.R., Thompson, M.D., Vermeulen, M.J., Meier, C. *et al.* (2007) 'Vitamin B12 and the risk of neural tube defects in a folic-acid-fortified population', *Epidemiology*, 18 (3): 362–6.

Reddy, S., Sanders, T.A. and Obeid, O. (1994) 'The influence of maternal vegetarian diet on essential fatty acid status of the newborn', *European Journal of Clinical Nutrition*, 48 (5): 358–68.

SACN/CoT (Scientific Advisory Committee on Nutrition/Committee on Nutrition/Committee on Toxicity) (2004) *Advice on Fish Consumption: Benefits and Risks*. London: The Stationery Office.

Sanders, T. (1995) 'Vegetarian diets and children', *Pediatric Clinics of North America*, 42: 955–65.

Sanders, T.A. (2009) 'DHA status of vegetarians', *Prostaglandins Leukotrienes and Essential Fatty Acids*, 81 (2–3): 137–41.

Schösler, H., de Boer, J. and Boersema, J.J. (2012) 'Can we cut out the meat of the dish? Constructing consumer-oriented pathways towards meat substitution', *Appetite*, 58 (1): 39–47.

Selhun, J. and Paul, L. (2011) 'Folic acid fortification: why not vitamin B12 also?' *Biofactors*, 37 (4): 269–71.

Stables, D. and Rankin, J. (2006) 'The haematological system-physiology of the blood'. In: *Physiology in Childbearing*. London: Elsevier, pp. 205–18.

Stuebe, A.M., Oken, E. and Gillman, M.W. (2009) 'Associations of diet and physical activity during pregnancy with risk for excessive gestational weight gain', *American Journal of Obstetrics & Gynaecology*, 201 (1): 58. e1–8.

Timko, C.A., Hormes, J.M. and Chubski, J. (2012) 'Will the real vegetarian please stand up? An investigation of dietary restraint and eating disorder symptoms in vegetarians versus non-vegetarians', *Appetite*, 58 (3): 982–90.

Torjusen, H., Lieblein, G., Næs, T., Haugen, M., Meltzer, H.M. *et al.* (2012) 'Food patterns and dietary quality associated with organic food consumption during pregnancy; data from a large cohort of pregnant women in Norway', *BMC Public Health*. [Epub ahead of print].

Urrutia, R.P. and Thorp, J.M. (2012) 'Vitamin D in pregnancy: current concepts', *Current Opinions in Obstetrics & Gynaecology*, 24 (2): 57–64.

Vegetarian Society (2012a) Statistics. Available HTTP: www.vegsoc.org/page.aspx?pid=750 (accessed 31 July 2012).

Vegetarian Society (2012b) Fats, Omegas and Cholesterol. Available at: www.vegsoc.org/page.aspx?pid=777 (accessed 12 January 2012).

Waldmann, A., Dörr, B., Koschizke, J.W., Leitzmann, C. and Hahn, A. (2006) 'Dietary intake of vitamin B6 and concentration of vitamin B6 in blood samples of German vegans', *Public Health Nutrition*, 9 (6): 779–84.

Waldmann, A., Koschizke, J.W., Leitzmann, C. and Hahn, A. (2004) 'Dietary iron intake and iron status of German female vegans: results of the German vegan study', *Annals of Nutrition & Metabolism*, 48 (2): 103–8.

Wang, Z.P., Shang, X.X. and Zhao, Z.T. (2012) 'Low maternal vitamin B (12) is a risk factor for neural tube defects: a meta-analysis', *Journal of Maternal, Fetal & Neonatal Medicine*, 25 (4): 389–94.

Watanabe, F. (2007) 'Vitamin B12 sources and bioavailability', *Experimental Biology & Medicine*, 232 (10): 1266–74.

Weaver, C.M. (2009) 'Should dairy be recommended as part of a healthy vegetarian diet?' *American Journal of Clinical Nutrition*, 89 (5): 1634S–1637S.

8

FOOD TALK WITH YOUNG PREGNANT WOMEN

Ruth Martis

'I had this old midwife talking to me about what I should eat and stuff. I could tell she was quite objectionable about my age. She thought I was quite young and I asked her a question about what to eat and about stretch marks and she just kind of fobbed me off. I thought, talk to me old woman . . .' Hannah, 16 years old.

(Martis 2005: 61)

Pregnancy is a life-changing event for any woman, regardless of age and whether the pregnancy was planned or unplanned. Evidence indicates that adolescents have very specific nutrient requirements, especially for calcium and iron, not because of pregnancy but because of the rapid growth and physiological changes that occur during this time (Table 8.1). Mary Story likens this rapid growth to that in the first year of life (Story 1992; Story and Stang 2000). According to Paul and Robinson (2012), during the teenage years young people gain about 20 per cent of their adult height and 50 per cent of adult weight. From birth to young adulthood, nutrition and physical growth are interrelated, requiring optimal nutrition in order to achieve full growth potential. Young pregnant women who are underweight and do not meet their nutritional requirements during their first pregnancy are at a higher risk of having a baby with a low birth weight (Scholl *et al*. 1991; Haas 2002; Nielsen *et al*. 2006).

Table 8.1 Nutritional requirements for young women

Calories	Due to rapid growth and activity, young women need around 2,200 calories per day. These can be obtained from lean protein, low-fat dairy, whole grains, and fruits and vegetables.
Protein	For the body to grow and maintain muscle, teens need 45–60g of protein per day. Most young women easily meet this requirement from eating meat, fish, and dairy, but vegetarians may need to increase their protein intake from non-animal sources such as soy foods, beans, and nuts.
Calcium	Many teens do not get sufficient amounts of the recommended 1,200mg calcium per day, leading potentially to osteoporosis later in adult life. Soda/sugary carbonated drinks and other overly sugary foods leach calcium from bones. Calcium is found in dairy, cereals, sesame seeds, and leafy greens like spinach.
Iron	Iron deficiency can lead to anaemia. Young women, who often lose iron during menstruation, need 15mg per day. Iron-rich foods include red meat, chicken, beans, nuts, enriched whole grains, and leafy greens like spinach and kale.

Source: Adapted from Helpguide.org, *Nutrition for Children and Teens*, www.helpguide.org/life/healthy_eating_children_teens.htm.

Pregnancy has been identified as a powerful 'teachable moment' for the promotion of healthy eating (Paterson 2012; Phelan 2010). Midwives and other health professionals when providing care for young pregnant women often take this to mean handing out a long list of 'don't eats' during the pregnancy, perhaps more so than for their older counterparts, without being able to communicate effectively. Health professionals, including midwives, may also make the assumption that all pregnant teenage women have unhealthy eating habits. As a result the young pregnant women is often confused, overwhelmed by the information (McLeish 2008), and will therefore not engage in the consideration of nutritional lifestyle changes. The quote at the beginning of this chapter highlights this well.

Midwives and other health professionals often assume that all teenage pregnancies are 'high risk', without actually contextualising this knowledge for each young woman individually. Additionally, they may not always consider that the health outcomes of concern listed below are potentially due to poverty, poor nutrition and social exclusion issues, rather than to actual maternal age (Smith and Pell 2001; Burchett and Seeley 2003).

It has been documented in the literature that pregnant teenage women do not seek early antenatal care, placing both the mother and the baby at greater health risk (Baker 1996; Wilson *et al.* 1996; Baddiley 1997; Quinlivan and Evans 2002). Young women who become pregnant may face increased health risks, including mental health issues, which may manifest in suicidal tendencies and postnatal depression (Panazarine *et al.* 1995); substance use effects on the baby, such as alcohol, drugs, and smoking (Quinlivan and Evans 2002); lower birth weight for gestational age (Malchodi *et al.* 2003; Kramer 1987); increase in prematurity (James *et al.* 1995); stillbirths (Ministry of Health 2003); anaemia; hypertension; toxaemia and cephalopelvic disproportion (James op. cit.); and sexually transmitted infections, especially chlamydia (Fraser *et al.* 1995). Additionally, pregnant teenagers in high-income countries often meet with judgemental attitudes and are pushed into isolation by society as well as by midwives and other health professionals (Baddiley 1997; Patterson 2003; Beckinsale 2003).

The list of risks highlighted above is potentially overwhelming for health professionals working with young pregnant woman to ascertain the most effective approach to food and nutrition advice. Communication, above all else, including the way that midwives and other health professionals talk to young pregnant women, is the key factor in enabling young pregnant women to effect nutritional changes in their lives (McLeish 2008). Therefore this chapter explores a developmental communication approach incorporating an assessment tool called HEADDS (Home, Health, Education, Employment, Activities, Drugs, Depression and Safety), which might be particularly helpful when considering food and nutrition conversations with young pregnant women.

The World Health Organization defines adolescence as the period between the ages of 12 and 19 years (Watson 2001). This is the most commonly accepted age definition; although some studies include pregnant women up to the age of 24 years and others include only those aged 15–19.

Psychosocial development

First and foremost, the midwife and other health professionals need to understand that just because the young woman is pregnant, this does not make her an adult. Her pregnancy, her subsequent mothering and parenting style, her food and nutritional attitude will reflect her developmental stage, which is that of adolescence, not of adulthood.

According to Erikson's eight psychosocial stages of man (*sic*), based on psychoanalytic theory, a child moves into the teenage years roughly at the ages of 12–18 (Erikson 1980). This is termed by Erikson as the fifth stage of man (*sic*) and is referred to as Identity vs. Role Confusion. Each psychosocial stage needs to be successfully negotiated in order for the individual to move on to the next stage. Becoming pregnant during the teenage years can either assist or hinder successful negotiation. In the fifth stage, Erikson identifies that young people begin to consider how other people think and feel and wonder what other people think of them. Peers, in particular for girls, are paramount in such deliberation. Physical maturation is taking place, with new feelings and bodily sensations occurring. As a result the teenager develops a multitude of new ways of looking at and thinking about the world. During this period teenagers are getting to know who they are, where they have been, and where they are going. Hence, on the positive spectrum, the teenager emerges with a focus on ego identity and, on the negative side, with a sense of role confusion (Erikson 1980). It is a huge achievement to bring together all of the aspects that young people learn about themselves, such as being a daughter, friend, pupil, part-time worker, and to bring these sometimes competing roles into a whole that makes sense of the person that she is (Elkind 1977). This is why young people during this stage appear to be egocentric, focused on themselves. They need to be, as this gives them the opportunity to get to know who they are. David Elkind (1967; 1976; 1978) refers to teenagers' egocentrism as the heightened self-consciousness of adolescents that is reflected in their belief in their personal uniqueness. The interesting fact about ego identity and the struggle to become independent is that the process is often too threatening for the young person to go through it alone (McCallum 1990; Dekovic and Meeus 1997). Therefore teenagers often choose to go through this process in the same way as others within their peer group, and thus they change together. I have been working with young pregnant women for many years, including setting up antenatal teenage support groups, and was privileged to observe at first hand how well young pregnant women can effect change together as a peer group, even though, paradoxically, being individually and egocentrically focused. I used to think of it as the individual young woman becoming a 'collective I', which means she eats the same foods as others in her group, drinks the same drinks, chews gum on the same side of her mouth, wears the same clothes, and hangs out in the same places.

However, becoming pregnant can also alter the 'collective I' feeling and isolate a young woman from other teenage women. This may affect her transitioning into adulthood. Kuykendall (1989) argues that the only viable approach to working with teenagers has to come from the developmental approach, which characterises what is happening to them socially, intellectually, emotionally, spiritually, physically, sexually and psychologically. This may be especially so for young people who are sick. An unintended pregnancy, whilst not an illness, will affect all developmental issues for the young woman, and Kuykendall (1989) encourages health professionals to embrace this understanding in providing effective advice and care. When engaging in conversation around food and nutrition with a young pregnant woman, it is critical to understand this development stage. This may encourage the young woman to engage in the process of making effective nutritional lifestyle changes and facilitate regular attendance at midwifery appointments. Both of these actions may affect the long-term health of both the woman and her baby in a positive way.

Table 8.2 provides a generalised summary of the key developmental behavioural descriptions of the teenage years, as well as some examples on how to initiate discussion around food and nutrition with a young pregnant woman. Please note that this is a generalised summary drawn from the literature. It is of great importance to remember that each young pregnant woman is

Table 8.2 Developmental stage summary with food and nutrition conversation examples for health professionals

Developmental behaviour	Behaviour description	Food and nutrition conversation examples
Egocentric	The universe revolves around 'me' (Erikson 1980)	Do not focus on the benefits for the baby of healthier eating; rather, frame the message around the mother (ego-focused message). For example: If you are able to eat two fruits and four vegetables a day your skin will look healthier (Jeffs 2012; Warren, Rance and Hunter). A good iron intake will help you to concentrate better (pass your tests at school) and you will feel less tired (can stay up later). If you eat bread, cereals, rice and pasta every day then not only your iron, but other necessary minerals and vitamins will be covered (Bowden and Tannies 2009).
Becoming independent	Seeking independence to learn who am I and where do I fit (Santrock 1996)	Get a group of your friends together and have a cook off. Who comes up with the best tasting and cheapest and fastest meal? What's your favourite vegetable? Ever thought of growing it?
Living in the here and now	Living for today, but slowly learning about tomorrow's consequences (Santrock 1996)	Discuss short-term consequence rather than long-term. For example: Consider reducing sugary drink intake, as it will make you less sleepy and enable you to stay up longer at night.
Learning to individualise within a collective 'I' peer group	Placing great importance on peers, learning about different kinds of relationships (Kuykendall 1989; Martis 2005)	Invite the young woman to bring her friends to appointments so that they can all participate in hearing and sharing the information around food and nutrition, as well as other areas. Collectively, they can change their nutritional lifestyle together. Brainstorming about where to get food that is reasonably priced, sharing cooking skills and tips and recipes can also start to change eating behaviour. For example, share ideas about what is a healthy affordable snack or which foods can increase calcium and protein intake, which can assist bone growth.
Learning about effective communication	Enjoying verbal logical dialogues that fluctuate between concrete thoughts, actual experiences and make-believe situations (Piaget 1954; 1972)	Use language that the woman and her friends can understand. Learning about communication can be difficult and, like learning to ride a bicycle, it requires practice. Expect some miscommunication or different choice of words. Comments such as 'I don't like this crap' might actually translate as 'I have no money to buy iron-rich foods'.
Body image	Placing great importance on self/body image, maturing their self-esteem (Kuykendall 1989)	Affirm, when appropriate, that stretch marks are concerning and putting on weight can be a worry. Discussions around the weight distribution, such as baby and placenta, might alleviate some of these concerns. Stress that eating plenty of fruit and vegetables will help, as they contain vitamins (A, B, C, E) that will help with stretch marks because they aid skin elasticity and firmness; together with drinking plenty of water.

Table 8.2 Continued

Developmental behaviour	Behaviour description	Food and nutrition conversation examples
Physically still developing and maturing	In great need of food and sleep (Story 1992; Elliott 1993; Story and Stang 2000)	This is a reminder to the midwife and other health professionals that, as stated in the introduction, young people need to eat more than adults because they are still developing physically. It can be reassuring to the young woman to comment on this and will enhance her understanding about eating regularly. Similarly with sleep. Physical growth and development require energy, which can be replenished with food and sleep. 'Sleeping in' is an expected phenomenon during adolescence because of this (combined with late nights). This is why midwifery or other clinical appointments made after lunch will attract better attendance.
Engaging in health-compromising risks	Perceiving themselves to be invincible, invulnerable and immune to the laws that apply to others (Elkind 1967; 1978; Arnett 1992)	Without being patronising, the following questions might guide discussion of health-compromising behaviour. For example: Did you know that when you smoke, the baby smokes? When you drink, the baby drinks? This includes any drug use too. Your baby is smaller in size; hence it will get more than you. It could also be said (loosely) that if you eat junk food, then the baby eats it too. It can mean that your baby will be smaller and less healthy once it is born, which might mean that you have to feed the baby more often or the baby might be more irritable (due to withdrawal symptoms) or cry frequently.

Source: Adapted from Martis (2005).

a unique person with her own needs and understanding of nutrition within the context of her developmental stage. Furthermore, the discussions in this chapter are from the perspective of a high-income country and may or may not be applicable to low- and middle-income countries.

In order for young people to negotiate their psychosocial developmental stage, 'feeling safe' is one of the aspects that will enable them to steer through this period and attain their identity (Maslow 1970; Erikson 1980). Midwives and health professionals need to engage the young pregnant woman in ways that build trust and partnership based on 'feeling safe', and this includes reassuring her of confidentiality. Information shared by the young pregnant woman should not be discussed with anyone else, including parents, unless with her consent. A small study of 30 pregnant teenagers discussing their antenatal education needs identified the importance of this in a number of focus groups (Martis 2005).

Participants identified clearly that feeling safe was a significant issue for them. Whilst they could not change an unsafe environment at home or in other areas of their lives, they wanted a teenage pregnancy support group where they could feel and be safe. The need to feel safe in such a group meant something different to different participants, but overall it was expressed as physical safety, no occurrence of physical abuse, and emotional safety. Feeling safe meant that participants could express verbally how and what they wanted, without needing to mod- ify their emotional or verbal expressions, and to be accepted for who they were, no matter what they had done or were perhaps continuing to do (Martis 2005). In a safe and nurturing environment, young pregnant women may be able to ask questions such as: How do I cook a nutritious meal? If I drink, does my baby drink? Does healthy equal yucky food? Where do I get such food? At teenage antenatal groups, instead of learning about the stages of labour, the participants could learn to cook a nutritious meal together. Whilst these findings related to antenatal groups, the principles may also apply to midwifery clinics and home visits.

Emotional needs

Internationally renowned parent educators and psychotherapists Ken and Elizabeth Mellor identified that the emotional needs of teenagers require 'regrowing', regardless of whether they are pregnant or not (Mellor and Mellor 2004; Allen 2003). Young people need to 'regrow' emotionally through all the younger stages of their lives, as this will enable them to get to know themselves. Figure 8.1 shows the regressed emotional ages and how they correspond to

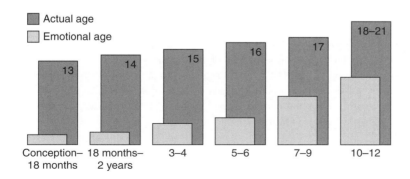

Figure 8.1 Actual physical age and emotional age of teenagers

Source: Mellor and Mellor (2004:17). Reprinted with permission from the authors and the publisher.

actual ages. According to Mellor and Mellor (2004), this means that if, for example, the young pregnant woman is 15 years old, her emotional 'regrowing' will be at the level of a 3- to 4-year-old. Therefore, an approach to discussing nutrition may benefit from revisiting how 3- to 4-year-olds react emotionally to food and nutrition, as illustrated in the following example.

> Your child may gobble down a particular food one day, and then push away the plate with the same food the next day. She may ask for a certain food for several days in a row, and then insist that she doesn't like it anymore. As irritating as it may be to have her turn up her nose at a dish she devoured the day before, it's normal behaviour for a pre-schooler, and best not to make an issue of it. Let her eat the other foods on her plate or select something else to eat.
>
> (www.healthychildren.org)

It is interesting to consider that parents, midwives and health professionals would tolerate this eating behaviour in a 3- to 4-year-old but not in a 15-year-old, developing, pregnant teenage woman.

Nurturing emotional and psychosocial development needs, which includes understanding of the 'regrowing' of emotional needs, may guide midwives and health professionals during conversations around food and nutrition. This is especially important during a time when a young pregnant woman may face relationship breakdowns with her parents, the father of the baby, his family, school teachers, class mates, friends, neighbours or community groups as a result of her unplanned pregnancy.

> 'I felt a bit down through my pregnancy because all my mates ditched me . . . My family rejected me at the start because I was pregnant . . . and at school I was told off that I was doing the wrong thing . . .' Sarah, 15 years old.
>
> (Martis 2005: 62)

Sarah's situation is not an isolated example. Many young pregnant women and men have shared with me their relationship breakdowns with family and friends around them. While the breakdowns are multifaceted, they are often due to judgemental attitudes or, for the parents of the young couple, the shock of becoming grandparents before their time and the aspirations and dreams they had for their daughter or son being shattered (Stevenson, Maton and Teti 1999). It is not surprising, then, that young pregnant women become stressed and sometime display emotional outbursts. Midwives and health professionals who find the emotional needs and psychosocial needs of young pregnant women difficult to relate to may need to refer them to someone who is better equipped to support them. Pregnant young women respond well to sincerity. They do not expect anyone to be perfect or right at all times, but they do expect honesty (Checkley 1990). Pregnant teenage women rapidly detect whether they are liked or not liked, or are being judged by a midwife or health professional, and as a result they may reject antenatal care and disregard any nutritional advice, thus abandoning any positive lifestyle changes (Martis 2005).

Body image

Body-image distortions during a young woman's pregnancy may develop as a result of emotional needs not being met (McGraw 2003; Micali 2010). This may greatly influence what a pregnant young woman will eat. Kuykendall (1989) and Erikson (1980) both describe the importance of body image development during the teenage years. This is part of the young woman's getting to know who she is and who she will become. During this stage a pregnant young woman can become obsessed with stretch marks, distressed about her growing abdominal size and breasts and becoming rounder in the face. The idea of having a small baby may be very appealing, and myths of eating less to make a little baby and fewer stretch marks are widespread (Maputle 2006; Mehta, Siega-Riz and Herring 2011; Newcombe and Hinkley 2012). Additionally, this can all be compounded by the many negative reactions from health professionals, family, friends, community and society when teenage women disclose their unplanned pregnancy or when they start to show physically that they are pregnant. This can create feelings of loss, loneliness and low self-esteem. It is not surprising, then, that the literature indicates that young people are at high risk of developing anorexia, bulimia or binge-eating disorders (Ministry of Health 2006). It is not within the scope of midwifery to diagnose and treat these disorders, but it is helpful to have some knowledge to ascertain when a referral is needed. Further information on the subject of eating disorders can be found in Chapter 6. Some of the questions identified in Boxes 8.1 to 8.3 might be a useful guide, once a trusting midwifery partnership has been established. The question guide should be used only if concerns have been identified, and not used routinely.

Box 8.1 Question guide: signs of anorexia

- Do you feel fat even though people tell you you're not?
- Are you terrified of gaining weight?
- Do you lie about how much you eat or hide your eating habits from others?
- Are your friends or family concerned about your weight loss, eating habits or appearance?
- Do you diet, compulsively exercise or purge when you're feeling overwhelmed or bad about yourself?
- Do you feel powerful or in control when you go without food, over-exercise or purge?
- Do you base your self-worth on your weight or body size?

Source: Adapted from www.helpguide.org/mental/anorexia_signs_symptoms_causes_treatment.htm.

Box 8.2 Question guide: signs of Binge Eating Disorder

- Do you feel out of control when you're eating?
- Do you think about food all the time?
- Do you eat in secret?
- Do you eat until you feel sick?
- Do you eat to escape from worries, relieve stress, or to comfort yourself?
- Do you feel disgusted or ashamed after eating?
- Do you feel powerless to stop eating, even though you want to?

Source: Adapted from www.helpguide.org/mental/binge_eating_disorder.htm.

Box 8.3 Question guide: signs of bulimia

- Are you obsessed with your body and your weight?
- Does food and dieting dominate your life?
- Are you afraid that when you start eating, you won't be able to stop?
- Do you ever eat until you feel sick?
- Do you feel guilty, ashamed, or depressed after you eat?
- Do you vomit or take laxatives to control your weight?

Source: Adapted from www.helpguide.org/mental/bulimia_signs_symptoms_causes_treatment.htm.

'HEADDS UP': food talk

Many midwives and health professionals find it challenging to engage pregnant teenage women in meaningful conversations. HEADDS has been identified in the literature as a helpful screening tool for identifying potential psychosocial factors that influence the well-being of young people (Goldring and Rosen 2004; Stephens 2006; Reitman 2007). HEADDS can be easily adapted for conversation about food and nutrition during pregnancy and I have found it to be an effective tool when providing midwifery care for young pregnant women. It is advisable not to use the full HEADDS tool for one antenatal visit, but instead to take one or two aspects to each appointment as a reminder of how to approach a given topic with open-ended questions. Closed questions are appropriate at times, but they tend to elicit monosyllabic answers, particularly at the beginning of the midwifery relationship. A question like 'Do you drink coke or frequently eat takeaway burgers?' requires a yes or no answer. This could also be easily interpreted as a judgemental question by the young pregnant woman and elicit a defensive answer. Asking about her favourite food or snack or what she enjoys eating when meeting up with her friends will elicit a far more honest answer and encourages conversation about how people enjoy different foods and how it might have become their favourite food. Eventually the conversation can be directed to discussion around nutrients and how they are important not only in pregnancy but also for staying healthy throughout life. This conversation might take place over a number of antenatal appointments, depending on how well rapport has been established. The following are examples of how food talks with pregnant women might be approached using the HEADDS tool. This is always in the context of the young pregnant woman's circumstances and the importance of understanding the challenges she may face when attempting to make nutritional lifestyle changes.

Home/Health

Conversations about Home/Health provide an opportunity to find out what happens at home with meals.

Such a discussion may enable the midwife to gather information and converse about healthy snack foods, drinking plenty of water, lifestyle changes around eating patterns, recipes, or even to have some healthy foods available to share. It can also be an opportunity to assess the woman for potential eating disorders (see Boxes 8.1 to 8.3). A midwifery col-

Prompt-question examples

Who cooks her meals?
Does she live at home?
How well does she get along with the people she lives with?
What foods are shared? Is there any cultural significance of the food that she eats?
Does she enjoy cooking?
What are her favourite meals?
Is she vegetarian or vegan?
How is her health in general?
How does she think her health could be improved?

league of mine always has cooled water with a slice of lemon available for her clients to drink during antenatal appointments. Many pregnant women have been surprised at how the lemon makes such a difference and this creates an effortless opening for discussion about food.

Education/Employment

Education/Employment provides opportunities to ascertain the woman's educational and financial situation. This then can be linked to nutritional knowledge and who buys and pays for the food in her life.

Prompt-question examples

What did you do at school/work today?
How was school/work today?
Where did you learn to cook?
Who buys and pays for the food at home?

Such questions can lead into the topics of where she learned or is learning to cook (e.g. at school or working in a restaurant) and how to read food labels. The cost of food is an important topic. When money is short, food shopping may be curtailed or healthy eating may be replaced with less healthy options. For example, it would seem that it is cheaper to buy a bottle of carbonated soft drink than it is to buy milk. Other examples include white bread, which is less expensive than wholegrain bread, or lettuce or other green vegetables, which can be more expensive than a bag of chips (McLeish 2008; Barrow 2013). It seems paradoxical that in many situations mineral and vitamin supplements are available free of charge or at very low cost on prescription but little provision is made in the form of food vouchers, for example, to support the purchase of 'real' food (Burchett and Seeley 2003). The midwife needs to have community support information available that might assist with food and finances, and to be able to refer appropriately, where necessary (McLeish 2008).

It should also be acknowledged that often the young woman is usually not in charge of food preparation or purchasing. The midwife needs to aim to involve those responsible for food and nutrition in the woman's life.

Activities

This topic should elicit information about what the young pregnant woman does in her spare time.

Prompt-question examples

What does she do to have fun?

Where and how does she socialise (hang out or chill) with her friends/peers?

Does she play a sport/exercise/musical instrument or love going to the movies?

While it appears that these questions have nothing to do with nutrition they actually can open many opportunities to discuss interest in food activities. There are numerous apps/resources available that can be downloaded to a smartphone, including recipes, weekly meal planners, themed healthy food parties, nutrition dictionaries, food label tools, nutrition games, watching the baby grow, exercises and how to grow food, including information on community gardens (Hanna and Oh 2000; Harris 2009; Smith 2009; 2011). Box 8.4 outlines additional nutrition activities and information resources.

Drugs

The letter D, for Drugs, is intended to trigger a conversation about the possibility of any substance use, including alcohol and tobacco. Binge drinking is the most common drinking pattern of alcohol consumption among young people (Miller, Naimi, Brewer and Everett Jones 2007; Lohmann 2013) and is strongly associated with a wide range of health risks, including depletion of essential nutrients. Similarly, tobacco use is common during adolescence and associated with serious long-term health risks (World Health Organization 2011; Hackshaw, Rodeck and Boniface 2011). Experimenting with designer drugs such as ecstasy has increased in the past decade (Fryar *et al.* 2009). The risk factors are well known to midwives and health professionals and it is recognised that stopping substance use is not an easy step to take. There is no one right way to approach this difficult topic, but making direct eye contact when asking open-ended questions will be most effective.

Prompt-question examples

Some of my clients tell me their friends sometimes try drugs and alcohol. What kind of things have your friends talked about trying?

It must be a challenge for you to be at a party where your friends are drinking. How do you deal with it when they offer you a drink, smoke, drug?

Some direct questions regarding smoking or alcohol intake can be normalised by the midwife or health professional stating that she/he is required to ask every pregnant women in her/his care if they smoke and drink, and how much. This enables the young pregnant woman to understand that this is a routine question and no personal judgement is involved. A link to food and nutrition could then be made in terms of the difficulty to remember to eat regularly when drinking too much alcohol and how it depletes nutrients in the body, as well as for the baby. Linking this message to body image and examples of nutritional needs (Table 8.1) can provide an impetus for changing substance use behaviour. Confidentiality must be assured, especially when the young woman requests a referral to professional services.

Depression

Nutrition can play a key role in the onset, as well as the severity and duration, of depression. Many of the easily noticeable food patterns that precede depression are the same as those that occur during depression. These may include poor appetite, skipping meals, a dominant desire for sweet foods or inability to sleep/go back to sleep once woken (Sathyanarayana Rao *et al.* 2008).

Prompt-question examples

What do you do to cheer yourself up?
Do you eat less when you are feeling sad?

It may be useful to explain that many young people during their teenage years, whether pregnant or not, have to deal with strong emotions that sometimes can make them feel 'out of control'. The hormonal changes during pregnancy may compound this feeling (Reitman 2007). Such an explanation may give clarity and offer a greater chance for the young pregnant woman to understand the importance of eating well. If, during the course of this conversation, the young pregnant woman identifies thoughts or self-harming or killing herself, an emergency referral to psychiatric services will be needed.

Safety

Safety is an area of which midwives and health professionals are acutely aware. This usually relates to family violence and sexual abuse, and discussion is prompted by questions like 'Are you feeling safe at home/school/work/with your friends?' In terms of nutrition, however, this would apply to food safety, preparation and hand hygiene. Pregnant women are more susceptible to food-borne illnesses than are non-pregnant women (Lund and O'Brien 2011). Often a pamphlet about food safety is handed to the young pregnant woman to read at home. This does not constitute contextualised care. The young pregnant woman might know already how to handle food safely, what foods to avoid, and hand hygiene, but has never thought about how long it is safe to store the cooked food in the fridge. This will become evident only if a conversation has been initiated around food safety. It also highlights the importance of acknowledging that the young pregnant woman has her own empirical knowledge and needs the opportunity to share this. Her self-esteem will be lifted as she shares what she knows and, through this empowering experience, becomes more open to further learning and willing to apply lifestyle changes by making healthy food and nutrition choices.

Conclusion

Working with young pregnant women and teenage mothers is a rewarding experience for many health professionals, despite some challenging situations. Establishing a relationship that is grounded in trust and respect, incorporating a psychosocial development approach (that of adolescent, not adulthood), and understanding the need for teenage women to emotionally 'regrow' enables effective food talk with young pregnant women. HEADDS is one helpful tool to guide and support health professionals in this. For Bahati, a 15-year-old young woman from Africa, it made a significant difference, and she expressed it like this:

> 'I find . . . when seeing the midwife . . . I feel like I am, I feel very honoured because I'm bringing a life into this world. I feel safe with her at her clinic, like an oasis. Chaos and desert outside, love and acceptance inside. But when I am going out . . . it is different. I've been a person who always put myself down but the midwife helped me to think and now I just feel wow, I'm actually doing something for me and my baby's health like you know [healthy eating]'. . .

(Martis 2005: 100)

Box 8.4 Nutrition activities and information resources

Nutrients for teenagers:

www.nutritionfoundation.org.nz/nutrition-facts/healthy-eating-for-all-ages/adolescents

Nourish interactive meal plan 2,200 calories for 9- to 18-year-olds:

www.nourishinteractive.com/nutrition-education-printables/254-older-children-daily-balanced-meal-plan-2200-calories
www.nourishinteractive.com/system/assets/free-printables/254/2200meal_plan.pdf?1341346058

Nutrition for children and teens:

www.helpguide.org/life/healthy_eating_children_teens.htm

Food-savvy kids:

www.foodsavvykids.com/

Nutrition for pregnancy and the early years:

webarchive.nationalarchives.gov.uk/+/www.dh.gov.uk/en/Publichealth/Nutrition/Nutritionpregnancyearlyyears/DH_127622

Growing vegetables in containers:

www.sparkpeople.com/resource/nutrition_articles.asp?id=1741

Best nutritional and food information app for iPhone:

www.imore.com/best-nutrition-and-food-information-app-iphone

References

Allen, E.J. (2003) 'Aims and associations of reducing teenage pregnancy', *British Journal of Midwifery*, 11 (6): 366–69.

Arnett, J. (1992) 'Reckless behaviour in adolescence: a developmental perspective', *Journal of Developmental Review*, 12: 339–73.

Baddiley, C. (1997) 'The afternoon group', *MIDIRS, Midwifery Digest*, 7 (2): 214–15.

Baker, T.J. (1996) 'Factors related to the initiation of prenatal care in the adolescent nullipara', *Nurse Practitioner*, 21 (2): 26–42.

Barrow, B. (2013) 'Food prices rise three times faster than wages as the cost of living 'crisis' continues', *Mail Online News*. Available at: www.dailymail.co.uk/news/article-2277798/Food-prices-rise-times-faster-wages-cost-living-crisis-continues.html (accessed 10 April 2013).

Beckinsale, C. (2003) 'Why choose motherhood? The older teenage client's perspective', *The Practising Midwife*, 6 (3): 10–13.

Bowden, J. and Tannies, A. (2009) *The 100 healthiest foods to eat during pregnancy*, Beverly, Massachusetts, USA: Fir Winds Press.

Burchett, H. and Seeley, A. (2003) *Good enough to eat? The diet of pregnant teenagers*, London, England: The Maternity Alliance and The Food Commission.

Checkley, G. (1990) 'Talking to teenagers', *Healthright*, 9 (4): 25–7.

Dekovic, M. and Meeus, W. (1997) 'Peer relations in adolescence effects of parenting and adolescents' self-concept', *Journal of Adolescence*, 20: 163–76.

Elkind, D. (1967) 'Egocentrism in adolescence', *Journal of Child Development*, 38: 1025–34.

Elkind, D. (1976) *Child development and education: a Piagetian perspective*, New York, NY, USA: Oxford University Press.

Elkind, D. (1977) 'Erikson's eight ages of man', in D. Hetzel (ed.) *Readings in human development: contemporary perspectives* (9th edn), New York, NY, USA: Harper and Rowe.

Elkind, D. (1978) 'Understanding the young adolescent', *Journal of Adolescence*, 13: 127–34.

Elliott, D.S. (1993) 'Health-enhancing and health-compromising lifestyles', in S.G. Millstein, A.C. Petersen and E.O. Nightingale (eds) *Promoting the health of adolescents*, New York, NY, USA: Oxford University Press.

Erikson, E.H. (1980) *Identity and the life cycle* (2nd edn), New York, NY, USA: Norton.

Fraser, A.M., Lockert, J.E. and Ward, R.H. (1995) 'Association of young maternal age with adverse reproductive outcomes', *New English Journal of Medicine*, 332: 1113–17.

Fryar, C.D., Merino, M.C., Hirsch, R. and Porter, K.S. (2009) *Smoking, alcohol use, and illicit drug use reported by adolescents aged 12–17 years: United States, 1999–2004*, 15(20 May) Centers for Disease Control and Prevention. National Center for Health Statistics. Online. Available at: www.cdc.gov/nchs/data/nhsr/nhsr015.pdf (accessed 27 September 2012).

Goldring, J. and Rosen, D. (2004) 'Getting into adolescent heads: an essential update', *Contemporary Pediatrics*, 21: 64.

Haas, A.V. (2002) 'Nutrition during pregnancy', *Having a Baby Today*, 5: 3–5.

Hackshaw, A., Rodeck, C. and Boniface, S. (2011) 'Maternal smoking in pregnancy and birth defects: a systematic review based on 173 687 malformed cases and 11.7 million controls', *Human Reproduction Update*, 17 (5): 1–10. DOI: 10.1093/humupd/dmr022.

Hanna, A.K. and Oh, P. (2000) 'Rethinking urban poverty: a look at community gardens', *Bulletin of Science Technology Society*, 20 (3): 207–16. DOI: 10.1177/027046760002000308.

Harris, E. (2009) 'The role of community gardens in creating healthy communities', *Australian Planner*, 46 (2): 24–7.

James, D.K., Steer, P.J., Weiner, C.P. and Gonik, B. (1995) *High risk pregnancy management*, London: W.B. Saunders and Co.

Jeffs, E. (2012) 'Weight, height and their potential impact on pregnancy care', paper presented at New Zealand College of Midwives Conference, Wellington, New Zealand, August 2012.

Kramer, M.S. (1987) 'Determinants of low birth weight: methodological assessment and meta-analysis', *Bulletin of the World Health Organization*, 65 (5): 663–737.

Kuykendall, J. (1989) 'Adolescence: teenage trauma', *Nursing Times*, 85 (27): 26–7.

Lohmann, R.C. (2013) 'Teen binge drinking: all too common', *Psychology Today*, published online 26 January. Available at: www.psychologytoday.com/blog/teen-angst/201301/teen-binge-drinking-all-too-common.

Lund, B.M. and O'Brien, S.J. (2011) 'The occurrence and prevention of foodborne disease in vulnerable people', *Foodborne Pathogens and Disease*, 8 (9): 961–73. DOI: 10.1089/fpd.2011.0860.

Malchodi, C.S., Oncken, C., Dornelas, E.A., Caramanica, L., Gregonis, E. and Curry, S.L. (2003) 'The effects of peer counselling on smoking cessation and reduction', *Journal of Obstetrics and Gynecology*, March 101 (3): 504–10.

Maputle, M. (2006) 'Becoming a mother: teenage mothers' experiences of first pregnancy', *Curationis*, 29 (2), 87–95.

Martis, R. (2005) 'Teenage and pregnant: an exploratory study of pregnant teenagers and their antenatal education needs in the Palmerston North Region', Palmerston North, New Zealand: Massey University, unpublished thesis.

Maslow, A.H. (1970) *Motivation and personality*, New York, NY, USA: Harper and Row.

McCallum, I. (1990) 'Growing pains', *Nursing Times*, 86 (34): 62–4.

McGraw, J. (2003) *The ultimate weight solution for teens. The 7 keys to weight freedom*, New York, NY, USA: Free Press.

McLeish, J. (2008) *Pregnant teenagers and diet*, London: Tommy's, The Baby Charity.

Mehta, U., Siega-Riz, A. and Herring, A. (2011) 'Effect of body image on pregnancy weight gain', *Maternal & Child Health Journal*, 15 (3), 324–332. DOI: 10.1007/s10995-010-0578-7.

Mellor, K. and Mellor, E. (2004) *Teenstages. How to guide the journey to adulthood*, Lane Grove, NSW, Australia: Finch Publishing.

Micali, N. (2010) 'Management of eating disorders during pregnancy', *Progress in Neurology & Psychiatry*, 14 (2) 24–26. DOI: 10.1002/pnp.158.

Miller, J.W., Naimi, T.S., Brewer, R.D. and Everett Jones, S. (2007) 'Binge drinking and associated health risk behaviors among high school students', *Paediatrics*, 119 (1): 76–85. DOI: 10.1542/peds.2006-1517.

Ministry of Health (2003) *Report on maternity 2000 and 2001*, Wellington, New Zealand: New Zealand Health Information Service.

Ministry of Health (2006) *Food and nutrition guidelines for healthy pregnant and breastfeeding women: a background paper*, Wellington, New Zealand: Ministry of Health.

Newcombe, L.J. and Hinkley, J.L. (2012), 'Understanding the experience of weight gain and body image during adolescent pregnancy', New Hampshire, USA: University of New Hampshire, unpublished thesis.

Nielsen, J.N., Gittelsohn, J., Anliker, J. and O'Brien, K. (2006) 'Interventions to improve diet and weight gain among pregnant adolescents and recommendations for future research', *Journal of the American Dietetic Association*, 106 (11): 1825–40. DOI: 10.1016/j.jada.2006.08.007.

Panazarine, S., Slater, E. and Sharps, P. (1995) 'Coping, social support, and depressive symptoms in adolescent mothers', *Journal of Adolescent Health*, 17: 113–19.

Paterson, H. (2012) 'Exploring women's experiences of eating during pregnancy', paper presented at New Zealand College of Midwives Conference, Wellington, New Zealand, August 2012.

Patterson, M. (2003) 'Case study: Queen Charlotte's one-to-one 'young mums' midwifery scheme', *Midwives, Journal of the Royal College of Midwives*, 6 (2): 63.

Paul, M.W. and Robinson, L. (2012) *Nutrition for children and teens*. Online. Available at: www.helpguide.org/life/healthy_eating_children_teens.htm (accessed 20 April 2013).

Phelan, S. (2010) 'Pregnancy: a 'teachable moment' for weight control and obesity prevention', *American Journal of Obstetrics and Gynecology*, Feb; 202 (2): 135. e1–8. DOI: 10.1016/j.ajog.2009.06.008.

Piaget, J. (1954) *The construction of reality in the child*, New York, NY, USA: Basic Books.

Piaget, J. (1972) 'Intellectual evolution from adolescence to adulthood', *Journal of Human Development*, 15: 1–12.

Quinlivan, J.A. and Evans, S.F. (2002) 'The impact of continuing illegal drug use on teenage pregnancy outcomes – a prospective cohort study', *British Journal of Obstetrics and Gynaecology*, 109: 1148–53.

Reitman, D.S. (2007) 'HEADDS up on talking with teenagers', *Pediatric Consultant Live*, 6 (9): 1–6 Online. Available at: www.pediatricsconsultantlive.com/display/article/1803329/11894 (accessed 24 April 2013).

Santrock, J.W. (1996) *Adolescence*, Dubuque, IA, USA: Brown & Benchmark.

Sathyanarayana Rao, T.S., Asha, M.R., Ramesh, B.N. and Jagannatha Rao, K.S. (2008) 'Understanding nutrition, depression and mental illnesses', *Indian Journal of Psychiatry*, 50 (2): 77–82. DOI: 10.4103/0019-5545.42391.

Scholl, T.O., Hediger, C.M.L., Khoo, C.S., Healey, M.F. and Rawson, N.L. (1991) 'Maternal weight gain, diet and infant birth weight: correlations during adolescent pregnancy', *Journal of Clinical Epidemiology*, 44: 423–28.

Smith, E.C. (2009) *The vegetable gardener's bible*, New York, NY, USA: Storey Publishing.

Smith, E.C. (2011) *The vegetable gardener's container bible: how to grow a bounty of food in pots, tubs, and other containers*, New York, NY, USA: Storey Publishing.

Smith, G.C.S. and Pell, J.P. (2001) 'Teenage pregnancy and risk of adverse perinatal outcomes associated with first and second births: population based retrospective cohort study', *British Medical Journal*, 323: 476–79.

Stephens, M.B. (2006) 'Preventative health counselling for adolescents', *American Family Physician*, 74 (7): 1151–56.

Stevenson, W., Maton, K.I. and Teti, D.M. (1999) 'Social support, relationship quality, and well-being among pregnant adolescents', *Journal of Adolescence*, 22 (1): 109–21. DOI: org/10.1006/jado.1998.0204.

Story, M. (1992) 'Nutritional requirements during adolescence', in E.R. McAnarney, R.E. Kreipe, D.E. Orr and G.D. Comerci (eds) *Textbook of adolescent medicine*, Philadelphia, PA, USA: W.B. Saunders, pp. 75–84.

Story, M. and Stang, J. (eds) (2000) *Nutrition and the pregnant adolescent: a practical reference guide*, Minneapolis, MN, USA: Center for Leadership, Education, and Training in Maternal and Child Nutrition, University of Minnesota.

Warren, L., Rance, J. and Hunter, B. (2012) 'Feasibility and acceptability of a midwife-led intervention programme called "Eat Well Keep Active" to encourage a healthy lifestyle in pregnancy', *Biomed Central Pregnancy and Childbirth*, 12 (27): e1–e6. DOI: 10.1186/1471-2393-12-27. *Online*. Available at: www.biomedcentral.com/1471–2393/12/27 (accessed 31 October 2012).

Watson, P. (2001) 'Adolescent health in NZ', *New Ethicals Journal*, February: 23–26.

Wilson, N., Clements, M., Bathgate, M. and Parkinson, S. (1996) *Using spatial analysis to improve and protect the public health in New Zealand*, Wellington, New Zealand: Ministry of Health.

World Health Organization (2011) *WHO report on the global tobacco epidemic. Warning about the dangers of tobacco*, Geneva, Switzerland: WHO.

Part III

DEBATES AND CONTROVERSIES

9

SUSTAINABILITY, FOOD AND CHILDBIRTH

Lorna Davies

We used to know how to make food that was healthy and natural, that was good for people, families and the environment. And we used to know how to help women birth. We must not allow those skills to be undervalued.

(Katz Rothman 2013: 22)

Introduction

The broad aim of this chapter is to stimulate thought and discussion around the significance of food and nutrition during the childbearing period in relation to the concept of sustainability.[1] This is a vast and complex area of focus that embraces issues at both local and global levels. It unearths a range of problems that may be difficult or even impossible to solve. Consequently, the discussion may create a series of both personal and professional challenges and leave us perhaps with more questions than answers. Nonetheless, it is important that we begin to engage with the issues at stake, as they are increasingly likely to influence our own lives and those of the women and families that we serve in the years ahead.

The chapter will begin with an overview to establish the generic relationship between food and sustainability from environmental, economic and social perspectives and will then proceed to make links with the childbearing period. Although there may be some ideas about applying some of the principles to midwifery practice, this is not the primary purpose of the chapter. The part that we can play as individual practitioners is something that we will need to address after having considered the issues at stake.

Food, health and the planet

Food forms part of our life-support system and is something that we should consistently give thanks for, and yet so frequently take for granted. In an age of convenience and of largely urban living we are often removed from the origins of our food. It is easy, therefore, to forget that our own health is reliant on the health of the food chain, which is dependent upon the health of the planet. The earth is believed to be currently in a state of serious malaise. Devastating occurrences such as mass soil erosion, the depletion of seas and oceans and the loss of biodiversity[2] are currently threatening the ecosystems of the planet (Giddens 2011). As a consequence of this disruption, the world's human food chain can be viewed as rapidly approaching a crisis point (Roberts 2008).

Environmental threats to the world's food supply have resulted in under-nutrition in many parts of the world (Black *et al.* 2008). Food shortages have led to escalation in the price of food grain in low-income countries, particularly since the 2008 global economic crisis (FAO 2012).This is contributing to mass levels of hunger and starvation in many areas of sub-Saharan Africa and Asia. It is estimated that over 900 million people on the planet are subsisting at starvation level (FAO 2012). In contrast to the problems of hunger and under-nutrition, high-income, Western-style countries are dealing with other food-related issues connected to over-nutrition and resulting in health-associated problems such as diabetes and coronary heart disease. Both under- and over-nutrition can be classified as malnutrition, and both result in micronutrient deficiencies (Brownell *et al.* 2005). Many of the problems associated with food production, distribution and end use can be directly linked to our current global ecological predicament (Chopra *et al.* 2002).

Global change and effect

In the course of the last fifty years the demands on the world's resources have been hugely intensified. The world's scientific community, with the exception of a small number of die-hard sceptics, is now persuaded that human-induced climate change is occurring and that weather patterns appear to be noticeably changing, with the effects of drought and adverse weather events taking their toll on world agricultural production (Giddens 2011). International attempts to curb carbon emissions globally have been consistently thwarted, meaning that the greenhouse effect has continued to gain momentum, which does not bode well for the future food supply. The world's population has also increased exponentially in the last fifty years, placing further demands on resources, and in particular on food supplies (Patel 2008). In 1960 the world's human population stood at 3 billion; in 1985 it was just below 5 billion; in 2011 it passed the 7 billion mark. If the current trajectory continues, then the world will have to support between 9 and 10 million people by 2050 (United States Census Bureau 2012). Additionally, life expectancy has increased overall in most countries, which also impacts on resource management (Shaw *et al.* 2005).

The argument for an overpopulated world as the root cause of threat to food security[3] is a convenient one. It would be easy to lay blame at the door of the world's poorest communities, where the birth rate continues to rise at a concerning pace, ostensibly producing more and more mouths to feed. However, in relative terms, resource use including food within poorer countries is considerably less than in high-income countries and the so-called developing economies such as India, Brazil and China. In fact it is estimated that it would take just 25 per cent of the food wasted in Europe each year to eliminate hunger in sub-Saharan Africa (Stuart 2009). Additionally, it is proposed that with good stewardship the earth should be able to produce adequate food for an estimated world population of up to 10 billion by 2050 (Godfray *et al.* 2010). Although such provision would mean measures such as relinquishing a heavy dependence on meat consumption eschewing the current drive for biofuels and dealing with the shameful issue of food waste (Stuart 2009; Foley 2011), this would result in significant changes to our present lifestyle and raises the point that the production of and access to food is currently grounded within a Western-based economic paradigm.

Neoliberalism and the food supply

The current globally focused capitalist economic hegemony is driven by an ideology which relies on success based on continuous economic growth of the free market via privatization, deregulation and decentralization (McGregor 2001). As a result of neoliberalism,[4] choice and consumerism have become a dominating if not the defining value of the postmodern world (Holzer 2006). The effects of choice and consumerism in relation to the broad area of food commodities are far reaching. In the last half century the industrialization of food production has taken us away from homemade and towards mass-produced food products that generate considerable energy requirements in the shape of manufacturing, packaging and transportation. At the end of their life cycle there is additional waste generated that is not always recyclable. This consumer-driven approach to food has a significant impact on our food purchasing and eating habits (Nestle 2002). Additionally, the vested interest of the food corporates in sponsoring health-related fields in order to gain direct contact with 'consumers' such as dieticians, doctors and midwives may compromise the integrity of these health professionals (Lappe 2013).

Working with women in pregnancy

At this point in reading the chapter, the following thought may arise: 'This is clearly important information, but what has this got to do with me as a health professional working with a childbearing population of women?' There are good reasons why it is important to have an overview of the issues at stake, but it is equally significant that we have a specific understanding relating to our own sphere of practice. The remainder of the chapter will endeavour to explore areas of food and sustainability that bear relation to midwifery practice.

The uterine ecosystem

A major component of the role of the midwife is to provide women with sound and contemporaneous information that will support them in providing the best possible uterine 'ecosystem' in which to grow their baby. In the last decade or so we have become increasingly aware of the importance of the uterine environment in relation to lifelong health outcomes, and here much of the focus is on maternal nutrition (Simmons 2011; Palmer *et al.* 2012; Ramakrishnan *et al.* 2012). The idea that we are what we eat is now being seriously challenged by the idea that we are the product of what our mother ate during pregnancy (Davies *et al.* 2013). If our food is contaminated, then so is the ecosystem of a pregnant woman's body and so is the baby growing within her (Steingraber 2003). By developing an understanding of the factors that may impact on this 'ecosystem', midwives may be able to support the woman in minimizing exposure to, or ameliorating the effects of, environmental toxins, for example, which are all too frequently present within the food chain (Mebs 1998).

Preconceptual discussion

In an ideal world much of this discussion would take place with the woman preconceptually, so that plans could be put in place to optimize the uterine environment in order to give the baby the best possible start in life. Yet, ironically, perhaps, this is an area which consistently fails to gather momentum in terms of preventative health measures. Midwives can be viewed as primary stakeholders because the information and support that they are able to offer women during this important period would ensure a healthier level of outcomes in terms of pregnancy, birth and the postnatal period. (See Chapter 14 for further information on preconceptual care.)

Modern food production and health

Many contemporary food production practices are believed to be impacting on the integrity of the uterine environment. Intensive farming methods employed globally have introduced chemical agents, hormonal growth promoters, antibiotics and other drugs into the food chain and the water table (Steingraber 2002). As long ago as the early 1960s, Rachel Carson, in her classic ecology-based text *Silent Spring* outlined the effects of excessive use of herbicides and pesticides on human health (Carson 2002). Her critique fell largely on deaf ears and agribusiness and corporate farming have subsequently continued to expand globally, adding further controversial elements into the mix such as intensive animal husbandry and the development of genetically modified organisms (GMO) – foods which, it is argued, bring with them the potential for health risks.

The situation has been compounded by modern food manufacturing practices such as the greater use of preservatives and other additives in processed foods (Baldwin 2012) or the use of fructose in food manufacturing in the form of corn syrup. This product, which was introduced on a large scale in the 1970s and 1980s is now associated with escalating levels of type 2 diabetes because high levels of non-fruit based fructose is difficult for the body to metabolize, the insulin response, it would seem, not being the same as that for sucrose (Goran, Ulijaszek and Ventura 2012). This may also have contributed to the increasing diagnosis of gestational diabetes and therefore has considerable significance for midwives and other health professionals working with pregnant women.

Pesticides and herbicides

Herbicides, fungicides and fumigants in every class of pesticide have been found to have one element or more which can be classified as an endocrine disruptor[5] either in laboratory animals or in humans (Frazier 2007). This means that they have the potential to impact on the reproductive function in one way or another. Although many of these substances are now banned from use in OECD countries, they are still being used widely in low-resource countries and thus may find their way into the food chain in countries where the substances are banned (Pesticide Action Network 2010). We should also consider those employed by the agricultural and horticultural industries who come into contact with endocrine disruptors in the course of their daily working lives.

In 2012 the Systematic Review of Pesticide Health Effects reviewed studies that were related to the effects of pesticides on human health over the last eight years. One of the areas of specific interest for the reviewers was that of reproductive health and pesticide exposure. The review concluded that there was evidence to suggest that non-organochlorine pesticides may cause serious reproductive outcomes (Sanborn *et al*. 2012). The strongest association would appear to be that between fetal growth outcomes and pesticide exposure. At a time when we are trying to establish more effective ways to identify babies at risk of perinatal mortality, many of whom are said to be growth restricted (Perinatal Institute 2011), it seems anomalous that the discussion around minimizing pesticide exposure is not at the forefront of discussion amongst health professionals and on a one-to-one basis with women preconceptually or in early pregnancy. Fetal growth restriction is only one of the many problems associated with the pesticide family of non-organochlorine and organochlorine agents, organophosphates, carbomates and pyrethroids. Other conditions that may result and may affect the fetus include neurological problems, intellectual challenge, autism spectrum disorder, pervasive developmental disorder and respiratory conditions such as asthma (Crain *et al*.

2008). We should remember that the placenta is a less than adequate filter when it comes to toxic chemicals. Pesticides that have a small molecular format are able to readily transfer from the mother to the baby. Ironically, those of a larger molecular structure are broken down to an extent by enzymatic action initiated by the placenta, but the transformation can render them even more toxic (Steingraber 2003).

A further associated aspect is that pesticides can enter the blood stream and can be passed to the baby via breast milk (Polder *et al.* 2009). This is not to suggest that it would be safer to feed a baby artificial baby milk, which also contains its fair share of toxins and contaminants. However, this fact should be borne in mind and efforts made to minimize the risk by, for example, ensuring that fruit and vegetables are washed thoroughly prior to consumption (Bartle 2010).

It should also be noted that while the impact of individual pesticides may be reasonably well documented, the combined effects of pesticides are not so well established. Because humans sit fairly high up on the food chain the risk of exposure is greater because the toxic effects accumulate at higher trophic levels (Baldwin 2012).

Minimizing exposure to pesticides from food

In order to minimize exposure to toxins from pesticides during pregnancy, there are a number of things that may be advised. The first line of defence in negating the effects may be to avoid pesticide deposits by eating organic food wherever possible. Organic produce has received a less than positive press in the last few years. A systematic review published by Stanford University, which received a considerable amount of media attention, drew the conclusion that there was little benefit to be had from eating organic over 'conventional' produce in terms of nutritional gain (Smith-Spangler *et al.* 2012). This has led to accusations of 'greenwash' over the higher costs of foods that do not contain any nutritional value over that produced by farmers using chemically based pest control methods (Danills 2013). However, the point that may be missed is that when people purchase organics it is not simply a matter of nutritional components. It is also about other factors present in non-organic food and the potential that they have to affect our health and well-being that leads people to use organic foods. We do not currently have the scientific evidence to demonstrate that pesticide exposure is safe for a baby *in utero* in terms of both short- and longer-term outcomes, and therefore it would make sense to proactively avoid them where possible.

Unfortunately, the higher price of organic foods may deter women on a limited budget from buying pesticide-free produce. However, a social movement seems to be gaining momentum, with people using their gardens to grow food in a way that hasn't been seen since the utilitarian days of the Second World War, when austerity demanded such practicality. Cities in the USA, such as Detroit, which have seen mass exodus of population in recent years and subsequent mass dereliction of property, are flourishing with the growth of community-based gardens and related businesses (Connors *et al.* 2011). The idea of the edible garden is an opportunity for people to grow their own organic foods. Small gardens, terraces and balconies are being utilized with the aid of vertical growing systems, and even pot-bound planting.

Transition towns and similar social initiatives[6] are working hard to introduce the idea of communal gardens and orchards, and even edible walkways (Transition Network 2012). A birthing unit in rural New Zealand has in its grounds the community garden for the nearby town, and this ensures that the local community is linked with the birthing community. This may seem a Utopian ideal, but it is exactly this sort of lateral thinking that is needed if we are to change the way in which we view the manner in which we produce and distribute our food.

For those without the means to buy or to grow their organic fruit and vegetables, there are ways of minimizing exposure to pesticides in non-organic produce. The US Environmental Working Group (EWG) analysed pesticide residue-testing data from the US Department of Agriculture and Food and Drug Administration and was able to produce ranking for a range of fruits and vegetables (Environmental Working Group 2012). It claims that it is more conducive of health to have a diet that contains ample amounts of fruit and vegetables even if they are what the EWG refer to as 'conventionally' grown, because the benefits of such a diet outweigh the risks of pesticide exposure. The EWG has developed a shoppers' guide to pesticides in produce that identifies which produce has the highest levels of pesticide residue. This enables shoppers to avoid what the EWG has called 'The Dirty Dozen' –foods that have high levels of pesticide residues. This could be a valuable approach for those who cannot afford organic produce. The guide is available to download or as a free app for Android phones and Apple iPhones. Although it does not specifically refer to women in pregnancy, it could be a useful and tool to which to direct clients.

Pesticide use is not restricted to food, and women may be subjected to risk from pesticides in other areas of their lives, such as in their working environments or even simply by using flea treatments on their pets. The risks imposed on the baby *in utero* make assessment of pesticide exposure critical, and a discussion about this takes place at the booking visit with all pregnant women (Gilden *et al*. 2010)

Genetically modified organisms

Another agricultural practice which may prove to have significance for women and their babies is the production of genetically modified or engineered foods (GMOs). GMOs are foods that have genes from other plants or animals implanted into their genetic codes. The sanctioning and marketing of GM foods varies from country to country. For example, in the USA, a stronghold of genetic modification, there is no legal requirement to label foods as GM produce, whereas in Europe the approach is more cautious, as regulators seem to be more sensitive to public opinion. EU regulations require the clear labelling of food products that contain GMOs (Tiberghien 2007).

From a world hunger perspective, GM foods have been heralded as a sustainable mode of food production that can offer the potential to ease global malnutrition problems by allowing crops to be grown in difficult conditions such as drought or flooding (Azadi and Ho 2010). However, that claim has been challenged and it has been suggested that working towards finding solutions to world hunger that employ social justice in the form of access to food and equity in distribution is a more tenable long-term solution (Godfray *et al*. 2010). Using a techno-industrial solution that reflects a quick-fix approach, when actually the problem in low-resource countries is often not food supply but food distribution (WHO 2013). Additionally, it is argued that if greater attention were paid to reproductive health by improving rights and providing education for girls and women, there would almost certainly be a positive impact on food security and nutrition. When women are able to plan child spacing and family size, they frequently have smaller families, which means having to find less food for the family, and healthier existing children (FAO 2013).

Closer to home, in countries where GMOs have been marketed for the last several decades, there are increasing concerns around the immunogenic effects of GMOs which it is believed may be contributing to dramatic increases in allergies, auto-immune conditions and a range of other chronic diseases, particularly those pertaining to the gastro-intestinal system. They have also been associated with antibiotic (AB) resistance (Union of Concerned Scientists 2013). AB resistance genes are used as markers in the genetic engineering of food, and it is argued that this could affect the efficacy of antibiotics because enzymes produced by resistant genes can break down antibiotics and resistance could be transferred to diseased organs, making it harder to treat them (Keese 2008).

Although these alleged effects may have ramifications for women in pregnancy, there is actually little data on the effect of GMOs on pregnant women and their babies. The exception to this is a recent Canadian study (Aris and Leblanc 2011) that reported that 93 per cent of blood samples taken from pregnant women and 80 per cent from umbilical cords tested positive for the insecticidal protein Cry1 Ab, which is built in to the DNA of some GM crops. The study has been criticized as having a number of methodological and interpretive limitations (FSANZ 2103), but its findings certainly highlight the need for further research. The effects of the presence of the toxin Cry1 Ab are not fully known, but it is believed that it causes damage to the integrity of the gut, which could, in theory, lead to allergies, autism and auto-immune conditions (Aris and Leblanc 2011). There have additionally been a number of laboratory experiments with mice and rats exposed to GMOs where reproductive problems such as infertility or reduced fertility, low birthweight of offspring and uterine and ovarian cancers have been recorded (Bernstein *et al.* 2003; Freese and Schubert 2004). There are currently no long-term studies of the effects of GMOs on humans (European Commission 2010).

An important matter to consider in relation to GM foods is the recognition that genes play only a limited role in the control of the biochemistry of organisms and that the part that epigenetics play may have much more far-reaching significance, because it emphasizes that there is no one-size-fits-all response in the way that our bodies respond to external stimuli at a physiological and pathophysiological level. It may be that the truth lies in the old adage 'we don't know what we don't know'. In light of this, it may be that a conversation around the presence of GM foods is something that we should all consider having with our clients during their pregnancy, if not earlier, where possible.

Food safety

Another threat to the uterine environment comes in the form of food-borne infections. In pregnancy, infections such as listeria and salmonella can cause congenital abnormalities and even fetal death. It is therefore clearly important that pregnant women are made fully aware of the risks of infection from contaminated food and of the means of avoiding them. This generally involves advising the woman to shun a number of identified foods, including soft cheeses, offal, processed meat, eggs (unless thoroughly cooked), chilled prepared food (ready meals) and certain fish and seafoods (see Chapter 14).

It is understood that food-borne infections are on the rise (Centers for Disease Control and Infection (CDC) 2012) and it would seem that that there are a number of reasons for this that are related to commercial food preparation and storage, including the storage, transportation and mass production of food (Akkerman *et al.* 2010). Only sixty years ago or less, meat, for example, was prepared by the village butcher, who purchased animals from neighbouring farms; the chain was short and local and the operation was small scale, such that little transportation or storage was involved. The same applied to most other fresh foods, such as dairy produce and eggs. Ready meals were introduced only in the 1960s, and chilled versions in the 1980s (Morton 2009). Prior to this, meals would have been produced at home using fresh food items. Nowadays, food production is predominantly carried out on a much larger, centralized scale with factory farming and cattle lots providing an economy of scale which would have been unheard of in our grandparents' days. Much of the food produced is purchased by supermarket chains with centralized depots and this has led to the need for longer periods of time in storage and transportation. This has increased the risk of pathogen multiplication and cross-contamination if levels of cleanliness or stringent temperature controls are not sufficiently adhered to (Vermeir and Verbeke 2006). This is not to say that when the meat business was small scale it was not without outbreaks of infection that could be traced to meat preparation, but the key issue can be considered to hinge around the economy of scale. As a result of operation from centralized sources, contamination at source has the potential to initiate disease in many individuals. A reliance on technology and a move away from manually processed food products such as meat means that many carcasses may be processed on a single piece of equipment during a single shift, and if one carcass is contaminated, then cross-contamination may easily result. In recent decades, as farming has moved towards an industrial model, specialization has occurred. If fewer farms are producing more poultry for the table, for example, and the birds are contaminated, the disease has the potential to be spread across a large proportion of the population (Ashdown 2011). Density of the livestock populations in farming practice has led to concerns about ground water contamination from animal faecal matter, which has the potential to create further spread of food-borne disease (Walls 2004). Finally, many factory-farmed or intensively reared animals are now treated prophylactically with antibiotics. It is believed that overuse of this practice may have led to microbial adaptation and there is concern that antibiotic resistance has become another cause of increasing pathogenesis in food production (Stein 2011),

Whose interests are represented?

It would seem that when it comes to food, nutrition and diet during pregnancy, questions need to be addressed such as what constitutes a healthy diet in pregnancy, who decrees what this should look like and whether the interests of those who decide are always objective. Some critics argue that such decisions are largely left to the mercy of the food industry, and perhaps the pharmaceutical industry, both of which could be viewed as being less than objective. The meat and dairy industries in particular have been exposed as having huge influence on US food policy and advice (Nestle 2009). The 'food pyramid' which for decades was used as the benchmark for good dietary intake was largely the product of the meat and dairy marketing boards in the USA. Notwithstanding, this model went on to inform dietetic practice universally, and without critique, for many years (Nestle 2002). On a similar theme, there is currently a concern about the increasing global drive for greater cattle numbers for both meat and dairy production. It is estimated that it takes between 16,000 and 100,000 litres of water to produce a kilogram of beef (Jane Goodall Institute 2008). The idea of encouraging a national meat-free day each week has been mooted in several countries, including the USA (Goodlife 2013). This small act could assist in reducing the amount of resources used and of methane produced – a notorious greenhouse gas. It would also provide a relatively painless way for women to cut down on their meat consumption during pregnancy and so reduce the amount of antibiotic and growth hormone that they would be vicariously providing to their baby.

A brief content analysis of much of the literature that is utilized for women during pregnancy reveals a huge input from the food industry, and it is critical that we keep a close watch on what materials we are presenting to women and perhaps consider the development of independent information resources so as to enable women to make informed decisions about what to eat during pregnancy, without fear of manipulation or bias. It may be that a greater level of activism as well as of awareness is required.

Birth and food as social movements

There is an analogous relationship between birth and food which may provide a compelling case for stepping up levels of sociopolitical awareness in both areas. In 2002, Michel Odent produced a book called *The Farmer and the Obstetrician* in which he drew on the analogy of intensive farming practices to draw parallels with what he described as the process of 'industrialized birth'. Odent suggested that by moving away from small, traditional farms and home-produced foodstuffs to corporate farms and agribusiness, we have alienated ourselves from our natural environment and compromised our whole ecosystem. Likewise, by allowing the transfer of childbirth from its traditional setting within the community to a medical processing system within healthcare institutions, we have relinquished the ownership of our birthing autonomy. Odent goes on to argue that either the former or the latter effect could place humanity at risk in the long run.

There is a rapidly developing sustainable food movement which has gained considerable momentum in the past decade (Nestle 2009; Katz-Rothman 2013). The rise of what is broadly referred to as the sustainable food movement came about largely as a result of the questionable ethics of mass industrial-style food production and marketing, as well as the potential effects on health. This movement, which is largely socially driven, advocates a move towards locally based, seasonal food production with less reliance on factory farming of animals; overfishing of the seas and oceans; GM foods, and more reliance on animal welfare and the production of organically grown plant-based foods. The sustainable food movement encourages involvement at a local as well as political levels. By eating sustainably, the individual can play an active part in changing unsustainable food-related practices, which, as we have already considered, are potentially damaging to both our health and our ecological landscape. This involves adopting an ethical approach to what we buy, grow and produce in terms of our food. The philosophy behind sustainable eating rests on encouraging the reduction of environmental damage caused by food production and processing. It is also believed that such an approach to food will tackle some of the associated health concerns in society. The sustainable food movement is a broadly based and eclectic movement that includes numerous organizations, initiatives and groups, including farmers' markets, local food activism and the slow food movement (Pollan 2009).

Birth activism has been evident in many different guises for the past half century or so. The arguments presented by groups representing the interests of both women using maternity services and health professionals working within them have pivoted primarily on the areas of promoting 'natural' or mother-friendly birth; campaigning for birthing environments that respect birth physiology; drawing attention to the problems associated with the medicalization of birth; and championing a woman's right to autonomy and the right to make informed choices about her childbearing experience. Recently the growth of social networking has led to a surge of online birth-related campaigns and groups, and in the last few years a spate of documentary films calling for greater birth autonomy have been released to a global audience. However, in spite of these advances, the data related to birth outcomes shows an ever-increasing trajectory of interventions such as caesarean section and induction of labour.

It has been suggested that both the food and the birth activist movements face tremendous challenges. The worlds of both food and childbirth provide for mass employment and the introduction of more humane approaches, such as producing barn-raised chickens instead of the factory-farmed variety; or by prettifying the delivery rooms in a tertiary hospital, simply reinforce a 'business as usual approach' and in doing so endorse the existing biomedical status quo. Such a move generally would not threaten the system and might even generate employment and revenue, which might justify the changes, however superficial. These types of measures can effectively lull us into a false sense of security by making us feel better about ourselves. However, they do not lead to the sort of major shift that might actually take both food production and childbirth back from corporate boardrooms and replace them into the hands of community, where, it is argued, they belong (Katz-Rothman 2013).

Perhaps the two movements need to be more collaborative and to campaign for safer food sources for women during pregnancy and breastfeeding. The sustainable food movement could provide alternative sources of information for women during pregnancy, to counter the consumerist approach that is currently the primary and, all too frequently, only option. Anecdotally, however, when suggestions around healthier diets in pregnancy have been mooted, the response seems to be characterized by the presentation of a series of stumbling blocks. For example, it is stated that 'organic food is twice the price of other food so women can't afford it', or 'farmers' markets are only for middle-class people who have choices in food buying', or that 'many women have to work through pregnancy and as a result do not have the time to indulge in "slow" food'. However, as a saying of indiscriminate origin states, 'if we are not part of the solution then we may be part of the problem'. There are several things that we ought to consider before we throw the whole matter into the 'too hard basket'.

Approaching the issues with women

During pregnancy, women may be open to accepting information about food and diet in a way that is unprecedented because, perhaps for the first time, the woman is really considering what she eats in relation to longer-term outcomes for her baby. This may be a time in their life when women are possibly more likely to change the types of foods they eat. This time may therefore offer a window of opportunity for midwives, and other healthcare workers who may encounter women in early pregnancy, to have a positive influence on outcomes relating to a specific pregnancy. More far-reaching, however, is the possibility of making a difference to how a woman views food, diet and nutrition, and the ripple effect that this may have on her family and within her community. Surprisingly, this does not require us to become experts in nutrition, simply to ensure that we have a foundation knowledge of the principles and that we are able to convey these in a way that makes the information accessible to women. We could do far worse than use the wisdom of the acclaimed critic Michael Pollan, whose food rules, when broken down into their component parts, identify that we should eat real food, mainly plant based, and not too much of it (Pollan 2009).

Conclusion

The growth and development of an individual from embryo to adulthood is dependent on the integrity of the interaction of genetic and environmental factors, and it would appear that nutrition takes a fairly central, if not the definitive, role in this tableau. It is alarming to contemplate that a child who is born today is likely to have a lower life expectancy than its parents because of the nutritional deficits and interferences of the current industrial approach to food production (Olshansky *et al*. 2005). As health professionals, we have an important part to play because, by virtue of our role, we are fulfilling an important public health function. Sustainability in health is now considered to be an important component of public health, and this is borne out in the burgeoning of academic papers and educational programmes around sustainability literacy in healthcare (Davies *et al*. 2010). We therefore have a professional responsibility to keep abreast of the issues relating to sustainability that may impact on the families that we work with, and this includes food and nutrition. Sadly, there are not the time and the space to address all of the related issues in a chapter of this length. Other areas which might have been included are the effects of environmental toxins on lactation, issues related to weaning, the importance of access to unadulterated water and the pollution of our seas and oceans. Notwithstanding, it is hoped that the chapter has given the reader 'food for thought' around the area of sustainable food and eating in the childbearing period and has offered an opportunity for reflection on food sustainability in practice.

Notes

1 It is appreciated that the term sustainability is a nebulous concept which is defined in many ways. For the purposes of this chapter it will be defined as the capacity to endure.
2 Biodiversity describes the variation of life forms within a given species, ecosystem, or an entire planet. Biodiversity is said to be a measure of the health of ecosystems.
3 The World Food Summit of 1996 defined food security as existing 'when all people at all times have access to sufficient, safe, nutritious food to maintain a healthy and active life'.
4 The term 'neoliberalism' refers broadly to an economic paradigm which is generally based on the classical liberal ideal of the self-regulating market, but it does function in a range of ways in a variety of contexts and to different degrees of intensity (Brown 2006).
5 The International Program on Chemical Safety defines an endocrine disruptor as an exogenous substance that alters the function(s) of the endocrine system and as a result can cause adverse health effects in an intact organism, or its progeny, or (sub)populations (www.who.int/ipcs/en/).
6 A Transition Initiative, which may be a town, village, university etc. is a community-led response which aims to address the pressures of climate change, fossil fuel depletion and economic contraction with a community-resilience approach.

References

Akkerman, R., Farahani, P. and Grunow, M. (2010) Quality, safety and sustainability in food distribution: a review of quantitative operations management approaches and challenges. *OR Spectrum* 32: 863–904.

Aris, A. and Leblanc, S. (2011) Maternal and fetal exposure to pesticides associated to genetically modified foods in Eastern Townships of Quebec, Canada. *Reproductive Toxicology* 31 (4): 528–533.

Ashdown, T. (2011) Poultry processing. In: *Food processing sectors*, Berkowitz, D.E. (ed.) *Encyclopedia of occupational health and safety*. Geneva: International Labor Organization.

Azadi, H. and Ho, P. (2010) Genetically modified and organic crops in developing countries: a review of options for food security. *Biotechnology Advances* 28: 160–168.

Baldwin, C.J. (2012) *Sustainability in the food industry*. Oxford: Wiley Blackwell.

Bartle, C. (2010) Breastfeeding and sustainability: loss, cost, 'choice', damage, disaster, adaptation and evolutionary logic. In: Davies, L., Daellenbach, R., and Kensington, M. (eds) *Sustainability, midwifery and birth*. London: Routledge.

Bernstein, J.A., Bernstein, L., Bucchini, L., Goldman, L.R., Hamilton, R.G. *et al*. (2003) Clinical and laboratory investigation of allergy to genetically modified foods. *Environmental Health Perspectives* 111: 1114–1121.

Black, R.E., Allen, L.H., Bhutta, Z.A., Caulfield, L.E., de Onis, M. *et al.* (2008) Maternal and child undernutrition: global and regional exposures and health consequences. *The Lancet* 371: 243–60. (Online) Available at: www.thelancet.com/journals/lancet/article/PIIS0140-6736(07)61690-0/ abstract [Accessed 22 January 2013].

Brown, W. (2006) American nightmare neoliberalism, neoconservatism, and democratization. *Political Theory* 34: 690–714.

Brownell, K.D., Puhl, R.B., Schwartz, M.B. and Rudd, L.C. (eds) (2005) *Weight bias: nature, consequences, and remedies*. New York: Guilford Press.

Carson, R. (2002) *Silent spring*. New York: Mariner Books [First published by Houghton Mifflin, 1962].

Centers for Disease Control and Infection (2012) *Foodborne illness. Foodborne disease*. (Online) Available at: www.cdc.gov/foodsafety/facts.html [5 January 2013]

Chopra, M., Galbraith, S. and Darnton-Hill, I. (2002) A global response to a global problem: the epidemic of overnutrition. *Bulletin of the World Health Organization*, 80: 952–958.

Connors, L., McInnes, M. and Schmid, M. (2011) *Urban roots*. Santa Monica, CA: Tree Media Productions.

Crain, D., Janssen, S.J. and Edwards, T.M. (2008) Female reproductive disorders: the roles of endocrine-disrupting compounds and developmental timing. *Fertility & Sterility* 90 (4): 911–940.

Danills, S. (2013) Americans still wary of 'greenwashing', including organic labels: Harris Poll. (Online) Available at: www.foodnavigator-usa.com/Markets/Americans-still-wary-of-greenwashing-including-organic-labels-Harris-Poll [Accessed 24 May 2013].

Davies, L., Daellenbach, R. and Kensington, M. (2010) *Sustainability, midwifery and birth*. London: Routledge.

Davies, L., Deery, R. and Katz Rothman, B. (2013) Pregnancy and food. In: Thompson, P. and Kaplan, D. (eds) *Encyclopedia of food and agricultural ethics*. SpringerReference (www.springerreference. com). Berlin Heidelberg: Springer-Verlag. DOI: 10.1007/SpringerReference_334988 2013-01-03 08: 16: 43 UTC.

Environmental Working Group (2012) *EWG's shopping guide to pesticides in produce*. (Online) Available at: www.ewg.org/foodnews/ [Accessed 12 December 2012].

European Commission, Directorate-General for Research (2010) *A decade of EU-funded GMO research*.

FAO (Food and Agriculture Organization of the United Nations) (2012) *The state of food insecurity in the world, 2012 :* Rome: Food and Agriculture Organization Economic and Social Development Department.

FAO (2013) *Food security*. (Online) Available at: www.fao.org/gender/gender-home/gender-programme/gender-food/en/ [Accessed 23 May 2013]

Foley, J. (2011) Can we feed the world and sustain the planet? *Scientific American* 305: 60–65. Published online 18 October 2011, DOI: 10.1038/scientificamerican1111-60.

Frazier, L.M. (2007) Reproductive disorders associated with pesticide exposure. *Journal of Agromedicine*, 12: 27–37.

Freese, W. and Schubert, D. (2004) Safety testing and regulation of genetically engineered foods. *Biotechnology & Genetic Engineering Review* 21: 229–324.

FSANZ (Food Standards Australia New Zealand) (2013) FSANZ response to studies cited as evidence of adverse effects from GM foods (Online) www.foodstandards.govt.nz/consumer /gmfood/safety/ documents/ [Accessed 20 August 2013].

Giddens, A. (2011) *The politics of climate change* (2nd edn) Cambridge: Polity.

Gilden, R.C., Huffling, K. and Sattler, B. (2010) Pesticides and health risks. *Journal of Obstetric, Gynecologic, and Neonatal Nursing* 39: 103–110.

Godfray, H.C.J., Beddington, J.R., Crute, I.R., Haddad, L., Lawrence, D. *et al.* (2010) Food security: the challenge of feeding 9 billion people. *Science* 327 (5967): 812–818.

Goodlife (2013) *Meat Free Mondays*. (Online) Available at: www.meatfreemondays.co.uk/ [Accessed 22 March 2013].

Goran, M.I., Ulijaszek, S.J. and Ventura, E.E. (2012) High fructose corn syrup and diabetes prevalence: a global perspective. *Global Public Health* 8 (1): 55–64.

Holzer, B. (2006) Political consumerism between individual choice and collective action: social movements, role mobilization and signaling. *International Journal of Consumer Studies* 30: 405–415.

Jane Goodall Institute (2008) *Project Blue Roots and Shoots Water Campaign*. (Online) Available at: www.janegoodall.ca/project-blue/FoodProductionandWater.html [Accessed 23 March 2013].

Katz-Rothman, B. (2013) Midwifery skills on expertise and craft. *Essentially MIDIRS* 4: 2.

Keese, P. (2008) Risks from GMOs due to horizontal gene transfer. *Environmental Biosafety Research* 7 (3): 123–14.

Lappe, A. (2013) Force-fed: how corporate sponsorship poisons nation's top group of nutritionists. (Online) Available at: http://grist.org/food/force-fed-how-corporate-sponsorship-poisons-nations-top-group-of-nutritionists/ [Accessed 23 February 2013].

McGregor, S. (2001) Neoliberalism and health care. *International Journal of Consumer Studies* 25: 82–89.

Mebs, D. (1998) Occurrence and sequestration of toxins in food chains. *Toxicon* 36: 1519–1522.

Morton, M. (2009) The shape of food to come. *Gastronomica: The Journal of Food and Culture* 9 (4): 6–7.

Nestle, M. (2002) *Food politics: how the food industry influences nutrition and health*. Berkeley, CA: University of California Press.

Nestle, M. (2009) Reading the food social movement. *World Literature Today*. January–February: 37–39.

Odent, M. (2002) *The farmer and the obstetrician*. London: Free Association Books Limited.

Olshansky, S.J., Passaro, D.J., Herslow, R.C., Layden, J., Carnes, B.A. *et al.* (2005) A potential decline in life expectancy in the United States in the 21st century. *New England Journal of Medicine* 352: 1138–1145.

Palmer, D.J., Metcalfe, J. and Prescott, S.L. (2012) Preventing disease in the 21st century: the importance of maternal and early infant diet and nutrition. *The Journal of Allergy and Clinical Immunology* 130 (3): 733.

Patel, R. (2008) *Stuffed and starved: the hidden battle for the world food system*. New York: Melville House.

Perinatal Institute (2011) *PEER Report – Q2, 2010/11*. (Online) Available at: www.pi.nhs.uk/pnm/maternitydata/Q2_2010-11_Perinatal_KPI_report.pdf [Accessed 12 April 2013].

Pesticide Action Network International (2010) *Communities in peril: global report on health impacts of pesticide use in agriculture*. (Online) Available at: www.pan-international.org/panint/files/PAN-Global-Report.pdf [Accessed 21 April 2013].

Polder, A., Skaare, J.U., Skjerve, E. *et al.* (2009) Levels of chlorinated pesticides and polychlorinated biphenyls in Norwegian breast milk (2002, 2006), and factors that may predict the level of contamination. *Science of the Total Environment*, 407: 4584–4590.

Pollan, M. (2009) *Food rules; an eater's manual*. London: Penguin.

Ramakrishnan, U., Grant, F. and Goldenberg, T. (2012) Effect of women's nutrition before and during early pregnancy on maternal and infant outcomes: a systematic review. *Paediatric and Perinatal Epidemiology* 26, Suppl. s1.

Roberts, P. (2008) *The end of food*. Boston and New York: Houghton Mifflin Co.

Sanborn, M., Bassil, K., Vakil, C., Kerr, K. and Ragan, K. (2012) *2012 systematic review of pesticide health effects*. Toronto: Ontario College of Family Physicians. (Online) Available at: www.ocfp.on.ca/docs/pesticides-paper/2012-systematic-review-of-pesticide.pdf [Accessed 23 January 2013].

Shaw, J.W., William, H. and Vogel, R. (2005) The determinants of life expectancy: an analysis of OECD health data. *Southern Economic Journal* 71 (4): 768–783.

Simmons, R. (2011) Epigenetics and maternal nutrition: nature v. nurture. *The Proceedings of the Nutrition Society*, 70: 73–81.

Smith-Spangler, C., Brandeau, M.L., Hunter, G.E., Bavinger, J.C., Pearson, M. *et al.* (2012) Are organic foods safer or healthier than conventional alternatives? A systematic review. *Annals of Internal Medicine* 157 (5): 348–366.

Stein, R.A. (2011) Antibiotic resistance: a global, interdisciplinary concern. *The American Biology Teacher* 73: 314–321.

Steingraber, S. (2002) *Having faith: an ecologist's journey to motherhood.* New York: The Berkley Publishing Group.

Steingraber, S. (2003) *The organic manifesto of a biologist mother.* (Online) Available at: www.organicvalley.coop/community/moo/mothers-for-organic/page-1/ [Accessed 12 December 2012].

Stuart, T. (2009) *Waste. Uncovering the world's food scandal.* London: Penguin.

Tiberghien, Y. (2007) *The gene revolution.* London: Earthscan.

Transition Network (2012) (Online) Available at: www.transitionnetwork.org [accessed 23 May 2013].

Union of Concerned Scientists (2013) *Risks of genetic engineering.* (Online) Available at: www.ucsusa.org/food_and_agriculture/our-failing-food-system/genetic-engineering/risks-of-genetic-engineering.html [Accessed 22 May 2013].

United States Census Bureau (2012) *US and world population clock.* (Online) Available at www.census.gov/popclock/ [Accessed 17 October 2012].

Vermeir, I. and Verbeke, W. (2006) Sustainable food consumption: exploring the consumer attitude and behavioral intention gap. *Journal of Agricultural and Environmental Ethics* 19: 169–194.

Walls, I. (2004) Microbial food-borne diseases. *Nutrition in Clinical Care* 7 (4): 131–133.

WHO (2013) Food Security (Online). Available at www.who.int/trade/glossary/story028/en/ [Accessed 20 August 2013].

10

BABY-LED FEEDING

The best start to life

Gill Rapley

Introduction

Healthy mammals of any age are equipped to feed themselves. At birth, a term baby is able to find his mother's nipple, attach and feed. Subsequently, his body tells him when he needs to eat and how much of his mother's milk to drink. These are essential survival skills that ensure the continuation of the species; but their existence should not surprise us. Non-human mammalian mothers do not know (in any cognitive sense) that their babies have to be fed, and they have no guides to tell them what or how much food to give. If it were up to the parent to *think* about what they should do, the baby's chances would be poor. Instead, mammalian mothers follow what their instincts and their hormones tell them – to keep their young close and let them nuzzle. The baby takes care of the rest.

Human babies are born with similar skills, and their parents, too, can take a baby-led approach to feeding their offspring – not just during the first few months of breastfeeding but throughout the introduction of solid foods, and beyond. Provided the foods offered are appropriate and in a suitable form, the baby will know what to eat, when and how much. As he becomes more independent, continuing to follow a baby-led approach ensures that breastfeeding winds down gradually, at a pace to suit the child and his mother, finally ending when it is no longer needed.

This chapter explains what baby-led feeding is and why it makes sense to support parents to implement this type of approach.

Baby-led breastfeeding: from birth onwards

The system that governs breastfeeding is remarkable. At birth, the primary hormone of labour – oxytocin – and the hormone of motherhood – prolactin – combine to bring about the onset of lactation. They also make the mother want to hold her baby close. The baby, meanwhile, is born with the instinct to search for his mother's breast. Held against her abdomen and chest, and attracted by the smell produced by the Montgomery's tubercles surrounding her nipples, he starts to explore her breasts. When he finds a nipple, he instinctively attaches and starts to feed.

The baby is stimulated to keep feeding because it soothes him, and because he recognizes and likes the taste of his mother's milk, having been exposed to similar tastes in the amniotic fluid that surrounded him in the womb. The mother is prompted to allow him to keep feeding because her circulating hormones give her a feeling of calmness and pleasure. As the feed continues, the baby's touch promotes the production of yet more maternal oxytocin and prolactin, strengthening the mother–infant bond and helping to ensure on-going milk production.

This system is secure, provided that the baby is held in way that allows him to feed, and provided that he is not separated from his mother in the first crucial hours after birth. Skin-to-skin contact in a warm, supportive and unhurried environment, and a laid-back maternal position have been shown to encourage and support the instincts of both mother and baby, so that breastfeeding becomes the natural fourth stage of labour (Anderson *et al.* 2007; Colson *et al.* 2008).

In the days and weeks that follow the birth, keeping her baby close and responding to his requests to be held and to feed ensure that the mother's milk production keeps pace with the baby's needs – both on a feed-by-feed basis and over time, as the baby grows. When the baby is supported to feed in the way that he wants, whenever he wants, for as long as he wants, breastfeeding proceeds naturally and the risk that things will go wrong is drastically reduced.

Babies breastfeed; not mothers. As any mother who has tried to persuade her baby to feed when he does not want to will testify, you cannot 'do' breastfeeding to a baby. The whole process is designed to be baby led. A breastfeeding mother is not someone who breastfeeds her baby, she is someone who makes herself available to her baby so that he can breastfeed.

A useful mnemonic, *FEEDS*, encapsulates the features of baby-led breastfeeding (Rapley and Murkett 2012):

Frequent: Breast milk is digested rapidly, so most babies want to feed frequently, both during the day and at night. This can easily mean twelve or more feeds in 24 hours. This is not a design fault – it helps to ensure that the mother stays near, as a source of comfort, warmth and security as well as of food and drink. Artificially soothing the baby with a dummy (pacifier) can mean fewer breastfeeds and reduced milk production.

Effective: Babies need to be held in a way that enables them to tilt their head back, scoop up a good mouthful of breast – with the nipple pointing at an angle towards the soft palate – and feed in a relaxed and rhythmic way, with deep, yawning sucks and audible swallows. To assist him to achieve this easily, the baby's body must be supported in close contact with his mother's, with his head and trunk in alignment, his nose opposite his mother's nipple and his head and arms free to move. A Biological Nurturing™ position (Colson *et al.* 2008), in which the infant lies prone on his mother's gently sloping abdomen, is ideal in the early days, and especially for the first breastfeed. Actions such as holding the baby's head, or trying to insert the breast into his mouth, or the use of an artificial teat or dummy (pacifier) interfere with the consolidation of babies' innate feeding skills, with potentially adverse consequences for both mother and infant.

Exclusive: Breast milk provides perfect and complete nutrition for at least the first six months of life (Butte *et al.* 2002; Kramer and Kakuma 2002). Exclusive breastfeeding ensures that the baby also receives a full complement of growth and protective factors, so maximizing his chances of optimal health and development. The vast majority of mothers can produce plenty of milk for their baby during this time, provided that the baby is allowed to put in the appropriate 'order'. If his appetite is dulled by formula, water, juices, teas or solid foods, diminished milk production may be the result. Exclusive breastfeeding is the key to maintaining flexibility in the balance of supply and demand.

On Demand: Allowing the baby to feed whenever he wants, for as long as he wants (from either or both breasts), ensures that the mother's body is stimulated to produce the amount and type of milk that the baby needs. If her breasts are uncomfortably full, she can offer him a feed before he asks. This flexibility to the needs of both not only ensures nourishment for the baby; it also minimizes the risk of complications such as damaged nipples, engorgement and mastitis for the mother.

Skin to skin: When the baby and his mother are skin to skin, their instincts and hormones are maximized, supporting effective feeding and milk production. Such close contact also enhances the baby's sense of security and allows his mother to learn to interpret his movements and signals, thus facilitating the development of a close bond between them. Skin-to-skin breastfeeding is especially valuable in the early weeks, when lactation is being established and the two halves of the new dyad are getting to know one another.

Unsurprisingly, this approach to feeding is what underpins the World Health Organization and UNICEF's Ten Steps to Successful Breastfeeding (UNICEF, 2012). Steps 4 to 9 deal specifically with the importance of:

- skin contact at birth (Step 4)
- effective breastfeeding (Step 5)
- exclusive breastfeeding (Step 6)
- keeping the baby and mother together, or 'rooming in' (Step 7)
- breastfeeding on demand (Step 8)
- avoiding teats and dummies (Step 9).

Baby-led breastfeeding ensures that the vast majority of mothers will be able to nourish their babies, without discomfort, for as long as they wish. Interfering with this natural process, for example by restricting the baby's free movement at the breast, introducing bottles or attempting to follow a schedule, is what triggers most of the problems that are nowadays all too common. Baby Friendly hospitals worldwide provide their staff with training to implement policies that support baby-led breastfeeding, thereby giving both mother and baby the best start to their feeding relationship.

The first two weeks have been found to be crucial for long-term milk production for mothers whose babies are born early (Jones and Spencer 2007). It seems likely that a focus on responding to the baby's requests and supporting him to become proficient at breastfeeding *for at least the first two weeks* would benefit mothers of term babies, too. Relatives and professionals can do much to support new parents, simply by encouraging them to invest time and effort in getting breastfeeding up and running during this important 'babymoon' phase.

Starting solid food: baby-led weaning

In many countries, the word 'weaning' (or its equivalent) is used to describe the end of breastfeeding – whether this occurs after only one or two breastfeeds, three or four months of breastfeeding or many years. Under this definition, a baby may be weaned 'off' the breast and onto either full formula feeding or a range of foods, depending on his age. In other countries (notably the UK) the word 'weaning' is more often used to refer to the introduction of solid foods, alongside milk feeds, for any baby, whether breast or formula fed.

Although, superficially, these two interpretations appear to be in conflict, a broader definition can comfortably incorporate them both: *Weaning is the gradual process by which a baby's total dependence on breast milk (or a suitable breast milk substitute) is transformed into complete independence of it, nutritionally speaking.* In other words, weaning begins with the first solid food and ends with the last milk feed – a process that can normally be expected to take at least six months, and quite possibly several years. It is in this sense that the term is used in this chapter.

When baby led, weaning is part of a natural continuum with breastfeeding, based on the abilities and instincts of all babies to feed themselves. The baby can be trusted to take the lead not only as breastfeeding ends but also at the very beginning of weaning, when solid foods are first introduced. However, in order to embrace a baby-led approach to weaning, we need to let go of some of our preconceptions about what the introduction of solid foods must entail.

Why baby-led solids?

The World Health Organization (WHO) currently recommends exclusive breastfeeding for the first six months of a baby's life (WHO/UNICEF, 2002), with complementary foods being added gradually from then on. The majority of countries have incorporated this into their own recommendations. As a result, many parents – encouraged by health professionals – circle on their calendar the date when their baby will be 26 weeks old, and make preparations for how they will manage this momentous event, without consulting their baby at all.

Most people would consider it a ludicrous idea to decide the date on which a baby should walk, and to introduce a 'walking programme' on that day. They would also consider it positively cruel to prevent a child from walking before the designated day arrived. Yet we have been happy to take exactly this type of adult-managed approach to introducing solid foods. It seems ironic that we should consider babies competent to know what they need and how to feed themselves when they are newborn – and at their most vulnerable – but incompetent to do these things half a year later. In fact, we need only to look at how babies develop to see that, by six months, they have all the skills they need to begin the transition to solid foods unaided.

The newborn baby relies mainly on smell and feel to locate the breast. Later, he begins to use his hands in a more focused way, to help him access the breast. As his postural control, hand–eye co-ordination and manual dexterity improve, he begins to use his hands and mouth to explore objects within his reach. At six months he can maintain an upright sitting position with minimal support, reach out easily to grasp interesting objects and take them to his mouth. By seven months he can usually chew on them. These are the skills he uses to learn about his environment – but they are also self-feeding skills. Their emergence indicates that the baby is ready to expand his eating experience into the world of solid foods. Unfortunately, their importance has not been widely recognized because of the genuinely held belief – prevalent for the last few generations – that breast milk alone could not be relied on to provide sufficient nourishment beyond the age of four months.

If we believe that the majority of four-month-old babies need foods other than breast milk, the fact that a six-month-old might be able to feed himself is an irrelevance; the challenge is how to get food into this younger baby, who can't. Spoons and purees are the obvious answer, which is why they have come to be seen as an integral part of feeding babies. But now that there is good evidence to support exclusive breastfeeding for six months, we need to take another look at just how much help a baby of this age needs when it comes to eating solid foods. Even a cursory look at the skills that he possesses will show that, in the same way that there is no rationale for 'doing' breastfeeding to a baby, there is nothing to justify 'doing' solid feeding to him, either.

All healthy, able-bodied babies roll over, sit up, crawl and walk when they are developmentally ready to do so, provided that they are given the opportunity. What tends to go unnoticed is quite how long the opportunity has been present, nor exactly how the baby has made use of it in the run-up to the milestone being achieved. The baby of two weeks who is put on the floor 'for a kick' is actually being given the opportunity to walk; only his level of development is holding him back. Every day he uses the opportunities he is given to practise new skills, in different combinations, until the day when he finds that he can stand, lift one foot and take a step. He does not just 'learn' to walk over a few days: he develops the strength, balance and co-ordination to enable him to walk, over many months.

In the same way, baby-led weaning relies on the baby being given an opportunity to practise his developing self-feeding skills, and this can follow a similarly gradual and barely noticeable path – as the following vignettes from the life of baby Jack illustrate.

Scene 1, one week old: Jack is lying in his mother's arms while she eats a meal. He is either breastfeeding or asleep. He is dimly aware of her eating, through the noises she is making. He is able, through her breast milk, to taste some of what she has eaten earlier that day, so he is already, in one sense, sharing her food.

Scene 2, two months old: Jack is being held in a sitting position on his father's lap while his parents eat a salad. Jack looks with interest at his mother, the plates, the colourful food and the cutlery, as well as other objects within his field of view. He responds excitedly when he is spoken to. He is 'joining in' the mealtime, if not the meal.

Scene 3, four months old: Jack is being supported in a sitting position on his father's lap while his parents eat spaghetti Bolognese. He watches as they twirl their spaghetti and lift it to their mouths, and he waves his arms enthusiastically. He reaches out towards his father's plate and gives the pile of pasta and sauce a hefty smack. He has made the acquaintance of his first solid food.

Scene 4, five months old: Jack is being supported in a sitting position on his mother's lap while his parents eat a roast dinner. He watches as she lifts food to her mouth and he tries to grab her hand. She puts some pieces of carrot on the table top in front of him. Jack looks at them, pushes them around, then picks one up, squeezes it and drops it. He brings his hand to his mouth and sucks his fingers. He has experienced a new texture and an interesting taste – but he has not eaten anything.

Scene 5, six months old: Jack is sitting in his high chair, with a rolled-up towel tucked around him for support. His parents are eating a chicken casserole. His mother puts a piece of potato, a broccoli floret and a chicken drumstick on his tray. Jack has a go at all three, doing a lot of squishing, squashing and banging, and occasionally biting off small amounts, which he chews, and which then fall out of his mouth. He experiences several different flavours and textures but does not swallow any measurable quantity of food.

Scene 6, seven months old: Jack is sitting in his high chair, sharing a meal of bread, avocado, cheese and fruit with his parents. By the end of the meal there is noticeably less food in his chair and on the floor than has been the case in the past. His parents have noticed that his stools have become darker and stronger-smelling in recent days, too, and that they contain occasional bits of partly digested food. They know Jack is eating some of what they offer him but they cannot say exactly when he swallowed his first mouthful.

As this sequence illustrates, with a truly baby-led approach, the move to solid foods is not identifiable as a single moment. Even when the opportunity to begin exploring solid food is not provided until the infant is six months old, there is commonly a time gap of several days or weeks between the moment the baby first meets solid food and the moment he first eats it. In this context, the phrase 'starting solids', like much of our other language around weaning, is almost meaningless (Rapley 2011). Parents who choose baby-led weaning do not decide when to 'start' their babies on solid foods, they simply decide when to begin providing the opportunity for their babies to do this themselves.

Allowing a baby to practise skills as soon as he shows readiness to do so is crucial to the optimal development of those skills (Illingworth and Lister 1964; Jindrich 1998). Indeed, children who are not introduced to lumpy foods at a relevant point in their first year can present with feeding problems later in childhood (Northstone *et al.* 2001). It follows that taking a skills-led approach to the introduction of solid foods is likely to maximize a child's eventual proficiency with food. By the same token, helping a baby to become familiar with a wide range of foods, and ensuring that eating is a pleasurable experience from the beginning, will tend to lead to a varied diet and a healthy relationship with food in later life.

As discussed in the early part of this chapter, the natural appetite of a breastfeeding baby can be relied upon to ensure an appropriate intake of food. There is no reason why this mechanism should become faulty when solid foods are introduced – provided that the baby himself is allowed to continue to make his own decisions about how much to eat, how quickly and how often. Thus, baby-led weaning may have implications in the fight against obesity, and there is already some evidence to support this (Townsend and Pitchford 2012).

Baby-led weaning may also have a part to play in preventing food refusal, which has been found to be common among older babies and toddlers (e.g. Young and Drewett 2000). Sharing mealtimes encourages babies to copy others, and to eat what they are eating (Nicklas *et al.* 2001). Babies who are spoon fed are often fed separately from the rest of the family. Even if they share the mealtime, their food is not the same in appearance as that of the other people present. So the opportunity to copy others is limited. In addition, being able to separate the ingredients of, say, a casserole, and to sample them individually, allows babies to identify foods they like or dislike in a way which is not possible when a complex dish is made into a single puree. If a disliked element cannot be isolated, the baby is likely to refuse the whole meal.

To date, we cannot be certain about the health outcomes of taking a baby-led approach to weaning but we cannot escape the fact that BLW (as it is known) has spread rapidly since the phrase was coined in 2002, chiefly by word of mouth among parents and via the internet. Its popularity can be explained by the reports of parents who say that it 'makes sense', prevents mealtime battles and enables them to enjoy feeding their babies (Rapley and Murkett 2008; Brown and Lee 2011). These are the everyday benefits that resonate with parents and encourage them to look beyond the conventional norms of solid feeding.

Baby-led solids: the practicalities

Baby-led weaning is more than just allowing babies to feed themselves when they are ready. It's a concept that revolves around shared mealtimes, where the whole family chooses from food that is nutritious, safe and, as far as possible, free from added salt, sugar, chemicals and other extras unsuitable for babies.

The baby is supported (if necessary) in an upright sitting position, either in a high chair or on an adult's lap, so that he can use his hands and arms freely. He is offered a few pieces at a time of the same food as everyone else (or a selection from it), in a shape and size that he can handle easily and of a consistency that is firm enough to grasp but soft enough to chew.

To start with, this will mean sticks or strips of food but, gradually, he will show that he can manage smaller pieces and a variety of consistencies.

The motivation for a baby to begin exploring solid food appears to be curiosity, not hunger. He therefore needs, when he joins in the mealtime, to be in a frame of mind to explore – not distracted by hunger or the need for a nap. Once at the table, the whole experience will be new and he may need help to focus on the food. For this reason plates and cutlery are often best omitted in the beginning; they will come into their own once the baby is more skilled. Water can be offered with the meal, although most breastfeeding babies will continue to quench their thirst at the breast for several weeks or months after they have started to eat solid foods. The digestive tract of a six-month-old is ready for solid foods, so there is no need to restrict him to one new food at a time. Indeed, the chance to experience a variety of flavours and textures is one of the things that makes this way of learning about solid foods so enjoyable. The exception is any foods which the family history suggests may be linked to allergy.

The principle behind baby-led weaning is a developmental one and this is closely linked to its safety as a feeding method. Allowing the baby to remain in control is the key. The normal sequence of oral skill acquisition in the period between five and seven months of age is as follows (Naylor, 2001):

1   bringing things to the mouth
2   biting and munching
3   chewing
4   purposeful swallowing.

It seems likely that progress through this sequence keeps pace with the development of the gut and the immune system, such that a baby who is not ready to digest solid foods will not be able to get them into his mouth in the first place. Similarly, if he is not able to bite off a piece of food, this suggests that he is not ready to chew. It is therefore important that no one attempt to 'help' the baby by putting pieces of food into his mouth for him.

The fact that the ability to chew develops before the ability to move a bolus of food to the back of the mouth for swallowing means that most early bites of food will fall forward, out of the baby's mouth. This protects his airway until he is mature enough to swallow safely. However, while safety is generally assured if the baby is in an upright position, common-sense rules should nevertheless be observed. Thus, whole nuts should not be offered, while small, round fruits should be stoned, if necessary, and cut in half.

Gagging (or retching) is common in the early stages of baby-led weaning. The gag reflex acts to prevent food from being pushed too far back in the mouth without having been chewed adequately, and it is particularly sensitive between six and eight months (Naylor 2001). As the baby matures, he becomes more adept at chewing and the point at which the reflex is triggered moves farther back in the mouth, so gagging occurs less often. Although gagging can appear alarming to parents, babies are rarely bothered by it and it may be that it has an important protective function during this learning period.

It is likely that, given the opportunity, the majority of babies will start feeding themselves spontaneously, at the time that is right for them (Wright *et al.* 2011). However, for a minority of babies this may happen too late to ensure adequate nutrition. Preterm infants, for instance, or those with developmental delay, may require additional nutrients before they are physically capable of feeding themselves. Usually, vitamin and mineral supplements will suffice, but some paediatricians may recommend that a start be made with pureed food. Provided that the baby is given the opportunity to handle pieces of food once he can sit upright, he will develop the necessary skills in his own time and the need for spoon feeding will gradually fade.

Baby-led weaning will be effortless if the family is already in the habit of eating foods that are suitable for a baby. Pregnancy provides an ideal opportunity for expectant parents to make any necessary adjustments to their diet, such as learning to cook with fresh ingredients and without salt, not only in order to optimize the health of mother and baby during and after the gestation but also so that the whole family will be able to share their meals easily once the baby is ready to join in.

Baby-led weaning: maintaining breastfeeding

We have seen that a baby's innate instincts and abilities are what equip him both to breast-feed and to begin to discover other foods, but it is the interplay of these two activities that makes baby-led weaning the ideal approach for a breastfed baby. In the past, the information given to parents about introducing solid foods commonly included instructions on how to cut out milk feeds and introduce other drinks as solid meals increased. The implied aim was that the changeover should be quick – to be completed, ideally, by the first birthday. Not only was this an unphysiological approach, which recognized neither the on-going importance of breast milk for older babies nor the baby's need to explore and handle food, but it assumed steady progress throughout and made no allowance for variations along the way.

Once solid foods have been introduced, breastfeeding can and should continue to be baby led. Complementary foods are intended to complement breast milk, not replace it. In the early weeks only very small amounts are needed, mainly to supply iron and zinc (Palmer 2011); not sufficient volume or calories to reduce the infant's appetite for milk. Indeed, it is unlikely that the baby's intake of breast milk will start to lessen noticeably until he is at least nine months old, so frequent breastfeeding will continue to be the norm during this time. Even when solid foods do begin to edge out the need for breast milk as a food, many breastfeeding babies continue to have all their drinks at the breast for several more months. Baby-led weaning thus ensures a much greater intake of breast milk over a longer period of time than does a managed approach, which aims to reduce milk feeds from the outset. This may have important implications for blood levels of nutrients such as iron.

The natural progress of the transition from total reliance on breast milk to total reliance on foods other than breast milk is gradual and slow. It can also be far from constant. Allowing the baby to continue to breastfeed whenever he wants, for as long as he wants, enables him to regulate his intake of food and milk on a daily basis, thus ensuring a well-balanced diet throughout. For example, if the baby is unwell or teething or simply 'off' solid foods for no apparent reason, he will naturally want to feed more at the breast. This will stimulate his mother's milk production, ensuring an abundance of easily digestible food and important protective factors. Once he is well again, his increased appetite for solid foods and dimin-ished appetite for breast milk will allow the breasts' output to settle back naturally to its previous level. This flexibility requires no calculations on the part of the mother – it is all under the control of the child.

Sometime after the baby's first birthday, solid foods will begin to take over from breast milk as his main source of nourishment. As the frequency of feeds and the amount of time spent at the breast decline, so milk production is gradually reduced. As this happens, the milk becomes more like colostrum again – packed full of antibodies but low in volume. This means that, although the nutritional role of breast milk may diminish, its relevance to the baby's health is still significant. Breastfeeding will also continue to play a part in his emotional well-being, and benefit his mother's long-term health, for as long as this special relationship exists.

Baby-led weaning: the natural end to breastfeeding

Biologically speaking, human babies are probably designed to breastfeed for six or seven years (Dettwyler 1995). This is the age when the baby's immune system can be said to be fully mature and, coincidentally (or perhaps not), when he begins to lose his 'milk' teeth. Commonly, it continues for at least two years. Provided that the mother is happy to follow her baby's lead, breastfeeding can continue to be baby led throughout this time, so that the last breastfeed happens when the baby is ready.

When the end of breastfeeding is chosen by the baby it can happen suddenly, with him pushing the breast away or proclaiming that he does not need it any more, or it can be a much more gradual process, with the last feed not being recognized as such by the mother, except in retrospect. Sometimes, as with the start of weaning, the end can be difficult to pinpoint, as when a toddler refuses the breast for a few weeks and then decides to resume breastfeeding as if nothing had happened.

Ironically, a baby-led end to breastfeeding does not necessarily mean that the baby is ready for it to cease. In some cases, circumstances arise that make stopping preferable to continuing. One of the most likely scenarios is that the mother is pregnant again. Pregnancy can make breastfeeding physically awkward for the child, because of the 'bump', but it can also alter the taste, quantity or flow of the milk in a way that he does not like.

To some children, the arrival of a new sibling renews their interest in breastfeeding or their need for 'mummy time', so that a period of tandem breast feeding follows naturally from the pregnancy. Others take the birth of a new baby as a sign that they are now 'grown up' and ready to explore more exciting activities. Either response can be encouraged or discouraged, while still allowing the decision to remain the child's. For older children, especially, it is not unusual for the end of breastfeeding to be something that is negotiated between them and their mother. Although not fully 'baby led', such an arrangement is nevertheless based on respect for the child's wishes and a willingness to allow him to share in such an important decision.

Baby-led feeding: the full picture

Baby-led breastfeeding has been around for as long as humans have existed; it has simply fallen out of favour – at least in the western world – in the last few hundred years. Baby-led weaning is probably equally old but has tended to be practised in secret, for fear that the (experienced) mother will be exposed as a lazy or undisciplined woman. The signs are now that a baby-led approach to the continuum of infant feeding is being seen as logical and natural by increasing numbers of parents, and that more and more professionals are willing and able to support it.

Most adults appreciate being able to choose what to eat, how to eat, how often, how much and how quickly. Why should babies not feel the same way, particularly if their instincts and abilities are driving them to want to make these decisions for themselves? Research strongly suggests that denying the very young the opportunity to make feeding choices has the potential to lead to serious consequences; we should be wary of interfering in matters about which babies probably do know best.

References

Anderson, G.C., Moore, E., Hepworth, J. and Bergman, N. (2007) Early skin-to-skin contact for mothers and their healthy newborn infants. *Cochrane Database of Systematic Reviews*, Issue 2. Art. No.: CD003519. DOI: 10.1002/14651858.CD003519.

Brown, A. and Lee, M. (2011) A descriptive study investigating the use and nature of baby-led weaning in a UK sample of mothers, *Maternal & Child Nutrition* 7 (1): 34–47.

Butte, N.F., Lopez-Alarcon, M.G. and Garza, C. (2002) *Nutrient Adequacy of Exclusive Breastfeeding for the Term Infant during the First Six Months of Life*, Geneva: WHO.

Colson, S.D., Meek, J.H. and Hawdon, J.M. (2008) Optimal positions for the release of primitive neonatal reflexes stimulating breastfeeding, *Early Human Development*, 84 (7): 441–449.

Dettwyler, K.A. (1995) A time to wean: the hominid blueprint for the natural age of weaning in modern human populations. In: Stuart-Macadam, P. and Dettwyler, K.A., *Breastfeeding: Biocultural Perspectives*, New York: Walter de Gruyter.

Illingworth, R.S. and Lister, J. (1964) The critical or sensitive period, with special reference to certain feeding problems in infants and children, *Journal of Pediatrics*, 65 (6): 839–848.

Jindrich, S. (1998) *How Do Children Develop?* Online. Available at: www.gdrc.org/kmgmt/learning/child-learn.html (Accessed 30 May 2013).

Jones, E. and Spencer, S.A. (2007) Optimising the provision of human milk for preterm infants, *Archives of Disease in Childhood: Fetal & Neonatal Edition*, 92 (4): F236–F238.

Kramer, M.S. and Kakuma, R. (2002) Optimal duration of exclusive breastfeeding. *The Cochrane Database of Systematic Reviews*, Issue 1. Art. No: CD003517. DOI: 10.1002/14651858.CD003517.

Naylor, A.J. (2001) Infant oral motor development in relation to the duration of exclusive breastfeeding. In: Naylor, A.J. and Morrow, A. (eds) *Developmental Readiness of Normal Full Term Infants to Progress from Exclusive Breastfeeding to the Introduction of Complementary Foods: Reviews of the Relevant Literature Concerning Infant Immunologic, Gastrointestinal, Oral Motor and Maternal Reproductive and Lactational Development*, Washington, D.C.: Wellstart International and the LINKAGES Project Academy for Educational Development.

Nicklas, T.A., Baranowski, T., Baranowski, J.C., Culen, K., Rittenbruy, L. and Olvera, N. (2001) Family and child-care provider influences on preschool children's fruit, juice and vegetable consumption, *Nutrition Reviews*, 59: 224–235.

Northstone, K., Emmett, P., Nethersole, F. and ALSPAC Study Team (2001) The effect of age of introduction to lumpy solids on foods eaten and reported feeding difficulties at 6 and 15 months, *Journal of Human Nutrition and Dietetics*, 14 (1): 43–54.

Palmer, G. (2011) *Complementary Feeding: Nutrition, Culture and Politics*, London: Pinter & Martin.

Rapley, G. (2011) Talking about weaning, *Community Practitioner*, 84 (8): 40–41.

Rapley, G. and Murkett, T. (2008) *Baby-led Weaning: Helping Your Child to Love Good Food*, London: Vermilion.

Rapley, G. and Murkett, T. (2012) *Baby-led Breastfeeding: How to Make Breastfeeding Work with Your Baby's Help*, London: Vermilion.

Townsend, E. and Pitchford, N.J. (2012) Baby knows best? The impact of weaning style on food preferences and body mass index in early childhood in a case-controlled sample. *BMJ Open* 2:1 e000298. DOI: 10.1136/bmjopen-2011-000298.

UNICEF (2012) www.unicef.org/programme/breastfeeding/baby.htm [accessed October 2012].

WHO/UNICEF (2002) *Global Strategy for Infant and Young Child Feeding*, Geneva: WHO.

Wright, C.M., Cameron, K., Tsiaka, M. and Parkinson, K.N. (2011) Is baby-led weaning feasible? When do babies first reach out for and eat finger foods? *Maternal & Child Nutrition*, 7 (1): 27–33.

Young, B. and Drewett, R. (2000) Eating behaviour and its variability in 1-year-old children, *Appetite*, 35: 171–177.

11

NUTRITION FOR LABOUR
AND BIRTH

Penny Champion

In 2002 I was joint editor of a book entitled *Eating and Drinking in Labour* (Champion and McCormick 2002) which brought together much of the research available at that time on this subject. Since then, I have continued to write and speak about the subject. With the increase in both free-standing and 'alongside maternity units' in the UK (NCT 2011: 7), it is probable that women do have more choice now about eating and drinking at the time of birth. There has not been a survey of UK practice since 1991, when Michael found that of the units that had a policy (79.5 per cent), 64.7 per cent allowed drinks only, 31.7 per cent allowed food and drink and 3.6 per cent did not allow any form of oral intake in labour (Michael *et al.* 1991). Powell Kennedy *et al.* (2010) acknowledge that women found that nourishment in labour helped them to feel their birth was normal. Parsons (2001) found that low-risk women were permitted to eat (and drink) as desired in 52 per cent of hospitals in New South Wales, Australia, high-risk women were permitted to eat and drink as desired in only 4 per cent of hospitals. The survey by Hawkins *et al.* (1998) of hospital practice across the United States with regard to oral intake in labour found that 88 per cent of responses permitted clear liquids in latent labour and 82 per cent in active labour, while 8 per cent permitted food intake in the latent phase and only one hospital (out of 740) permitted food in the active phase.

The issue of whether women should have the choice of eating and drinking what they would like to in labour remains a contentious one. The hospital environment where most women give birth is an institution, which in many cases mitigates choice and individualised care. The institution often demands control and homogeneity of care, which means that standards should be maintained, but also means that it is more difficult to facilitate choice. It is against this backdrop that midwives and medical practitioners who care for women in childbirth are working, trying to offer women informed choice and to facilitate 'normal' birth.

This chapter will give you a picture of the issues which surround eating and drinking in labour and will include: an exploration of why we impose limitations on women's oral intake in labour; the physiology relating to labour, birth and appetite; how the interventions that we use can affect the physiology of birth and the adaptation of the newborn; and how we can facilitate evidence-based practice and woman-led eating and drinking around the time of birth.

Why do we restrict the oral intake of women when they are in labour?

Food and drink are culturally important substances. They are associated with pleasure and positive emotions; with sharing and being sociable; and with the ability to sustain and strengthen us. The growing market in supplementary foods such as vitamins demonstrates an increasing public awareness of the value of food. It seems strange, then, that such a significant commodity which sustains life should be restricted during the time of childbearing, a time when both physical and psychological strength are required.

If we look at anthropological work in the field of birth practices, Laderman (1988) notes the importance of considering the 'custom' of restricting eating and drinking in labour within the context of society as a whole. There are many factors which impose upon women's activity in labour, and these include the role of the midwife and medical practitioner, the position of the woman in relation to the team of carers and the relative power of all these people in the childbearing process.

Laderman (1988) highlights the issue of autonomy and how Western women are often divested of their autonomy as they enter the care setting, with midwives and obstetricians taking lead roles. She also considers the effect that maternal morbidity and mortality has on our practice. Whilst it is a laudable aim to try to identify ways to prevent deaths among the childbearing population, this means that we impose universal restrictions which 'sacrifice the comfort of many in order to (possibly) preclude the death of a few' (Laderman 1988: 87). Not only do these kinds of restrictive practices erode the autonomy of women, they also erode the autonomy of midwives and obstetricians trying to provide physiological care.

Broach and Newton (1988) revealed an amazing diversity of practices relating to oral intake in labour. Food was used both as sustenance and as medicine, to ease pain, hasten labour, strengthen contractions and promote relaxation. The foods used varied, but included alcohol, herbal concoctions, raw eggs and tea made from human hair and gunpowder. Historical texts relating to American obstetric practice (DeLee 1904) indicate that food and drink were positively encouraged in order to preserve the woman's strength and keep her hydrated, and this is supported in British midwifery textbooks up to 1980 (Towler and Butler-Manuel 1980).

The 1940s saw the beginning of the use of general anaesthesia (GA) during childbirth. Many women were anaesthetised during the second stage of labour as a routine practice (Broach and Newton 1988). Around this time medical practitioners also began to suspect that the process of labour might have a delaying effect upon gastric emptying, although their research findings present a confusing picture, with different measurement methods used and no firm conclusion being reached (Wilson 1978). These two factors, along with increasing medical interest in the causes of maternal mortality and the increase in institutional birth, prompted the study of gastric aspiration by Mendelson (1946) and Parker (1956).

Mendelson's Syndrome

Mendelson (1946) undertook a huge retrospective study of 44,016 pregnancies of women who attended the New York Lying-in Hospital from 1932 to 1945. The incidence of aspiration of stomach contents was 0.15 per cent (66 women). The women who suffered from aspiration had a slightly higher incidence of prolonged labour (30 hours or more) and the details reveal a spontaneous birth rate of only 44 per cent, a caesarean section rate of 21 per cent and an instrumental delivery rate of 35 per cent. Slightly more than half of the women who aspirated had operative intervention which required longer and greater depth of anaesthesia than those who delivered spontaneously. The birth details state that all the women who aspirated were anaesthetised to some degree during the second stage of labour and the anaesthetic was a mixture of gas, oxygen and ether. Mendelson does not describe the routine practices in the hospital, such as whether all women were anaesthetised for the second stage, if women ate and/or drank in labour and whether the women who attended the hospital could be classified as high risk, as might be suspected if they were attending hospital for birth in 1946.

Of the 66 women who aspirated, Mendelson managed to record the nature of the aspirate for 45 women. Only two died because they suffocated on solid material in the trachea. Three more women managed to cough up obstructive material and the remaining 40 aspirated liquid material and developed aspiration pneumonitis. All these women recovered. It is not known if these women ate or drank during labour.

Despite the imperfections in his work Mendelson's paper went on to have a very significant impact upon current midwifery, obstetric and anaesthetic care. In fact, the impact of his work bears a remarkable resemblance to the changes in practice resulting from the Term Breech Trial (Hogle *et al.* 2003).

In the UK, Parker published a paper in 1956 about the mortality of women in the Birmingham (UK) area from aspiration asphyxia. His mortality rate for aspiration was 1:27,000 births. The women who died are described in detail and would be considered high risk by today's standards. He does not record whether they ate or drank during labour. He noted that where instrumental deliveries were performed at home with the aid of chloroform or ether no aspiration occurred, but of those women who had instrumental delivery in hospital four died of aspiration asphyxia. Parker made some recommendations about preventing anaesthetic-related deaths: skilled, readily available anaesthetists, use of local analgesia where possible and use of cuffed endotracheal tubes. These were taken on board by the medical profession and in 1956 Crawford published a series of articles in the *British Journal of Anaesthesia* about the anaesthetic care of childbearing women and the issue of vomiting. Whilst Crawford suggested that the starving of women might prevent vomiting, he was not keen to introduce this practice, and instead suggested a semi-liquid diet that could be easily aspirated if necessary. Some thirty years later Crawford (1986: 920) commented: 'Is it not intriguing that, in England and Wales, the number of maternal deaths from acid aspiration apparently rose only after the appearance of Parker's 1956 paper led to severe dietary restriction in labour, amounting in most units to almost starvation?' Even more interesting is that Parker's paper made no recommendations about dietary restriction.

What the work of these authors did was to confine the risks of acid aspiration syndrome to the use of general anaesthesia. Even though the restriction in food and fluid intake were applied almost universally, the risk is present only when general anaesthesia is performed.

Since 1952 there has been a triennial review and report of all maternal deaths in England and Wales and this is now overseen by Mothers and Babies: Reducing the risk though audit and confidential enquiries (MBRRACE). The report has been influential in changing practice and has made recommendations which have changed practice with regard to the anaesthetic care of childbearing women.

The specific recommendations are:

- skilled anaesthetic staff available at all times;
- use of cricoid pressure at the time of intubation and the use of cuffed endotracheal tubes;
- antacid therapy in labour;
- reducing the volume of stomach contents;
- skilled post-operative care.

It is assumed that women are not fed whilst they are in labour, as noted in the 2000–2002 report (Lewis 2004: 124): 'The widely adopted policy of limiting oral intake during labour has ensured that relatively few women are anaesthetised with a genuinely full stomach.'

This has not been a specific recommendation since the 1979–81 report (Department of Health 1986), which stated very clearly that no food or fluid should be given in labour to any labouring woman. Since 1991 the number of women who died from gastric acid aspiration in the UK has been no more than one in any of the triennia considered, making the risk of death from acid aspiration 1:2,291,493 maternities in the 2006–8 report (CMACE 2011). The anxieties of anaesthetists are summed up in the following response to a research paper looking at the effect of food intake during labour: 'what is predictable is that; non fasted obstetric patients have a much greater risk of gastric aspiration than the fasted normal population' (Windsor 2009: 784). Windsor also highlights the fact that obstetric patients (his word) have a ten-fold risk of failed intubation when compared to the general population, and this risk is exacerbated by the reduced exposure of trainee anaesthetists to obstetric general anaesthetics.

Another consideration is the increased use of regional anaesthesia for obstetric operations. Using data from the Hospital Episode Statistics (HES), between 1989 and 1990, 8 per cent of women had GA and 17 per cent had regional anaesthesia. Between 2010 and 2011, 2.6 per cent of women had GA and 32.4 per cent had regional anaesthesia. This not only highlights the rise in caesarean section rates, necessitating the need for anaesthesia from 11.3 per cent in 1989–90 to 24.6 per cent in 2008–9, but also the reduction in numbers of women having GA before or during delivery.

The reason why oral intake has been limited, sometimes severely, for women in labour is to prevent them dying from acid aspiration syndrome (Mendelson's Syndrome) (Table 11.1); however, the combination of the very small risk of acid aspiration and very low numbers of general anaesthetics being performed leads us to question the need to routinely restrict oral intake for all labouring women.

What happens when we restrict the oral intake of women who are in labour?

Empty stomach

The idea behind starving women is to ensure that they have an empty stomach, so that they are less likely to vomit or regurgitate gastric contents during obstetric anaesthesia.

Table 11.1 Maternal mortalities resulting from Mendelson's Syndrome 1973–2008

Year	Total number of maternities	Total maternal deaths known to Enquiry	Number of deaths attributed to aspiration of gastric contents
1973–75	1,921,568	390	13
1976–78	1,748,851	325	11
1979–81	1,923,725	268	8
1982–84	1,888,753	209	7
1985–87	2,268,766	223	1
1988–90	2,360,309	238	2
1991–93	2,315,204	228	1
1994–96	2,197,640	268	0
1997–99	2,123,614	242	0
2000–2	1,997,472	261	1
2003–5	2,114,004	295	0
2006–8	2,291,493	261	1

Sources: Department of Health (1986; 1989; 1991; 1994; 1996; 1998); Lewis (2001; 2004; 2007); CEMACE (2011).

Ludka and Roberts (1993: 199) stated that 'attempting to keep the stomach empty appears to be an impossible task'. Roberts and Shirley (1976: 611) concluded a study of the gastric contents of labouring women by stating that 'no time interval between the last meal and the onset of labour guaranteed a stomach volume of less than 100mls. There is an increased risk of mortality and morbidity if the gastric contents are of a volume greater than 0.4mls/kg which is about 28mls for a 70kg woman' (Moir and Thorburn1986).

Neutral pH

The other factor of significance in mortality and morbidity is the pH of the gastric contents, the risks being greater if the pH is less than 2.5 (Moir and Thorburn1986)

The major stimulus to acid secretion is ingestion of food. However, acid secretion continues in the absence of food at about 5–10% of the maximum rate. Roberts and Shirley (1976) found that four out of six women whose last meal was more than 20 hours prior to delivery had an aspirate with a pH below 1.8. So, it cannot be assumed that fasting will result in gastric contents with a pH of greater than 2.5. The use of antacids to try to counteract this acidity is common. A combination of H2 receptor antagonists (to reduce acid production) during labour, with the addition of IV Metoclopramide (to induce stomach emptying) and oral sodium citrate (to neutralise any residual stomach contents), should caesarean section become necessary, is thought to be an effective regime to prevent acid aspiration. However, even with this medication and the addition of IV ranitidine a woman (in the 1985–1987 report, Department of Health 1991) was noted to have died following acid aspiration syndrome.

Current NICE (2007: 84) guidelines for intra-partum care state:

Neither H2-receptor antagonists nor antacids should be given routinely to low risk women.

Either H2-receptor antagonists or antacids should be considered for women who receive opioids or who have or develop risk factors that make a general anaesthetic more likely.

Will the woman have enough energy?

Humans store glycogen in the liver and muscles, which has a calorific potential of around 3000kcal. In addition, pregnant women generally accrue body fat. A woman weighing 60kg at the start of pregnancy will carry about 12kg of storage fat, which has an energy potential of 90,000kcals (Hill 1992). With a daily requirement of 2140kcal, an average woman should have enough calories to manage 42 days of fasting! However, the body's response to fasting is not that straightforward.

The actual energy requirement of a woman who is in labour is debatable. Ludka and Roberts (1993) suggest 700–1000kcals per hour. Lewis (1991) and Hazle (1986) both refer to labouring women as marathon runners and suggest that they need adequate oral intake to sustain this energetic event. Odent (1994), Anderson (1998) and McNabb (2002) feel that the uterus, being a smooth muscle, works more efficiently than skeletal muscle and does not make huge energy demands at all. The uterus is also able to utilise fatty acids and ketone bodies readily as an energy source. When a woman is in active physiological labour she tends to become withdrawn from higher cerebral activity and her skeletal muscles are at rest and this minimises her calorific requirement.

Ketone bodies

If a non-pregnant woman is starved, within 48–72 hours glycogen stores which generate glucose are depleted and the body begins to utilise fats in the form of fatty acids. The brain and nerve cells still need glucose to function and this is generated from amino acids released from muscle protein. These stores last for a few days before nervous tissues begin to adapt and utilise ketone bodies, which are formed in the liver from fatty acids. When the level of ketone bodies rises, they spill over into the urine, taking large quantities of sodium and potassium with them, which may decrease the pH of the blood, resulting in dehydration.

In pregnant women the response to fasting appears to be accelerated. Felig *et al.* (1972) found ketone bodies in the blood of non-labouring pregnant women in the third trimester of pregnancy after only 12–18 hours of fasting.

Something which we see quite commonly in labour is the presence of ketones in the urine. In the pathological paradigm we associate urinary ketones with the keto-acidotic state of insulin-dependent diabetes, where the lack of insulin causes the body to burn fat, the by-product of which is ketones. This is most certainly a pathological condition for a non-pregnant diabetic person. There has been interest in a therapeutic diet that induces ketosis and can help in the control of epilepsy (Kossoff *et al.* 2011), but which has also been advocated for effective weight loss by Taubes (2011). The diet includes proteins, fats and vegetables/fruit but no carbohydrate, which forces the body to use its own fat reserves for energy. The ketotic state created by this 'diet' is not sustainable for the long term, but does not appear to be harmful for short-term weight loss.

Pregnant women are known to convert up to 90 per cent of glucose to fat during pregnancy and this becomes the fuel for use during labour and breast-feeding (Anderson 1998). Ketosis is a sign that this fuel is being utilised. We know that rising oxytocin levels during labour will cause the maternal and fetal blood glucose to be low; the maternal body responds by breaking down the adipose tissue to release fatty acids and glycerol. One of the byproducts of this process is the formation of ketone bodies. The placenta is known to be permeable to ketones. The fetus is able to utilise the increasing concentrations of ketones for energy, as is the mother (Anderson 1998).

Ketosis in labour is such a common occurrence that we have to question whether it is pathological. In fact, with our knowledge of physiology, we can see that as labour progresses and the maternal blood sugar level falls, so the levels of fatty acids and ketones will rise, and this is exactly what we see if we observe the ketone concentration in the urine during labour.

Another interesting finding is that increased ketonuria is found when skeletal muscles are not relaxed and adrenaline levels are high. Women who are fearful will have a higher incidence of ketonuria.

There is no doubt that ketonuria concerns us, but our concern may be the result of applying non-pregnant parameters for body chemistry to labouring women. Pregnant women are not in a diabetic keto-acidotic state (generally); they are in a finely balanced physiological state which facilitates both their own and their baby's well-being.

Fluid balance

A normal, healthy pregnant woman who is at full term has an abundance of water – at least 2 litres in her expanded extracellular space. This should be sufficient to sustain her through an unprolonged labour and birth. If fluid intake is restricted, i.e. the woman is prevented from drinking when she wishes to during labour, there is some evidence to suggest that one of the

146

first signs of dehydration is fatigue. Greenleaf *et al.* (1983) showed that a 5 per cent water loss can reduce normal physical work capacity by 20–30 per cent and this has implications for labour and birth. Dumoulin and Foulkes (1984) suggest that severe maternal ketosis together with starvation and dehydration can lead to inefficient uterine action.

Mendelson (1946) suggested substituting oral feeding with parenteral administration (intravenous fluids). Midwives and obstetricians observe the urine of labouring women for ketones and use their presence as an indicator of the need for fluid replacement. The wisdom of doing this is certainly questionable and care needs to be taken when choosing the replacement fluid. Johnson *et al.* (1989) reveal several disadvantages to the use of IV (intravenous) glucose solutions for rehydration and prevention/treatment of ketonuria. The rise in maternal blood glucose is accompanied by a rise in serum insulin and there is a corresponding effect in the fetus. This can lead to hyperinsuleamia and subsequent hypoglyceamia in the newborn.

There are significant implications of drinking too much water in labour. Johansson *et al.* (2002) discuss four case histories where newborn infants and the mother of one of them suffered seizures because they were hyponatraemic (lacking in sodium), secondary to water intoxication caused by excessive oral intake. Johansson suggests that 'if the woman in labour has an apparently high intake of water, the volume should be monitored and restricted if it exceeds 150–200mls/hour'. It appears that the practice of 'encouraging' women to keep themselves well hydrated in labour is considered an intervention by Michel Odent (Davies 2012). He suggests that the production of both oxytocin and vasopressin, which occurs naturally in labour, protects a woman from dehydration, as both of these hormones are anti-diuretic. Johansson *et al.* (2002: 813) point out that this protective mechanism will 'reduce the intrinsic ability of the mother to compensate for an acute water surplus', resulting in water intoxication if a woman drinks excessive amounts. Further work by Scrutton *et al.* (1999: 333) suggests that 'isotonic drinks which have been shown to be rapidly emptied from the stomach and absorbed by the gastro intestinal tract may provide an alternative nutritional strategy in labour'. These types of fluids may also help to reduce water intoxication (Johansson *et al.* 2002: 814).

The 'pregnant stomach'

In order for acid aspiration syndrome to occur, three factors must be present:

- The stomach contents must be of a volume and nature to cause lung damage.
- The stomach contents must reflux or be vomited, in order to reach the pharynx.
- The stomach contents must enter the lungs.

There are certain factors which increase the probability of vomiting in a pregnant woman and these include delayed gastric emptying, which may be exacerbated by narcotic analgesia, emotional strain and vomitable material in the stomach. Work by Scrutton *et al.* (1999) paid particular attention to the volumes vomited by women (N=56) who had eaten a light diet in labour. Women who had eaten were twice as likely to vomit at some point in their labour, although just fewer than 50 per cent of them did so after the administration of intramuscular syntometrine. The volumes vomited were significantly larger than those vomited by women who had water only. Both groups of women vomited volumes which were more than the danger level of 0.4ml/kg, but the pH of the vomit was not measured.

The physiology of pregnancy is such that reflux appears to occur more readily, as evidenced by some 80 per cent of women reporting symptoms of heartburn (Bainbridge *et al.* 1983). This may be because of the rise in intragastric pressure caused by the volume of the pregnant uterus and/or because of the reduced muscle tone at the lower oesophageal sphincter, which may be as a result of the effect of progesterone (Smith and Bogod 1995). Other factors which increase the likelihood of passive regurgitation during anaesthesia are: large volumes of fluid in the stomach with a pH of less than 3, raised intra-abdominal pressure and relaxation of the cricopharyngeal sphincter caused by muscle relaxants.

In summary

- A woman in labour who does not eat cannot be guaranteed to have an empty stomach.
- Fasting does not guarantee stomach contents with a pH of more than 2.5.
- Antacid medication can be used to minimise acid production, neutralise acidic stomach contents and encourage gastric emptying.
- The calorific demand of labour and birth is not known, but a healthy woman has bodily reserves which will sustain her through the process and adaptive mechanisms to provide additional energy for herself and her baby.
- The presence of ketones in the urine does not necessarily indicate a pathological reaction.
- If dehydration is suspected, the replacement fluid should be an isotonic solution.
- Pregnant women have an altered physiology which makes vomiting and regurgitation of gastric contents more likely and which necessitates adjusted anaesthetic technique when using general anaesthesia.

How does the process of birth affect appetite and metabolism?

In a detailed account of the neuro-hormonal changes in maternal appetite around the time of birth McNabb (2002: 46) makes the following key points:

- Pregnancy itself has a significant effect upon maternal appetite and metabolism, so that the baby is provided with a constant level of nutrients. The placenta is permeable to ketone bodies, which provide energy to the baby during maternal fasting. The baby can use ketone bodies effectively in the brain as well as in other tissues.
- The hormone oxytocin regulates appetite, thirst and ingestive behaviours. Oxytocin is responsible for stimulating prolactin production in late pregnancy and early labour. It also decreases maternal appetite and gastrointestinal activity during active labour. The raised prolactin levels in early labour may stimulate maternal appetite at this time. Around two hours before the birth prolactin levels fall and oxytocin levels rise, and this seems to suppress the maternal appetite in active labour.
- The hormonal changes in labour also stimulate a fall in maternal and fetal blood glucose levels.
- Evidence (Ktorza *et al.* 1981; Martin *et al.* 1981; Girard *et al.* 1992; Chen *et al.* 1998) suggests that the ability of the baby to metabolise lipids following birth is stimulated by transplacental supplies of ketones and inhibited by elevated concentrations of glucose.

All these factors indicate that the physiology of a healthy pregnant woman and her baby are finely balanced to facilitate the transition from intra-uterine to extra-uterine life. This knowl-

148

edge also supports the view that, as midwives and obstetricians caring for women who are in labour, the only way that we are going to know whether it appropriate to offer food and fluid to women is to ask them.

What does the evidence we have say about oral intake in labour?

There is only one piece of recent primary research about oral intake in labour, by O'Sullivan *et al.* (2009: 5), which concluded: 'We found that eating during labour did not influence neonatal or obstetric outcomes, including the rates of spontaneous and operative delivery and the duration of labour.'

This trial was unable to show evidence of harm, as it was not powered to do so, given the low prevalence of aspiration, and this question of harm is unlikely to be answered in clinical trials because of the extremely low incidence of acid pulmonary aspiration. The greatest evidence for safety is probably related to the lack of aspiration-related morbidity in recent years, in spite of an increasing trend to feeding in labour over the past decades. Aspiration pneumonitis/pneumonia is significantly associated with intubation and ventilation. In modern obstetric practice it is the use of regional anaesthesia, thereby avoiding intubation, rather than fasting regimens that is likely to have reduced mortality from aspiration.

There has been one relevant Cochrane review which looked at five randomised and quasi-randomised controlled trials comparing freedom and restriction to eat and drink in labour (Singata *et al.* (2010: 2), which concluded: 'Since the evidence shows no benefits or harms, there is no justification for the restriction of fluids and food in labour for women at low risk of complications. No studies looked specifically at women at increased risk of complications; hence there is no evidence to support restrictions in this group of women.'

The literature review from King *et al.* (2011) supports this conclusion, using the professional responsibility to use evidence-based practice to strengthen the argument. 'For over 15 years, the evidence has indicated that it is acceptable for women who have low risk pregnancies and who are not at increased risk of requiring a caesarean section to partake of oral nutrition in labour . . . all health care practitioners have the responsibility to ensure that their practice is current by being aware of recent and reliable evidence.'

The current context of care, as highlighted by O'Sullivan *et al.* (2009), is very different from that in Mendelson's time. The skills of anaesthetists are finely honed to meet the needs of childbearing women, and the increased use of regional anaesthesia has minimised the risk of acid aspiration syndrome. There are always going to be obstetric circumstances when women who would have been considered low risk need urgent delivery which requires general anaesthesia, such as ante partum haemorrhage and cord prolapse. For these circumstances it is essential that the anaesthetic staff are informed as soon as possible about the circumstances and have the skills to manage potentially difficult airway intubation at speed (Sia *et al.* 2010).

How can we use the knowledge and evidence we have to the benefit of women in labour?

Recent literature reviews on this subject by King *et al.* (2011) and Sharts-Hopko (2010) call for multidisciplinary teams to revise policies which are restrictive in terms of oral intake for low-risk women. Sharts-Hopko (2010) mentions the WHO recommendation that healthcare providers should not interfere in women's eating and drinking during labour when no risk factors are present.

From the knowledge and evidence that we have, it would seem appropriate to have a guideline for practice which included the following:

- Women who are deemed low risk should be able to eat and drink *as they wish* during the course of labour.
- Care should be taken to inform women that isotonic drinks may be more beneficial than water if dehydration is suspected.
- If a decision has been made to transfer to theatre for any operative procedure, then the woman should be kept nil by mouth
- A record should be kept of the nature and volume of food/fluid consumed and if an anaesthetist becomes involved in the woman's care, she/he should be informed of this intake.
- The following cases may be assessed to have an increased chance of requiring an operative intervention and general anaesthesia and should be advised to refrain from eating food during labour:

  - Women with a BMI of >40 at booking (refer these women for anaesthetic review antenatally because they are at greater risk of failed intubation and aspiration, Roofthooft 2009)
  - Multiple pregnancy
  - Breech
  - Oxytocin augmentation
  - Pathological cardiotacograph
  - Significant meconium staining of liquor
  - Opiate usage
  - Known intrauterine growth restriction
  - Vaginal birth after caesarean section
  - Pregnancy Induced Hypertension
  - Known placenta praevia
  - Known anaesthetic problem (the woman should be identified and seen antenatally by the anaesthetist, Tambe and Charlton 2012: 214).

- For the above cases 6-hourly oral ranitidine 150mg should be considered.
- Documentation of the discussion between the woman and the midwife regarding dietary restriction and the need for prophylactic antacids.

Conclusion

Eating and drinking in labour is a symbolic issue in midwifery care because it is a way of normalising the care of childbearing women. As practitioners in maternity care, our common goal is to offer women choice, using appropriate evidence, and to achieve the best outcomes. We can do this only by working together, with women, recognising each other's skills and acknowledging each other as equal partners in care.

It is vital to use a woman-centred approach when developing guidelines such as those for nutrition in labour. Our experiences of the births we attend have very different meanings to us than they do to the women involved. If we do not involve women in the development of guidelines and in decision making, we create policies that have unknown implications.

The work of Mendelson (1946) which prompted the creation of restrictive policies and much of the work that supports them was undertaken using a quantitative, positivistic approach. Such an approach produces reliable information but often takes no account of the feelings and views of the subjects involved. It is important to use a more humanistic approach as well, in order to illuminate the experience of the women who are subject to the guidelines.

Having an awareness of the physiology of appetite during childbirth helps us to consider the implications of our restrictions or, indeed, our interventions upon the transition to extra-uterine life. It should also humble us, because our lack of understanding of such complex processes often leads us to make some very inappropriate interventions.

The answer to the question whether women who are in labour should eat and drink must be considered on an individual basis, using the evidence we have, but with an overriding emphasis on what the woman herself feels is the right thing for her.

References

Anderson, T. (1998) Is ketosis in labour pathological? *Practising Midwife* 1 (9): 22–6.

Bainbridge, E.T., Temple, J.G. and Nicholas, S.P., (1983) Symptomatic gastro-esophageal reflux in pregnancy: a comparative study of white Europeans and Asians in Birmingham. *British Journal of Clinical Practice* 37: 53–7.

Broach, J. and Newton, N. (1988) Food and beverages in labor. Part 1: Cross cultural and historical practices. *Birth* 15 (2): 81–5.

Champion, P. and McCormick, C. (2002) *Eating and Drinking in Labour*. Oxford: Books for Midwives.

Chen, D.C., Nommsen-Rivers, L., Dewey, K.G. and Lonnerdal, B. (1998) Stress during labour and delivery and early lactation performance. *American Journal of Clinical Nutrition* 68: 335–44.

CMACE (Centre for Maternal and Child Enquiries) (2011) *Saving Mothers' Lives: reviewing maternal deaths to make motherhood safer: 2006–08*. The Eighth Report on Confidential Enquiries into Maternal Deaths in the United Kingdom. BJOG 2011; 118 (Suppl. 1): 1–203.

Crawford, J.S. (1956) Some aspects of obstetric anaesthesia. *British Journal of Anaesthesia* 28 (146–54): 201–7.

Crawford, J.S. (1986) Maternal mortality from Mendelson's syndrome. *Lancet* I (19 April): 587.

Davies, L. (2012) Sitting next to Nellie: bladder care. *Essentially Midirs* 3 (3): 38–42.

DeLee, J.B. (1904) *Notes on Obstetrics*. Chicago: Kenfield, pp. 104–5.

Department of Health (1975) *Report on Confidential Enquiries into Maternal Deaths in England and Wales, 1970–72*, ed. H. Arthure *et al*. London: HMSO.

Department of Health (1979) *Report on Confidential Enquiries into Maternal Deaths in England and Wales, 1973–75*, ed. J.S. Tomkinson *et al*. London: HMSO.

Department of Health (1982) *Report on Confidential Enquiries into Maternal Deaths in England and Wales, 1976–79*, ed. J.S. Tomkinson *et al*. London: HMSO.

Department of Health (1986) *Report on Confidential Enquiries into Maternal Deaths in England and Wales, 1979–81*, ed. A. Turnball *et al*. London: HMSO.

Department of Health (1989) *Report on Confidential Enquiries into Maternal Deaths in England and Wales, 1982–84*, ed. A. Turnball *et al*. London: HMSO.

Department of Health (1991) *Report on Confidential Enquiries into Maternal Deaths in the United Kingdom, 1985–87*, ed. J.S. Tomkinson *et al*. London: HMSO.

Department of Health (1994) *Report on Confidential Enquiries into Maternal Deaths in England and Wales, 1988–90*, ed. J. Drife and G. Lewis. London: HMSO.

Department of Health (1996) *Report on Confidential Enquiries into Maternal Deaths in the United Kingdom, 1991–93*, ed. B.M. Hibbard *et al*. London: HMSO.

Department of Health (1998) *Report on Confidential Enquiries into Maternal Deaths in England and Wales, 1994–96*, ed. G. Lewis *et al.* London: HMSO.

Dumoulin, J. and Foulkes, J. (1984) Ketonuria during labour (commentary). *British Journal of Obstetrics and Gynaecology* 91: 97–8.

Felig, P., Kim, Y., Lynch, V. and Hendler, R. (1972) Amino acid metabolism during starvation and pregnancy. *Journal of Clinical Investigation* 51, 1195–202.

Girard, J., Ferre, P., Pegorier, J.P. and Duee, P.H. (1992) Adaptations of glucose and fatty acid metabolism during perinatal period and suckling-weaning transition. *Physiological Reviews* 72 (2): 507–62.

Greenleaf, J.E., Brock, P.J., Keil, L.C. and Morse, J.T. (1983) Drinking and water balance during exercise and heat acclimation. *Journal of Applied Physiology: Respiratory, Environmental and Exercise Physiology* 54: 414–19.

Hawkins, J.L., Gibbs, C.P., Martin-Salvaj, G., Orleans, M. and Beaty, B. (1998) Oral intake policies on labor and delivery: a national survey. *Journal of Clinical Anesthesia*, 10: 449–51.

Hazle, N.R. (1986) Hydration in labour: is routine intravenous hydration necessary? *Journal of Nurse Midwifery* 31: 171.

Hill, G.L. (1992) *Disorders of Nutrition and Metabolism in Clinical Surgery*, Part 1. London: Churchill Livingstone: pp. 7–8.

Hogle, K.L., Kilburn, L., Hewson, S., Gafni, A., Wall, R. and Hannah, M.E. (2003) Impact of the international term breech trial on clinical practice and concerns: a survey of centre collaborators. *Journal of Obstetrics and Gynecology* 25 (1): 14–16.

Hospital Episode Statistics, www.hesonline.nhs.uk.

Johansson, S., Lindow, S., Kapadia, H. and Norman, M. (2002) Perinatal water intoxication due to excessive oral intake during labour. *Acta Paediatrica* 91: 811–14.

Johnson, C. *et al.* (1989) Nutrition and hydration in labour. In: Chalmers, I. *et al.* (eds) *Effective Care in Pregnancy and Childbirth*. Oxford: Oxford University Press, pp. 827–32.

King, R., Glover, P., Byrt, K. and Porter-Nocella, L. (2011) Oral nutrition in labour: 'Whose choice is it anyway?' A review of the literature. *Midwifery* 27 ; 674–86.

Kossoff, E., Freeman, J., Millicent, R.D., Kelly, T. and Freeman, J.B. (2011) *Ketogenic Diets. A Treatment for children and others with epilepsy.* 5th edn. New York: Demos Health.

Ktorza, A., Girard, J., Kinebanyan, M.F. and Picon, L. (1981) Hyperglycaemia induced by glucose infusion in unrestrained pregnant rat during last three days of gestation: metabolic and hormonal changes in the mother and the fetus. *Diabetologia* 21: 569–74.

Laderman, C. (1988) Cross-cultural perspectives on birth practices. *Birth* 15 (2): 86–7.

Lewis, G. (ed.) (2001) *Why Mothers Die: 1997–99*. The Fifth Report on Confidential Enquiries into Maternal Deaths in the United Kingdom. London: RCOG.

Lewis, G. (ed.) (2004) *The Confidential Enquiry into Maternal and Child Health (CEMACH). Why Mothers Die – 2000–2002*. The Sixth Report on Confidential Enquiries into Maternal Deaths in the United Kingdom. London: RCOG.

Lewis, G. (ed.) (2007) *The Confidential Enquiry into Maternal and Child Health (CEMACH). Saving Mothers' Lives: reviewing maternal deaths to make motherhood safer – 2003–2005*. The Seventh Report on Confidential Enquiries into Maternal Deaths in the United Kingdom. London: CEMACH.

Lewis, P. (1991) Food for thought: should women fast or feed during labour? *Modern Midwife* July/August: 14–17.

Ludka, L.M. and Roberts, C.C. (1993) Eating and drinking in labor. *Journal of Nurse-Midwifery* 38 (4): 199–207.

Martin, A.T., Benito, C.M. and Medina, J.M. (1981) Regulation of glycogenolysis in the liver of the newborn rat in vivo, inhibitory effect of glucose. *Biochemistry Biophysics Acta* 672: 262–7.

McNabb, M. (2002) Changes in maternal food appetite and metabolism in labour and the shift from fetal to neonatal metabolism. In: Champion, P. and McCormick, C. (eds) *Eating and Drinking in Labour*. Oxford: Books for Midwives Press, pp. 46–110.

Mendelson, C.L. (1946) The aspiration of stomach contents into the lungs during obstetric anaesthesia. *American Journal of Obstetrics and Gynecology* 52: 191–205.

Michael, S., Reilly, C.S. and Caunt, J.A. (1991) Policies for oral intake during labour. A survey of maternity units in England and Wales. *Anaesthesia* 46: 1071–3.

Moir, D. and Thornburn, J. (1986) *Obstetric Anaesthesia and Analgesia*. London: Balliere Tindall.

NCT (2011) *Policy Briefing MS2/MN Midwife-led Units, Community Maternity Units and Birth Centres*. (Online) Available at: www.nct.org.uk/sites/default/files/related_documents/Midwife-led%20 units%2C%20community%20midwifery%20units%20and%20birth%20centres.pdf [Accessed 24 May 2013].

NICE (2007) *Intrapartum Care Clinical Guideline September 2007*. London: RCOG Press, P84.

Odent, M. (1994) Labouring women are not marathon runners. *Midwifery Today* 31: 23–51.

O'Sullivan, G., Liu, B., Hart, D., Seed, P. and Shennan, A. (2009) Effect of food intake during labour on obstetric outcome: a randomized control trial. *British Medical Journal* 338: 784.

Parker, R.B. (1956) Maternal death from aspiration asphyxia. *British Medical Journal* 7 July: 16–19.

Parsons, M. (2001) Policy or tradition: oral intake in labour. *The Australian Journal of Midwifery* 14 (3): 6–12.

Powell Kennedy, H., Grant, J., Walton, C., Shaw-Battista, J. and Sandall, J. (2010) Normalizing birth in England: a qualitative study. *Journal of Midwifery and Women's Health* 55 (3): 262–9.

Roberts, R.B. and Shirley, M.A. (1976) The obstetrician role in reducing the risk of aspiration pneumonitis with particular reference to the use of oral antacids. *American Journal of Obstetrics and Gynecology* 124: 611–17.

Roofthooft, E. (2009) Anesthesia for the morbidly obese parturient. *Current Opinion in Anaesthesiology* 22 (3): 341–6.

Scrutton, M.J.L., Metcalfe, G.A., Lowy, C., Seed, P.T. and O'Sullivan, G. (1999) Eating in labour. *Anaesthesia* 54 329–34.

Sharts-Hopko, N.C. (2010) Oral intake during labor: a review of the evidence. *The American Journal of Maternal and Child Nursing* 35 (4): 197–203.

Sia, A.T.H., Fun, W.L. and Tan, T.U. (2010) The ongoing challenges of regional and general anaesthesia in obstetrics. *Best Practice and Research Clinical Obstetrics and Gynaecology* 24: 303–12.

Singata, M., Tranmer, J. and Gyte, G.M.L. (2010) *Restricting Oral Fluid and Food Intake during Labour*. Cochrane database of Systematic Reviews. Issue 9.

Smith, I.D. and Bogod, D.G. (1995) Feeding in labour. *Balliere's Clinical Anaesthesiology* 9 (4): 735–47.

Tambe, K. and Charlton, J. (2012) Antacid prophylaxis in obstetrics. In: Calvin, J.R. *Audit Recipe Book Raising the Standard*. 3rd edn. London: Royal College of Anaesthetists, p. 214.

Taubes, G. (2011) *Why We Get Fat: and What To Do About It*. New York: Anchor.

Towler, J. and Butler-Manuel, R. (1980) *Modern Obstetrics for Student Midwives*. London: Lloyd-Luke Ltd, p. 317.

Wilson, J. (1978) Gastric emptying in labour: some recent findings and their clinical significance. *Journal of International Medical Research* 6 (Supplement 1): 54–60.

Windsor, D.R. (2009) Effect of food intake during labour on obsteric outcome. A rapid response. *British Medical Journal* 338: b784.

12

CHILDBIRTH IN A FAT-PHOBIC WORLD

Clara Miriam

Women's bodies are wonderful

As a midwife I bear daily witness to the beauty, resilience, creativity and variety of women's bodies. These bodies achieve tremendous physical transformations throughout the menarche, menstrual cycle, menopause and reproductive life. They can grow, birth and feed whole new human beings, and have done so successfully for hundreds of thousands of years, throughout the globe. I am privileged to attend beautiful births where women are amazed at their own strength and power. Frequently, I also bear sad witness to women feeling ashamed of their bodies and themselves. The shame takes many forms, often based around feeling in some way faulty: not visually pleasing enough, not healthy enough, not functional or clever enough to bear and feed their children. Often I see women deeply ashamed about being fat.

It is broadly accepted within the maternity professions that fatter women, and their babies, are more likely to experience a wide range of difficulties leading to morbidity and/or mortality in the antenatal, intrapartum and postnatal periods. Prospective and retrospective studies demonstrate associations between higher Body Mass Index (BMI)[1] and specific complications such as venous thromboembolism, gestational diabetes, hypertensive disorders, shoulder dystocia and birth by caesarian section (CS) (CMACE/RCOG, 2010). At the same time, anecdotal evidence and qualitative research indicate that big-bodied women report negative experiences of maternity care in relation to their body size. I wish to stimulate thought and debate about the apparent associations between fatness and poor maternity outcomes.

I begin with an exploration of anti-fat prejudice. What is it and what are its connections with the medical model of childbirth and social control of women? Having given some socio-cultural context to the medicalized idea of 'obesity', I briefly introduce the current critique of 'obesity science' and go on to take a critical look at national guidelines that influence maternity care, focusing on the issues of maternal mortality and CS rates amongst women with BMIs $\geq 30 \text{kg/m}^2$. I then turn to big-bodied women's experiences of maternity care; stories that reveal their perceptions of the impact of healthcare professionals' (HCPs') attitudes towards women's physical and mental well-being. Finally, I suggest how the power of compassion may be one of the most useful midwifery tools for relieving shame and improving outcomes in this group of women.

Anti-fat prejudice

The word 'fat' is layered with meaning. Adipose tissue, subcutaneous fat and structural fats are fundamental to the healthy human body (Kapit *et al.*, 2000). Fats are essential foods, sources of nutrition and comfort (Pitchford, 2002). Some cultures, such as those of Fiji,

Jamaica, Puerto Rico and Niger, traditionally associated fat with beauty, generosity, social standing and fertility. However, this is changing, as previously fat-positive cultures assimilate thin body norms and fat stigma via westernizing media and corporate activity (Bordo, 2003; Brewis *et al.*, 2011). In contemporary western capitalist societies the word 'fat' is frequently used pejoratively to describe a person's body shape and size.[2] Fat people are stereotyped as ugly, unlovable, sexless, lonely, lazy, lacking self-discipline, greedy, dirty, shameful, needy, uncooperative, unhappy, unhealthy, diseased, irresponsible and, increasingly, a burden on society (Crandall, 1994; Murray, 2008; Puhl and Heuer, 2009; LeBesco, 2010; Whitley and Kite, 2010; Brewis *et al.*, 2011; Lupton, 2013). These harmful stereotypes are produced and magnified in profit-driven media and marketing (Bordo, 2003; see also Unnithan-Kumar and Tremayne, 2011; All Party Parliamentary Group on Body Image, 2012). For instance, Fat Activist and writer Charlotte Cooper (2007) highlights the print-media habit of picturing fat people with their heads, faces or eyes excluded; stripping their identity and insinuating guilt and shame. Cooper is part of a counter-discourse, rooted in feminist, body-positive traditions, which seeks to reclaim the word 'fat' as a neutral or positive adjective, and promotes fat pride and fat acceptance (Cooper, 1998; Saguy and Riley, 2005; Murray, 2008).

Fat is indeed a feminist issue, as Susie Orbach proposed in 1978 (Orbach, 2006). Commonly, the midwives and women with whom I work express shame about being fat. This is unsurprising; the patriarchal 'tyranny of slenderness' (Bordo, 2003, p. 22) has been shaping western women's lives through media-fuelled social norms for many decades now (see Unnithan-Kumar and Tremayne, 2011). Increasingly, society's expectations of women and mothers (including of course their own expectations of themselves) are also informed by a medico-moral discourse based around constructs like the 'obesity epidemic', fat as a disease, weight management as the responsible route to health and fatness as something that mothers inflict on their offspring (Keenan and Stapleton, 2010; McNaughton, 2010; Lupton, 2013). Bordo (2003) and other feminists continue to argue that the slenderness ideal and anti-fat prejudice are inextricably entangled with misogyny and the on-going oppression of women.

Birth is also a feminist issue. Leading thinkers in midwifery, anthropology and sociology have suggested that the medical model of childbirth, too, is implicated in the patriarchal control and subjugation of women (Oakley, 1993; Murphy-Lawless, 1998; Fahy, 2008; Davis-Floyd, 2001). Anthropologist Robbie Davis-Floyd (2001, p. S5) coined the term 'the technocratic paradigm' of medicine and childbirth to describe an approach that arises from western, patriarchal, techno-scientific, capitalist culture. The technocratic paradigm stresses mind–body separation, treats the body as a combination of potentially faulty parts and promotes the use of standardized techno-scientific intervention in order to fix and control nature. According to Davis-Floyd (2001), the childbearing female body symbolizes uncontrollable nature and unacceptable uncertainty and risk, ultimately of death.

Bordo (2003) describes how the body–mind duality that originated with philosophers such as Augustine and Descartes conceptualizes the body as alien from self, heavy, disgusting, prison like, appetite driven, faulty and immoral. In contrast, the mind is identified as the locus of self, lightness, beauty, freedom, will, control and spirituality. Bordo (2003, p. 139) believes that food-related psychopathologies such as anorexia and bulimia reflect 'some of the central ills of our culture', such as the deep-rooted disdain for the body and the modern fear of loss of control over our destiny. She also reminds us that within western ideologies of mythology, religion, philosophy and science, 'woman' represents 'body' and 'man' represents 'mind'. Within this dualistic outlook, bodies, women, physical appetites, birth and fatness come to represent a terrible and a feared thing; nature out of control; think 'obesity epidemic!'. In a similar vein, feminist midwifery authors Davis and Walker (2010) assert that the distrust of the childbearing female body is rooted in patriarchal Cartesian dualism. I propose that, within the Cartesian split, both the fat female body and the pregnant or breast-feeding body pose a challenge to patriarchy by taking up physical space and stating female hunger, sexuality and creative power. I ponder whether the technocratic approaches to birth and to fatness share an origin in attempts to control women and all they symbolize – such as nature and the shifting cycles of life and death. If so, the fast-increasing medicalization of fat women in maternity opens a new chapter in this long-standing power struggle.

As I will argue, anti-fat prejudice is a significant force in women's health. For midwives to avoid discriminating against those in our care, to 'treat people as individuals and respect their dignity', as required by our regulating body (NMC, 2008, p. 3), and to avoid iatrogenesis through stigmatization and discrimination, it is necessary to pay attention to anti-fat prejudice (Wray and Deery, 2008; Deery and Wray, 2009). We must understand the influence that it has in the world and reflect on its presence within ourselves, colleagues, women and their communities, as well as within the guidelines and policies that influence midwifery.

Critiquing the 'obesity epidemic' rhetoric

The overwhelming majority of epidemiological studies of the relationship between BMI and life expectancy show either no increase or reduced mortality amongst people in the 'over-weight' category as compared with the 'normal weight' or 'underweight' classes (Farrell *et al.*, 2002; Engeland *et al.*, 2003; Flegal *et al.*, 2007; Orpana *et al.*, 2010). Additionally, when studies include covariates such as cardiorespiratory fitness (CRF) (Wei *et al.*, 1999; Farrell *et al.*, 2002; Lyerly *et al.*, 2009) or healthy lifestyle habits (not smoking, moderate alcohol, exercise, healthy eating) (Matheson *et al.*, 2012), the differences between life expectancy in the 'obese' (BMI≥30kg/m^2) grouping and the other groups is vastly reduced or elimi-nated. Yet these confounding factors are frequently overlooked in the 'obesity' research that informs practice. 'Obesity science' critic Meadows (2012) argues that the mainstream of healthcare research and policy sees fatness through 'obesity goggles', a world-view made of deeply normalized fat-negative attitudes and prejudices – and that this outlook skews the science and how it is reported.

Current conventional maternity discourse follows the broader 'obesity epidemic' rhetoric of the government, national health bodies and the media. The repeated messages are: that an alarming increase in overweight and obesity is causing death and disease, that HCPs must address the risks, and that individuals can and should take responsibility for their health by managing their weight through diet and exercise (Heslehurst *et al.*, 2011; Gardner, 2012). This rhetoric proclaims itself as both scientific *and* 'common sense'. However, there is a growing, multi-disciplinary, critical chorus exposing the harm done to fat people in the name of common sense and questioning the validity of 'obesity science' (Ernsberger and Koletsky, 1999; Gard and Wright, 2005; Evans, 2006; Bacon and Aphramor, 2011; Meadows, 2012).

Critics of the 'obesity epidemic' concept highlight persistent research issues regarding the confusion of causation with correlation and disregard for major potential confounding factors. This leads to spurious conclusions about fatness *causing* ill-health, when all that have been proved are statistical correlations between BMI status and health, without describ-ing whether the one is caused by the other, both result from a shared root-cause or both are related to other factors altogether and the association is complex or even coincidental (Wray and Deery, 2008). Aside from CRF and healthy lifestyle habits, other factors that have been shown to confound the BMI–health relationship include socio-economic status (Muennig *et al.*, 2007; Raphael *et al.*, 2010), dieting/weight cycling (Ernsberger and Koletsky, 1999; Schulz *et al.*, 2004) and stigma.

Anti-fat stigma and body dissatisfaction have been found to correlate with and cause reduced well-being, such as physical and psychological stress, days off work, low self-esteem, depression, body dysmorphia and eating disorders (Muennig *et al.*, 2008; Puhl and Heuer, 2010). Muennig (2008, p. 129) has examined 'stigma-induced psychological stress' as a possible cause of much of the disease commonly attributed to 'obesity'. He challenges the 'adiposity hypothesis': the idea that 'obesity' diseases, such as diabetes, hypertension, heart disease and immune dysfunction, are caused by excess visceral fat secreting pro-inflammatory and pro-thrombotic compounds. In the light of current debate as to whether or not adipose cells have the functionality to secrete these compounds, he proposes a complementary explanation: that the compounds are actually produced by immune cells. He critically reviews four lines of evidence: 'that BMI is predictive of blood-borne stress biomarkers; that stress and obesity correlate with the same diseases; that sub-group body norms leading to weight-related stigma are predictive of mortality and morbidity amongst fat people; and that independent of actual BMI, weight dissatisfaction correlates negatively with health status' (Miriam, 2011, p. 162). Muennig concludes that stress plausibly explains some of the BMI–health association and that social constructs around body-image norms may be contributing to 'obesity' disease. Muennig's findings suggest that experiences of internalized and external stigma are important covariates for valid 'obesity' research. If this is true, within the current climate of anti-fat stigma it is impossible to tease out the effects of obesity independent of this potential confound. Social epidemiologists also propose that stigma, discrimination, low status and resultant chronic physiological stress act as mediators of health inequalities (Marmot and Brunner, 2005).

Critiquing the 'maternal obesity' rhetoric

National 'maternal obesity' discourse

Over the last decade, national reports and guidelines have dramatically increased their focus on maternal obesity (Heslehurst, 2011). The Clinical Negligence Scheme for Trusts (CNST) maternity standards stipulate various biometric and biomedical requirements, including ensuring that obese women are informed of the extra risks they run in childbearing (NHS Litigation Authority, 2012). Recent Centre for Maternal and Child Enquiries and Royal College of Obstetricians and Gynaecologists (CMACE/RCOG) (2010) and National Institute for Clinical Excellence (NICE) (2010) guidelines for care in maternity strive to address deeply concerning findings around death and serious harm occurring more frequently amongst childbearing women with bigger bodies. The available evidence demonstrates *associations* between higher maternal BMI and higher incidence of 'miscarriage, gestational diabetes, pre-eclampsia, venous thromboembolism, induced labour, caesarian section, anaesthetic complications, wound infections . . . stillbirth, congenital anomalies, prematurity, macrosomia and neonatal death' (CMACE/RCOG, 2010, p. 4).

McGlone and Davies (2012, p. 14) describe the CMACE/RCOG, NICE and CNST documents as working from a biomedical and 'absolute risk' perspective. The guidelines cleave to a reductive fat=pathology dogma. They pinpoint maternal BMI as the problem and, in an effort to improve outcomes, endorse individual lifestyle changes to control weight, and standardized medical surveillance to control risk. The guidelines are directive, despite scanty evidence around causal relationships or the benefits versus risks of the interventions. Of the 38 CMACE/RCOG practice points, over two-thirds are based on evidence level 'D – non-analytical studies; e.g. case reports, case series and expert opinion/formal consensus . . . or extrapolated evidence from . . . case control studies' (CMACE/RCOG, 2010, p. 26). Only one practice point (regarding suturing technique for CS) has evidence level A, 'High quality meta-analysis, systematic reviews . . . or randomized controlled trials with a very low risk of bias' (CMACE/RCOG, 2010, p. 26). All bar one of the practice points fit within the technocratic paradigm of childbirth, as described by Davis-Floyd (2001). The instruction that 'Women with BMI ≥40 who are in established labour should receive continuous midwifery care' is a more humanistic approach. However, the rationale provided entirely overlooks the evidence regarding the importance of relational support in labour (Hodnett et al., 2012), stating only an increased need for surveillance and vigilance with regard to pressure area care, labour progress and fetal heart rate.

Maternal mortality rates

A major impetus for the CMACE/RCOG joint guideline was 'Saving Mothers' Lives' (CMACE, 2011), which reported 261 direct and indirect maternal deaths (a rate of 11.39 per 100,000 maternities) in the UK for the triennium 2006–8. Of the 227 mothers who died for whom BMI data was available, we know that 27 per cent had a BMI ≥30kg/m². In 2006–8 the Health Survey for England (NHS Information Centre, 2011) classified 21 per cent of women aged 16–44 as having a BMI ≥30 kg/m². These figures do suggest a possible relationship between elevated BMI and maternal mortality. However, the CMACE report does not offer a breakdown of the overlap between the other potentially significant characteristics of women who died. It is unclear how many of the mothers falling into the 'obese' category also had social care involvement (36 per cent total deaths), had no partner (36 per cent total deaths), were from a non-white ethnic group (31 per cent total deaths), smoked (28 per cent total deaths) or were subject to domestic abuse (12 per cent total deaths). Quite rightly, CMACE (2011) highlights the associations found between increased BMI and maternal mortality, particularly in deaths from venous thromboembolism and cardiac disease. However, the report does not constitute sound evidence that 'overweight' or 'obesity' pose a risk per se.

Another factor that potentially confounds the relationship between BMI and maternal death is fat discrimination within healthcare. Such discrimination can be due to inadequate facilities, equipment or practitioner skills and knowledge, anti-fat attitudes amongst staff, or self-exclusion due to previous experiences of discrimination in healthcare (Puhl and Heuer, 2009, 2010). In a survey of healthcare students in Nottingham using the Fat Phobia Scale (F-scale) and Beliefs about Obese People (BOAP) Scale, Swift and colleagues (2012) found that only 1.4 per cent of students expressed fat-neutral or fat-positive attitudes and 10.5 per cent expressed high levels of fat-phobia. Nyman and colleagues heard big-bodied women's testimonies of humiliating, offensive and dismissive encounters with midwives and doctors, whom they perceived to be 'rude, angry, moody, abrupt and bitter' (Nyman et al., 2010, p. 427). Late antenatal booking correlates positively with high BMI (Sebire et al., 2001), which may be a result of larger women wishing to such avoid negative encounters. Both survey findings (Thompson and Thomas, 2000) and anecdotal evidence identify fat patients' frequent experiences of HCPs attributing unrelated ailments to 'obesity' and 'prescribing' weight-loss as the cure-all, some examples being a 28kg ovarian tumour (McDermott, 2012), hypothyroidism (Benesch-Granberg *et al.*, 2012) and a broken toe (Chastain, 2012). Such medical fat-scapegoating shames, alienates and endangers patients. Gabriel and colleagues' (2006) retrospective investigation of post-mortem examinations of adults (including obstetrics-gynaecology patients) found that those falling into the 'obese' category were 1.65 times more likely than those in other categories to have a missed diagnosis leading directly to death. Such findings underline the urgency of distinguishing between women with high BMI being an *at risk group* in maternity and fatness *causing* maternal death. It could mean the difference between actually making maternity safer for bigger women by addressing the root causes of poor outcomes, or causing even greater harm through misdiagnosis and other iatrogenic consequences of anti-fat discrimination.

Caesarian section rates

CMACE/RCOG (2010) instructs practitioners to advise all 'women of childbearing age with a BMI ≥30 . . . about the risks of obesity during pregnancy and childbirth'. One of the listed risks is an increased chance of CS. CS of course has implications for a raft of maternal and neonatal sequelae also associated with fatness, such as venous thromboembolism, sepsis, artificial feeding and neonatal unit admissions. A meta-analysis of 11 prospective and 22 retrospective cohort studies found fatness to be associated with about a one-and-a-half- to three-fold chance of CS birth (Chu *et al.*, 2007). The findings withstood meta-regression analysis of covariates including study year and design, geographical location, parity and the CS rate amongst women classified as 'normal weight'. The authors note that a possible publication bias against studies without significant results may have resulted in an overestimation of the risks amongst high BMI groups. Yet they conclude that CS rates could be reduced by getting women to lose weight, thereby groundlessly inferring causality from correlation.

Sebire and colleagues (2001) conducted the only UK study included in Chu and colleagues' US-dominated meta-analysis. One of the largest studies, it retrospectively examined maternal BMI and pregnancy outcome for 287,213 singleton pregnancies and found that women with a BMI ≥30kg/m² were approximately twice as likely to have their baby via CS. Logistic regression analyses showed that this relationship was generally independent of a range of confounding factors, namely ethnic group, parity, age, history of hypertension, placental abruption, placenta praevia, gestational diabetes (GDM), pre-existing diabetes (DM), pre-eclampsia and breech presentation. However, the validity of these findings is compromised through omission of confounders that have elsewhere been found to mediate the apparent relationship between fatness and ill-health. As previously discussed, confounding factors such as CRF, healthy lifestyle choices, socio-economic status, history of weight cycling and social stigmatization have notable effects on fatness=disease findings, frequently making the relationship disappear. It is reasonable to speculate that these factors also affect maternity outcomes. Midwives' and obstetricians' attitudes and practice are potentially huge confounders. Some of these are difficult to measure, such as the subtle but powerful impact of a midwife 'sizing up' a woman she is attending and saying to herself 'she's going to be a c-section'. This kind of negative predictive thinking can also compromise research through outcome assessment bias.

Attitudes are particularly important in trials comparing culturally loaded variables such as BMI, where practitioners may be socialized to have a low index of suspicion for pathology and intervention requirements. However, physical interventions are easier to measure than thought processes. In a Canadian cohort study of 11,922 women, Abenhaim and Benjamin

(2011) found that the association between higher BMI and increased rates of CS was markedly attenuated by adjusting for the different labour management that larger women receive. For example, with increasing BMI, oxytocic augmentation and epidural anaesthesia were more common and fewer instrumental deliveries occurred. Higher BMI was also positively correlated with earlier decision for CS. The reason for these interventions is not clear; however, all of these practice decisions, particularly for epidural, are open to the influence of local policies and attitudes and beliefs of practitioners and women about the ability of a big woman to birth safely and autonomously. Early intrapartum epidural anaesthesia is promoted within the technocratic approach to 'management' of women with BMIs $\geq 40 \text{kg/m}^2$. This intervention may play a key role in generating a need for further interventions, due to the epidural's inhibitory impact on the endogenous oxytocin system, mobility and birth mechanics (Tamagawa, 2012).

Whilst the associations between body size and maternity outcomes highlighted by CMACE/ RCOG (2010), CMACE (2011) and NICE (2010) merit careful attention, the guidelines for best practice appear to be based on potentially harmful conclusions about causality that are skewed by the technocratic birth paradigm and by cultural prejudice against fat.

Big-bodied women's experiences of maternity care

Two women with BMIs of over 35kg/m^2 kindly shared their birth stories with me (I have used pseudonyms). I include the examples not because they are novel, but because they give some clues to big-bodied women's perspectives on how maternity care practitioners can dramatically help or hinder their birth processes. With her first birth, Lou had a CS, for labour dystocia after synthetic oxytocin augmentation with her baby in an occipito-posterior (OP) position. She 'found the whole experience of [my first] pregnancy dehumanising and stressful'. After a long second stage of labour, Lou was given the choice of CS or instrumental delivery and felt that CS was 'presented as the easiest and most preferable option'. Afterwards she regretted the surgery (the risks of which she felt were not communicated), she judged that the Syntocinon at 6cm dilatation had prevented her baby from turning effectively and she was distressed by her painful and fearful experiences of augmentation and narcotics within an environment that felt unsafe. Lou acquired a CS wound infection and suffered from postnatal PTSD. Consequently, she planned not to have any more children.

In her first pregnancy Chris felt pressured into having an induction at 42 weeks when, given the choice, she would have opted for planned CS in order to avoid the 'cascade of intervention'. She was told only on arrival at hospital that she could not use the birth pool, due to her BMI. After 10 hours of OP labour, she chose to have an epidural. She felt 'they were thinking this woman can't do it . . . [she's] overweight'.

Both Lou and Chris went on to have positive physiological birth experiences with their second babies: at home and in water. They both describe a process of self-empowerment that prepared them for making their own decisions the second time around. They then managed to build relationships with midwives (NHS and independent) who could give them continuity of care. Some of the midwifery interventions that they valued included:

- antenatal-intrapartum-postnatal continuity;
- community/home-based care;
- debriefing of previous birth trauma;
- individualized, holistic care; 'Never judge a book by its cover'(Chris);

- positive support for their choices regarding interventions;
- reassurance, positivity and trust; 'I felt so happy that I had a midwife who completely trusted me, a woman who had never birthed naturally before, to just go with my body and do my own thing' (Lou);
- help with making positive nutritional changes 'focused on health and feeling good rather than weight' (Lou);
- referral to an osteopath to help with pelvic alignment and pelvic girdle pain;
- use of hydrotherapy and mobility for birth.

'I credit [my midwife] with helping me to heal from my first birth . . . The two experiences were as different as night and day. My first one made me feel like I was being punished for being large. My second helped me to realise that my body is normal and that my size didn't stop it from working exactly the way it needed to!'

(Lou)

These testimonies are anecdotes from a self-selecting sample of two. Nonetheless, their suggestions chime with much of the research into physiological and psycho-social factors that inhibit/promote safe and positive childbearing for women of *all* sizes. Their experiences echo some of those found in the qualitative research into big-bodied women's encounters with maternity care that I will now describe.

Medicalization and surveillance

In a meta-synthesis of six qualitative explorations of fat women's experiences of maternity care Smith and Lavender (2011) found that, as with Chris and Lou, women reported that increased medicalization led to depersonalized care, with the increased surveillance (e.g. ultra-sound scanning) and risk discourse (e.g. risk of macrosomia) sparking elevated anxiety and guilt. Similarly to Chris, other women were informed late on in pregnancy that birthing options such as water-immersion, offered in earlier pregnancy and available to smaller-bodied women, were not available to them, due to their BMI. Participants said that this last-minute 'snatching away' of options elicited feelings of anguish, loss of control and a disengagement from decision-making processes.

Vulnerability in pregnancy

Rather than pregnancy being experienced as a relief from body-size norms, Furber and McGowan's (2011) semi-structured interviews and field notes revealed that anti-fat stigma persisted throughout pregnancy, and that women with BMIs >35kg/m² described maternity care as being provided in ways that stereotyped and increased their body shame and embarrassment at being fat. An exploration of the experiences of mothers who were classified as 'obese' in pregnancy (carried out in 2006–8) found that women were faced either with silence and avoidance of the subject or negative comments and/or assumptions based on their body size, particularly from more senior HCPs, friends and family and the media. This negative attention appeared to intensify postnatally, when scrutiny was extended to include them and their child (Keenan and Stapleton, 2010). In a Swedish phenomenological study, women with BMIs over 30kg/m² reported feeling self-conscious, visually exposed, scrutinized, ignored, disbelieved and humiliated in interactions with midwives and doctors, who were found to be negative/insensitive about their body size (Nyman *et al.*, 2010). The women spoke of shame, guilt and fear in relation to their fatness and the perceived risk of morbidity and mortality for themselves and their babies. They described worrying about being less valued and receiving less adequate care than smaller-sized women. The wish to avoid expressing concerns about offensive or inappropriate care appeared to be compounded by low self-esteem and the fear of conflict leading to further negative attitudes amongst caregivers, resulting in even worse care and increasing risk of harm to their babies (Nyman *et al.*, 2010).

Avoiding the subject

In a qualitative study of midwives and doctors, Heslehurst and colleagues (2007) highlight embarrassment and fear of alienating large women from maternity services as barriers to communication. Frequency of discussions around BMI may have increased since these studies were conducted, as midwives are increasingly directed to discuss 'the risks associated with obesity in pregnancy' (CMACE/RCOG, 2010, p. 6). However, underlying issues around social awkwardness due to wider fat-stigma, wanting to avoid harming the baby through weight loss and the importance of maintaining the midwife–woman connection are likely to have endured. Aversion to being weighed in pregnancy has been reported by women and their midwives (Nyman *et al.*, 2010; Olander *et al.*, 2011). Keenan and Stapleton (2010, p. 374) found that HCPs had avoided talking about 'obesity' or associated risks, but one interviewee stated 'Yeah, I think they probably did [think it], but they never said anything'. Few women were able to broach issues around their body size with HCPs, and some felt frustrated and patronized by professionals' avoidance.

Protection from fat-stigma

Smith and Lavender's (2011) meta-synthesis also found that pregnancy is perceived by some women to be protective against the social pressure to be thin, to increase body-acceptance/positivity, and to draw their attention to health and well-being. Women in Olander and colleagues' (2011) exploration of views around gestational weight gain expressed relief at being able to eat what they wanted and not worry about weight gain until after the birth. Nyman and colleagues (2010) found that some affirming encounters occurred with midwives who were fully present, positive, humorous and celebratory. These encounters relieved the discomfort of the prevalent anti-fat stigma and stimulated feelings of joy, pride, strength and power.

Compassionate relationships: the importance of love

It may seem that, as midwives, we are stuck between a rock and a hard place – damned if we do address body size and damned if we don't. Big-bodied mothers do appear to be suffering more physiological and psychological harm within a society that is deeply uncomfortable with fat and a maternity culture that pathologizes fatness. How do we manage to provide salutary midwifery when we are part of this culture? One way out of the conundrum is through building compassionate relationships of love and trust with women. The fields of neuro-endocrinology and psychology inform our understanding of how attending to the quality of our relationships can be a powerful tool for midwives.

Neuro-endocrinology

Oxytocin is sometimes referred to as 'the hormone of love'. It is a prime reproductive hormone, secreted by the pituitary gland; it engenders and is engendered by loving, trusting relationships (Foureur, 2008). It is also a midwife's best friend. By working with and promoting endogenous oxytocin production in women, we give them the best chance of a smooth and satisfying pregnancy, birth and postnatal period (Robertson, 2004; Foureur, 2008). The study of the oxytocin system is part of every British midwife's training. However the social/relational aspects of oxytocin deserve fresh attention when we are searching for ways to improve big-bodied women's experience of maternity care and ensure that we are not preventing them from achieving physiological births.

Endogenous oxytocin allows women to translate the normal stress of pregnancy and birth into a 'calm and connection' response which directs energy towards social cohesion, healing, growth, sleeping, digestion and successful sexual reproduction (Uvnäs Moberg, 2003, p. xi). Lack of oxytocin contributes to uterine inertia and fetal distress, impairs breast milk production and delivery and leaves women more sensitive to pain and feelings of disconnection (Foureur, 2008). The oxytocin system can be disrupted at many levels. Amongst midwives it is widely accepted that fear, mediated by adrenalin, reduces oxytocin flow. Wuntakal and Hollingworth (2010) hypothesize that a hormone known as leptin is an oxytocin antagonist that is higher in fatter women and contributes to the greater prevalence of prolonged pregnancy, slow labour, emergency CS, post-partum haemorrhage and reduced breastfeeding rates that we see in these groups. Leptin is produced in human adipose tissue and has been shown *in vitro* to cause quiescence in lower segment myometrium, thus decreasing both spontaneous contractions and those brought about with artificial oxytocin (Moynihan *et al.*, 2006). The evidence around this theory comes from the reductionist 'faulty body' school of science. Nonetheless, it stimulates interesting questions about endogenous oxytocin systems in women with high proportions of body fat, and perhaps adds weight to the argument that 'courting' oxytocin in these women is of extra importance. Many of the obstetric interventions that women with BMIs of $\geq 30 kg/m^2$ are more likely to experience may be performed in order to treat the actual or predicted consequences of low endogenous oxytocin, such as labour dystocia. Ironically, they may also hinder labour, breastfeeding and bonding through an inhibitory effect on the endogenous oxytocin system. These anti-oxytocin factors include medicalized environments and relationships, use of synthetic oxytocic labour induction/augmentation, epidural and CS (Foureur, 2008; Tamagawa, 2012). Many interventions could well be avoided through attending to a woman's own oxytocic flow earlier in the proceedings (Robertson, 2004). This is where the midwife's attention to relationships is of utmost importance. Feeling scrutinized, exposed, humiliated, abused, ignored or in any way emotionally unsafe may inhibit the oxytocin system. Equally, relating compassionately can stimulate oxytocin to flow (Foureur, 2008). This might be through felt or expressed love, smiling, comforting/rhythmic consensual touch, appropriately timed eye contact or just being present as a 'known (trusted) and pleasant companion' (Foureur, 2008, p. 71).

Psychology

Shame and the closely related feelings of humiliation and guilt are recurring themes in fat women's negative experiences of maternity. Shame is a near-universal experience and a core element of many mental health issues, including common addictions, such as those related to food. It has the capacity to keep a person frozen in her protective shell, desperately angry or wishing to conform and unable to develop or connect (Whitfield, 1991). These effects can impede the processes of new motherhood, as they demand epic physical and psychological transformations.

Psychologists have proposed that shame arises when a person's 'core' self has been violated or exposed to non-empathic treatment (from either themselves or others) (Firman and Gila, 1997). Conversely, empathy, for instance, in the form of self-acceptance or compassionate words or touch, is a cure for shame (Mollon, 2002). Because midwives and obstetricians are present at times of great exposure and vulnerability for women, they have many opportunities to offer the empathy that can help to heal shame. When a fat pregnant woman with body shame experiences non-empathic treatment, such as a critical gaze, cruel comment or denial of her choices, needs or feelings, her shame becomes even deeper and more toxic (Mollon, 2002).

Previously, I have argued that fatness itself does not necessarily cause disease, and that for many people fatness is a natural manifestation of size diversity. Nonetheless, it does appear that, just as thinness can indicate problems such as hypothyroidism or anorexia nervosa, fatness too can be a symptom of underlying imbalance, whether it be endocrinological, metabolic, emotional or spiritual. To take some psychological examples: calorie-rich foods are one of the many substances that people use addictively, and weight-gain can result from trauma such as abuse. If a woman brings these kinds of issues to her midwifery appointments, she should be offered signposting to further (preferably fat-friendly) psychological support, whilst receiving empathy to avoid further shaming.

Use of empathy and compassion can help health professionals to navigate the shame-ridden waters of fatness in maternity, to avoid causing further harm and to increase opportunities for women to heal their own shame from past trauma. It is possible that offering empathy and reducing shame may also help to optimize the oxytocin cycle, thereby reducing the need for medical intervention in childbirth. In order to do so, it is necessary to build relationships of mutual respect and trust. The argument has been made many times over for the salutary effects of both continuity of carer and continuous support in labour (Hodnett et al., 2012; Sandall, 2012). Perhaps women classed as having BMIs $\geq$30kg/m^2 could particularly benefit from these models of midwifery care, which make it easier to develop relationships.

Conclusion

Anti-fat prejudice is widespread in western and westernized cultures. Based on a range of negative stereotypes and perpetuated through the media, it negatively impacts upon fat people's lives in both intimate and public contexts. I argue that the 'obesity epidemic' and the technocratic birth paradigm are intertwined, that they share a common origin in patriarchal Cartesian dualism, function as protection against the fear of woman/nature out of control and contribute to the continuing subjugation of women. A brief look at some criticisms of the evidence behind the 'obesity epidemic' highlights frequent confusion of correlation with causation and lack of attention to key covariates (such as CRF, healthy lifestyle choices, socio-economic status, weight cycling and anti-fat stigma itself) when considering the relationship between fatness and health. A review of current national maternity guidelines for big-bodied women reveals a medicalized 'absolute risk' approach, founded on evidence that is compromised in similar ways to 'obesity science' in general, such as overlooking the context and complexity of statistical relationships. These guidelines focus on risk avoidance through increased medicalization and surveillance and fail to address the issue of how to increase women's chances of achieving safe, positive, physiological childbirth. Big-bodied women's testimonies regarding experiences of maternity care reveal high levels of medical- izing, discriminatory, shaming and alienating treatment and a frustrating combination of negative communication and evasive/embarrassed silence. What also emerge are the joyful, transformational effects that women attribute to having positive, trusting interactions with their midwives. With reference to the physiology of endogenous oxytocin and the psychology of shame, I suggest that midwifery practice emphasizing compassionate, empathic relation- ships may be the key to breaking the 'cascade of interventions' for a group of women who have for too long borne the brunt of their culture's negative attitudes towards fat bodies.

Notes

1 Body Mass Index (BMI) is simply a person's weight in kilograms divided by the square of her height in metres. It takes no account of the proportion of the weight which is fatty tissue, nor of its distribu- tion within the body. WHO (2000) classifications are as follows: 'underweight' (BMI <18.5kg/m²); 'normal range' (often referred to as 'normal weight' or 'healthy weight') (BMI 18.5–24.9 kg/m²); 'preobese' (often referred to as 'overweight') (BMI 25–29.9 kg/m²); obese class I (BMI 30–34.9 kg/ m²); obese class II (BMI 35–39.9 kg/m²); and obese class III (often referred to as 'morbidly obese'). The medicalized and arbitrary nature of these terms makes them ethically problematic; however, I make use of them in order to refer to the existing literature.
2 I use the terms 'fat', 'fat person' and 'fat woman' in my writing. Terms such as 'overweight' and 'raised BMI' are often utilized as acceptable/sanitized alternatives to 'fat'. Anecdotal evidence from fat women is that these terms are not necessarily more acceptable to them, as they impose a negative value judgement, whereas 'fat' is simply descriptive and can be meant and interpreted as negative, neutral or positive. It is in the neutral/positive sense that I use the word fat.

References

Abenhaim, H. A. and Benjamin, A. (2011) Higher caesarean section rates in women with higher body mass index: are we managing labour differently? *Journal of Obstetrics and Gynaecology Canada: JOGC = Journal d'obstetrique et gynecologie du Canada: JOGC*, 33 (5): 443–448.

All Party Parliamentary Group on Body Image (2012) *Reflections on body image* [online] London: YMCA. Available from: www.ymca.co.uk/bodyimage/report [accessed 26 November 2012].

Bacon, L. and Aphramor, L. (2011) Weight science: evaluating the evidence for a paradigm shift, *Nutrition Journal*, 10 (1): 1–13.

Benesch-Granberg, B., Harding, K., Richardson, R., Fillyjonk and Vesta44 (2012) *First do no harm; real stories of fat prejudice in health care* [online]. No geographical location: WordPress.com. Available from: http://fathealth.wordpress.com/ [accessed 16 December 2012].

Bordo, S. (2003) *Unbearable weight; feminism, western culture and the body*, 2nd edn, Berkeley: University of California Press.

Brewis, A., Wutich, A., Falletta-Cowden, A. and Rodriguez-Soto, I. (2011) Body norms and fat stigma in global perspective, *Current Anthropology*, 52 (2): 269–276.

Chastain, R. (2012) *Dances with fat. Just like you – only bigger* [online] Los Angeles: WordPress. com. Available from: http://danceswithfat.wordpress.com/2012/10/16/just-like-you-only-bigger/ [accessed 16 December 2012].

Chu, S. Y., Kim, S. Y., Schmid, C. H., Dietz, P. M., Callaghan, W. M., Lau, J. and Curtis, K. M. (2007) Maternal obesity and risk of cesarean delivery: a meta-analysis, *Obesity Reviews*, 8 (5): 385–394.

CMACE/RGOG (Centre for Maternal and Child Enquiries and Royal College of Obstetricians and Gynaecologists) (2010) *CMACE/RCOG Joint Guideline Management of Women with Obesity in Pregnancy*, London: CMACE and RCOG.

CMACE (2011) Saving Mothers' Lives: reviewing maternal deaths to make motherhood safer:

2006–08. The Eighth Report on Confidential Enquiries into Maternal Deaths in the United Kingdom. *BJOG: An International Journal of Obstetrics & Gynaecology*, 118 (Suppl. 1): 1–203.

Cooper, C. (1998) *Fat and proud: the politics of size*, London: The Women's Press.

Cooper, C. (2007) '*Headless Fatties*' [online] London: Charlotte Cooper. Available from: www.charlottecooper.net/docs/fat/headless_fatties.htm [accessed 25 December 2012].

Crandall, C. S. (1994) Prejudice against fat people: ideology and self-interest, *Journal of Personality and Social Psychology*, 66 (5): 882–894.

Davis, D. L. and Walker, K. (2010) Re-discovering the material body in midwifery through an exploration of theories of embodiment, *Midwifery*, 26 (4): 457–462.

Davis-Floyd, R. (2001) The technocratic, humanistic, and holistic paradigms of childbirth, *International Journal of Gynecology & Obstetrics*, 75, Supplement 1(0): S5–S23.

Deery, R. and Wray, S. (2009) 'The hardest leap': acceptance of diverse body size in midwifery, *The Practising Midwife*, 12 (10): 14–16.

Engeland, A., Bjorge, T., Selmer, R. M. and Tverdal, A. (2003) Height and body mass index in relation to total mortality, *Epidemiology May*, 14 (3): 293–299.

Ernsberger, P. and Koletsky, R. J. (1999) Biomedical rationale for a wellness approach to obesity: an alternative to a focus on weight loss, *Journal of Social Issues*, 55 (2): 221–260.

Evans, B. (2006) 'Gluttony or sloth': critical geographies of bodies and morality in (anti)obesity policy, *Area*, 38 (3): 259–267.

Fahy, K. (2008) Power and the social construction of birth territory. In: K. Fahy, Foureur, M. and Hastie, C. (eds) *Birth territory and midwifery guardianship; theory for practice, education and research*, Edinburgh: Butterworth Heinemann Elsevier.

Farrell, S. W., Braun, L., Barlow, C. E., Cheng, Y. J. and Blair, S. N. (2002) The relation of body mass index, cardiorespiratory fitness, and all-cause mortality in women, *Obesity*, 10 (6): 417–423.

Firman, J. and Gila, A. (1997) *The primal wound: a transpersonal view of trauma, addiction and growth*, New York: State University New York Press.

Flegal, K. M., Graubard, B. I., Williamson, D. F. and Gail, M. H. (2007) Cause-specific excess deaths associated with underweight, overweight, and obesity, *Journal of the American Medical Association (JAMA)*, 298 (17): 2028–2037.

Foureur, M. (2008) Creating birth space to enable undisturbed birth. In: K. Fahey, Foureur, M. and Hastie, C. (eds) *Birth territory and midwifery guardianship; theory for practice, education and research*, Edinburgh: Butterworth Heinemann Elsevier.

Furber, C. M. and McGowan, L. (2011) A qualitative study of the experiences of women who are obese and pregnant in the UK, *Midwifery*, 27 (4): 437–444.

Gabriel, S., Gracely, E. J. and Fyfe, B. S. (2006) Impact of BMI on clinically significant unsuspected findings as determined at postmortem examination, *American Journal of Clinical Pathology*, 125 (1): 127–131.

Gard, M. and Wright, J. (2005) *The obesity epidemic: science, morality and ideology*, London: Routledge.

Gardner, S. (2012) Safeguarding against maternal obesity, *British Journal of Midwifery*, 20 (10): 688.

Heslehurst, N. (2011) Identifying 'at risk' women and the impact of maternal obesity on National Health Service maternity services, *Proceedings of the Nutrition Society*, 70 (04): 439–449.

Heslehurst, N., Bell, R. and Rankin, J. (2011) Tackling maternal obesity: the challenge for public health, *Perspectives in Public Health*, 131 (4): 161–162.

Heslehurst, N., Lang, R., Rankin, J., Wilkinson, J. R. and Summerbell, C. D. (2007) Obesity in pregnancy: a study of the impact of maternal obesity on NHS maternity services, *BJOG: An International Journal of Obstetrics & Gynaecology*, 114 (3): 334–342.

Hodnett, E. D., Gates, S., Hofmeyr, G. J. and Sakala, C. (2012) *Continuous support for women during childbirth*, Chichester: John Wiley and Sons, Ltd.

Kapit, W., Macey, R. I. and Meisami, E. (2000) *The physiology coloring book*, 2nd edn. San Francisco: Addison Welsey Longman.

Keenan, J. and Stapleton, H. (2010) Bonny babies? Motherhood and nurturing in the age of obesity, *Health, Risk & Society*, 12 (4): 369–383.

LeBesco, K. (2010) Neoliberalism, public health, and the moral perils of fatness, *Critical Public Health*, 21 (2): 153–164.

Lupton, D. (2013) *Fat*, London: Routledge.

Lyerly, G. W., Sui, X., Lavie, C. J. and Church, T. S. (2009) The association between cardiorespiratory fitness and risk of all-cause mortality among women with impaired fasting glucose or undiagnosed diabetes mellitus, *Mayo Clinic proceedings*, 84 (9): 780.

Marmot, M. and Brunner, E. (2005) Cohort profile: the Whitehall II study, *International Journal of Epidemiology*, 34 (2): 251–256.

Matheson, E. M., King, D. E. and Everett, C. J. (2012) Healthy lifestyle habits and mortality in over-weight and obese individuals, *Journal of the American Board of Family Medicine*, 25 (1): 9–15.

McDermott, K. (2012) *Doctors remove 28kg tumour which filled a WHEELBARROW from woman diagnosed as being obese* [online] London: Associated Newspapers Ltd. Available from: www.dailymail.co.uk/home/article-1227210/Contact-Us.html [accessed 16 December 2012].

McGlone, A. and Davies, S. (2012) Perspectives on risk and obesity: towards a 'tolerable risk' approach? *British Journal of Midwifery*, 20 (1): 3–17.

McNaughton, D. (2010) From the womb to the tomb: obesity and maternal responsibility. *Critical Public Health*, 21 (2): 179–190.

Meadows, A. (2012) *Why your fat back and bingo wings aren't going to kill you any time soon: debunk-ing the obesity science dogma*, Health At Every Size (HAES) UK/Fat Studies Conference, London: School of Oriental and African Studies (SOAS), University of London.

Miriam, C. (2011) Fat as deviancy: providing ethical midwifery care to women of all sizes in the UK, *MIDIRS Midwifery Digest*, 21 (2): 161–166.

Mollon, P. (2002) *Shame and jealousy; the hidden turmoils*, London: H. Karnac (Books) Ltd.

Moynihan, A. T., Hehir, M. P., Glavey, S. V., Smith, T. J. and Morrison, J. J. (2006) Inhibitory effect of leptin on human uterine contractility in vitro, *American Journal of Obstetrics and Gynecology*, 195 (2): 504–509.

Muennig, P. (2008) The body politic: the relationship between stigma and obesity-associated disease, *BMC Public Health*, 8 (1): 128–138.

Muennig, P., Jia, H., Lee, R. and Lubetkin, E. (2008) I think therefore I am: perceived ideal weight as a determinant of health, *American Journal of Public Health*, 98 (3): 501–506.

Muennig, P., Sohler, N. and Mahato, B. (2007) Socioeconomic status as an independent predictor of physiological biomarkers of cardiovascular disease: evidence from NHANES, *Preventive Medicine*, 45 (1): 35–40.

Murphy-Lawless, J. (1998) *Reading birth and death: a history of obstetric thinking*, Cork: Cork University Press.

Murray, S. (2008) *The 'fat' female body*, Basingstoke: Palgrave Macmillan.

NHS Information Centre (2011) *Health Survey for England: 2010, Trend tables* [online] Leeds: Avail-able from: www.ic.nhs.uk/pubs/hse10trends [accessed 16 December 2012].

NHS Litigation Authority (NHSLA) (2012) *CNST Maternity Standards: 2012–13* [online] Lon-don: NHSLA. Available from: www.nhsla.com/Pages/Publications.aspx?library=safety|standards [accessed 26 December 2012].

NICE (National Institute for Clinical Excellence) (2010) *Dietary interventions and physical activity interventions for weight management before, during and after pregnancy*, London: NICE.

Nursing and Midwifery Council (NMC) (2008) *The Code: Standards of conduct, performance and ethics for nurses and midwives*, London: NMC.

Nyman, V. M. K., Prebensen, Å. K. and Flensner, G. E. M. (2010) Obese women's experiences of encounters with midwives and physicians during pregnancy and childbirth, *Midwifery*, 26 (4): 424–429.

Oakley, A. (1993) *Essays on women, medicine and health*, Edinburgh: Edinburgh University Press.

Olander, E. K., Atkinson, L., Edmunds, J. K. and French, D. P. (2011) The views of pre- and post-natal women and health professionals regarding gestational weight gain: an exploratory study, *Sexual & Reproductive Healthcare*, 2 (1): 43–48.

Orbach, S. (2006) *Fat is a feminist issue*, 2nd edn, London: Arrow Books.

Orpana, H. M., Berthelot, J.-M., Kaplan, M. S. and Feeny, D. H. (2010) BMI and mortality: results from a national longitudinal study of Canadian adults, *Obesity (Silver Spring, Md.)*, 18 (1): 214–218.

Pitchford, P. (2002) *Healing with whole foods. Asian traditions and modern nutrition*, 3rd edn, Berkeley: North Atlantic Books.

Puhl, R. and Heuer, C. (2009) The stigma of obesity: a review and update, *Obesity*, 17: 941–964.

Puhl, R. M. and Heuer, C. A. (2010) Obesity stigma: important considerations for public health, *American Journal of Public Health*, 100 (6): 1019–1028.

Raphael, D., Lines, E., Bryant, T., Daiski, I., Pilkington, B. *et al.* (2010) *Type 2 diabetes: poverty, priorities and policy, the social determinants of the incidence and management of type 2 diabetes* [online] Toronto: York University School of Health Policy and Management and School of Nursing. Available from: http://tinyurl.com/ycysb9l [accessed 27 December 2012].

Robertson, A. (2004) *The midwife companion; the art of support during birth*, Camperdown: Birth International.

Saguy, A. C. and Riley, K. W. (2005) Weighing both sides: morality, mortality, and framing contests over obesity, *Journal of Health Politics, Policy & Law*, 30 (5): 869–921.

Sandall, J. (2012) Every woman needs a midwife, and some women need a doctor too, *Birth*, 39 (4): 323–326.

Schulz, M., Liese, A. D., Boeing, H., Cunningham, J. E., Moore, C. G. and Kroke, A. (2004) Associations of short-term weight changes and weight cycling with incidence of essential hypertension in the EPIC-Potsdam Study, *Journal of Human Hypertension*, 19 (1): 61–67.

Sebire, N. J., Jolly, M., Harris, J. P. and Wadsworth, J. (2001) Maternal obesity and pregnancy outcome: a study of 287 213 pregnancies in London, *International Journal of Obesity and Related Metabolic Disorders*, 25 (8): 1175–1182.

Smith, D. and Lavender, T. (2011) The maternity experience for women with a body mass index ≥ 30 kg/m2: a meta-synthesis, *BJOG: An International Journal of Obstetrics & Gynaecology*, 118 (7): 779–789.

Swift, J. A., Hanlon, S., El-Redy, L., Puhl, R. M. and Glazebrook, C. (2012) Weight bias among UK trainee dietitians, doctors, nurses and nutritionists, *Journal of Human Nutrition and Dietetics*, 26 (4): 1–8.

Tamagawa, K. (2012) Analysing adverse effects of epidural analgesia in labour, *British Journal of Midwifery*, 20 (10): 704–708.

Thompson, R. and Thomas, D. (2000) A cross-sectional survey of the opinions on weight loss treatments of adult obese patients attending a dietetic clinic, *International Journal of Obesity and Related Metabolic Disorders*, 24 (2): 164–170.

Unnithan-Kumar, M. and Tremayne, S. (eds) (2011) *Fatness and the maternal body*, Oxford: Berghahn Books.

Uvnäs Moberg, K. (2003) *The oxytocin factor: tapping the hormone of calm, love and healing*, Cambridge: Da Capo Press.

Wei, M., Kampert, J. B., Barlow, C. E., Nichaman, M. Z., Gibbons, L. W. *et al.* (1999) Relationship between low cardiorespiratory fitness and mortality in normal-weight, overweight, and obese men, *Journal of the American Medical Association (JAMA)*, 282 (16): 1547–1553.

Whitfield, C. (1991) *Co-dependence; healing the human condition*, Florida: Health Communications, Inc.

Whitley, B. and Kite, M. (2010) *The psychology of prejudice and discrimination*, 2nd edn, Belmont: Wadsworth.

World Health Organization (WHO) (2000) *Obesity: preventing and managing the global epidemic*, Geneva: WHO.

Wray, S. and Deery, R. (2008) The medicalization of body size and women's healthcare, *Health Care for Women International*, 29 (3): 227–243, DOI: 10.1080/07399330701738291.

Wuntakal, R. and Hollingworth, T. (2010) Leptin: a tocolytic agent for the future? *Medical Hypotheses*, 74: 81–82.

RELATING FOOD AND BODIES
TO HEALTH AT EVERY SIZE (HAES)
IN MIDWIFERY

Jennifer Brady, Lucy Aphramor and Jacqui Gingras

Introduction

The anthropologist Megan McCullough gives a first-person account of what it was like to be fat and pregnant in North America: she speaks of attitudes of disgust and blame among healthcare providers who saw her/her body as shameful, a problem and caused by lack of will-power. The sense of being judged, surveilled and viewed as an inconvenience, or worse, as less deserving of their care and respect, permeated her experience with the health system:

> What happens in these small acts is that the fat maternal body is made more visible – as out of the 'normal' range and this is performed and emphasized at each weigh-in. I have on occasion gotten on the scale and turned my back to the numbers. I wanted to embody my pregnancy and feel where I was and not deal with the numbers. This choice on my part usually invited scorn and scolding or if not scolding, then biting comments. For example, 'So we are not dealing with things today are we?'

McCullough reminds us that while anthropometric and biomedical readings have a place in global and personal pregnancy care, their impact can also be harmful:

> The effect of this emphasis on measurement, for me at least, is that the complexities and emotional experiences of fatness is diminished, deemed less relevant or perhaps seen as something too messy to deal with during a weigh in and yet it is these times when fat people are very vulnerable. Seeing and communicating with the 'whole' person and not just his or her numbers could be an opportunity for further communication in medical settings and respectful treatment invites a patient 'in' to their own care rather than judges them for somehow failing at it.
>
> (McCullough, under review)

McCullough's experience suggests that fat women in western healthcare settings are being unhelpfully micromanaged during pregnancy. A feminist midwifery perspective may express that fatter mothers are (symbolically) punished for their fatness. That is, that they are less likely to negotiate a midwifery model of care where the emphasis is on shared decision making and more likely to be 'managed' in a doctor-led system where they become disembodied receptacles for their babies (Griew, personal communication). As a result, the woman becomes disengaged from her care provider and experiences loss of control, a diminished sense of agency and disenfranchisement. An alternative scenario in which women are allocated an active voice within practice guidelines preferentially serves the interest of all parties within the healthcare relationship (Freeman and Griew 2007).

The current biomedical approach to maternity care creates the need to pathologize pregnant women and set up the maternal body in opposition to the baby (Griew, personal communication). A woman's agency is then linked to how she performs as a good mother, a role strongly tied to compliance with prescriptive expectations around medication, healthy eating and weight gain, for example (Katz Rothman 2000). In this scenario, a woman considered underweight would re/gain agency with care providers as she gained weight to standard levels. It is no surprise that the same discourse readily demonizes pregnant women who smoke: the smoker is deemed to be selfishly enacting evil on her baby and is treated accordingly; that is, with no recognition of any of the struggles that she may be living through or awareness that smoking may be her best option among others that is available at that moment. The absence of attention to context makes for a very dictatorial approach, resignifying a plethora of power imbalances that serve to normalize inequality in part by silencing everyday narratives of resilience and endurance.

As dietitians, we have witnessed at first hand the harm that has been inflicted on fat bodies. The nutritional advice offered by health professionals can be inconsistent and prescriptive, reflecting professional, personal and social mores about fat and food. In the context of maternity care, the impact of fat hatred exacts a particular toll on pregnant women that is layered with gendered ideas about health and what it means to be a woman, a mother and fat. In this chapter we wish to explore alternative possibilities for women accessing maternity care that are respectful of and compassionate toward all women with bodies of any size. We propose a Health at Every Size approach informed by relational-cultural theory (RCT) as one such alternative. We will first outline the principles of HAES as we understand them, before exploring RCT and how this connects to HAES. Next, we compare and contrast pregnancy-related guidelines for health practitioners involved in the care of pregnant women that are published by the National Health Service (NHS) in the UK and Health Canada (HC) in Canada.

Health at Every Size

A growing literature draws attention to the misrepresentation of weight science in mainstream policy and unearths significant flaws in the research on which weight-loss recommendations are based (Campos *et al.* 2005; Gard and Wright 2005; Aphramor 2010). To illustrate our claim, we will explore the evidence behind three assumptions that underpin a weight-reduction agenda. Each of these assumptions must be true for weight loss to be ethically justifiable as a health intervention. For the sake of clarity we will confine our example to a discussion of the evidence regarding people in the 'overweight' BMI category.

A core assumption precipitating intervention is that being overweight poses a significant health risk. In fact, it is well documented that overweight people typically live longer than people in the ideal weight category:

Analysis of the National Health and Nutrition Examination Surveys I, II, and III, which followed the largest nationally representative cohort of United States adults, determined that greatest longevity was in the overweight category [32]. As per the report, published in the Journal of the American Medical Association and reviewed and approved by the Centers for Disease Control and Prevention and the National Cancer Institute, '[this] finding is consistent with other results reported in the literature.' Indeed, the most comprehensive review of the research pooled data for over 350,000 subjects from 26 studies and found overweight to be associated with greater longevity than normal weight [36].

(Bacon and Aphramor 2011)

A second assumption throughout weight-loss literature is that when people adhere to a calorie deficit, through either reduced calorie intake, increased calorie expenditure or a combination of both, they will lose weight. Yet this is not supported by the evidence: a long-term trial involving 20,000 women that was designed to test this energy-balance hypothesis robustly disproves the assumption. Participants in this trial, known as the Women's Health Initiative, maintained a calorie deficit averaging 360 calories per day for nearly eight years and significantly increased their activity levels. After following this regime there was almost no change in weight (a loss of 0.1 kg from starting point), and average waist circumference had increased slightly (Howard *et al.* 2006). An accurate reading of the evidence shows that short-term weight loss can be achieved, but there is no research documenting successful weight loss in the long term.

A third assumption is that the most effective way for unhealthy overweight people to improve their health is by losing weight. However, there is abundant evidence that indicates that health benefits arise from improved self-care, including diet and activity patterns, which happen independently of weight loss. Put another way, sound nutrition and active living contribute to enhanced well-being, whether or not someone loses weight.

It quickly becomes apparent that there are serious scientific shortcomings in taken-for-granted assumptions about weight, health and dieting, and that these shortcomings invalidate key arguments used to promote weight loss. We would urge the reader to become more familiar with the critical-weight literature because of its enormous implications for the recommendations we make across all areas of practice concerned with weight and food and, relatedly, its significance to ethics. The problem of systemic sizeism in policy means that it is not sufficient for practitioners to accept guidelines on weight management at face value: instead, in order to provide acceptable healthcare we will need to interrogate our work through a critical lens. Jette and Rail (2012) use this critical stance to specifically explore the implications of sizeism in pregnancy.

Fat activists have used this critical lens to challenge some of the fundamental outrages of fat prejudice on fat people's rights. Documented activism has included, but is not limited to, an eclectic mix of performance, protest, support groups, fat swims and films; a recently available timeline gives a fuller picture of the movement (Cooper 2011). Fat activist writing ranges from an early feminist publication *Shadow on a Tightrope* (that includes chapters on critical weight science) (Schoenfielder and Wieser 1983) through zines and blogs to two more recent texts signalling a shift in academic attention to the field, *The Fat Studies Reader* (Rothblum and Solovay 2009) and *Fat Studies UK* (Tormley and Naylor 2009). Where fat activism engages with health, practitioners find allies in critical weight studies and the Health at Every Size (HAES) movement. The HAES philosophy expounds a compassionate and weight-neutral approach to self-care that explicitly seeks to challenge size discrimination and other forms of oppression, highlighting the role of structural factors, such as discrimination, on well-being.

In a clinical situation where a client seeks nutritional advice for eating or weight concerns, HAES offers both client and practitioner an effective alternative to a conventional weight-centred approach. As HAES practice is weight-neutral, effectiveness is assessed in terms of changes in a person's relationship with food, improvements in dietary intake, enhanced psychological well-being and improved physiological measurements of metabolic fitness, such as blood pressure and HDL cholesterol. Effectiveness extends to absence of adverse effect, including weight cycling, depression, reduced self-esteem and loss of bone mass, all of which are found with a weight-centred approach. HAES researchers are also concerned about health as a relational construct, and self-care more generally, and are finding ways to evaluate the impact of HAES interventions beyond the clinic. An open access article providing a comprehensive summary of the evidence base for claims made in HAES science is a useful adjunct to this section (Bacon and Aphramor 2011).

HAES practitioners work within a framework that embraces several hallmark tenets. The first is that a HAES approach is premised on promoting respect for everybody, whatever their size, fitness level, health, smoking status or attitudes towards self-care. This tenet is put into practice by teaching acceptance, often beginning with exploring size acceptance. Here, rather than encouraging clients to focus on altering their weight (a strategy that relies on the judgement that they should not accept themselves at their current weight), the focus is on helping people to value themselves and the bodies they have right now. Critics express concern that size acceptance is damaging because it tacitly lends people permission to give up on the pursuit of health. There are two obvious flaws in this reasoning: it assumes that the current approach effectively promotes health, when it is in fact detrimental; and it assumes that size acceptance results in decreased self-care when it is in fact associated with improvements in well-being.

A second characteristic of HAES practice is promoting reliance on internal regulation. As compared to a conventional dieting approach that relies on cognitive restraint to change people's eating habits in order to meet (external) dietary guidelines, a HAES approach encourages people to make food choices informed by internal signals of appetite, taste preference and fullness. It also teaches people how to identify emotional prompts to eat and how to enhance their menu of self-care options. Nutritional knowledge has its place in HAES practice when it can augment people's understanding of the link between what they eat and how they feel, rather than being taught as stand-alone, disembodied 'facts'. Another aspect of HAES practice that supports intuitive eating is that of legitimizing all food, so getting away from diet-mentality thinking that labels food as good/bad or healthy/unhealthy. Recognizing that food choices meet a range of needs, be they nutritional, cultural, psychological, emotional, religious, budgetary and so on, further helps people to make choices from a place of internal regulation rather than external prescription.

A third feature of a HAES approach that extends the rationale for encouraging intuitive eating is active embodiment. As with food choices, this means that people are taught how to engage in active living so as to maximize their feelings of well-being, as opposed to undertaking physical activity according to externally imposed targets. Reliance on embodied knowledge can also inform decisions around sleep, meditation and other avenues for compassionate self-care, such as pain management.

Fourth, a HAES philosophy recognizes the impact of material and non-material psychosocial and structural determinants of health and seeks ways to integrate this knowledge into practice in and beyond the clinic (McKibbin 2009; Aphramor 2011). Material factors have to do with the impact of poverty on health and well-being, for example, the restriction on food choices that this brings, the health impact of living in damp houses or polluted neighbourhoods; non-material factors concern the impact that living with chronic stress – from stigma, discrimination or poverty – has on neuroendocrine and hormonal pathways linked to increased disease prevalence. HAES thinking thus challenges the construction of health as an individualistic body project and recognizes that people's personal and political lived realities have physiological consequences. There is considerable support for this approach in the biomedical literature. Consider, for example, the finding that people's position in society more strongly impacts upon their health outcomes than do their health behaviours or economic standing, possibly via pathways mediated through the stress hormone cortisol. So, for example, black American men can expect to live nine years less on average than Cuban men, despite earning approximately four-fold the Cuban men's wage (Marmot 2006).

HAES practice thus offers people a radically different way of relating to food, health and their own and others' bodies. The point of intervention is to promote compassionate self-care that, in turn, typically helps people to develop a healthy relationship with food and fosters growth-promoting relationships.

A relational-cultural frame

Within this chapter we seek to conflate the emerging critical weight science with perhaps revised, but more ethically robust, evidence-based practices in midwifery care. After providing an appraisal of the HAES literature, we will explore the application of a theoretical framework through which to view this concept from the perspective of midwifery practice. The framework used to translate this new knowledge into ethical practice is relational-cultural theory (RCT).

RCT originated among a group of feminist psychologists and psychoanalysts in the mid 1980s and was marked by the publication of *Toward a New Psychology of Women* (Miller 1986), which put forth the possibility that developmental theories premised on growing more autonomous and independent did not fully explain the human growth process. Since then, the Jean Baker Miller Training Institute (www.jbmti.org) has researched and published extensively in Relational Theory and what eventually expanded into RCT.

RCT provides an alternate explanation for human psychological development. That is, human beings grow in relation to one another, interdependently, not independently. Recent work in brain science has provided fascinating insights into how human relationships embedded in complex cultural contexts influence and are influenced by neurotransmitters (dopamine, serotonin and opioids) in direct contact with the 'relationship centre' (orbitofrontal cortex) of the brain (Banks 2011). As Banks (2011) states,

> The human brain is profoundly vulnerable to the environment and to early relationships in its first stages of development. When connected with an early caretaker who is responsive, the human brain develops toward close, differentiated relationships. When early caretaking relationships are abusive or unresponsive or if the environment is chaotic and stressful, the human brain shapes itself to protect the person from future destructive relationships and physical harm.

What we intend to make clear by this description is that an environment that is sizeist or oppressive to a fat, pregnant or post-natal female body has the real potential to shape the brains of that mother and her infant through powerful waves of neurotransmitters – those responsible for attachment and pleasure. We do not imply by this observation that individuals are solely responsible for changing their environment and therefore their health, since to do so would be healthist (Crawford 1980). What we do intend is that, like all healthcare professionals, we encourage a turning of our attention to seeking and offering ways to create discursively healing environments with our words and language as much as with our other more practical and visible healing instruments.

As is to be expected, relationships are not always in a state of blissful connection; disconnection is a natural occurrence, but it is how the disconnections are responded to that is most instructive. In a traditional, perhaps biomedical setting, disconnections between 'patient' and 'expert' abound (see Chapter 1). From the humiliation of exposing intimate details of the body (questions regarding eating and activity patterns with the assumption that these patterns should influence body weight) to exposing the body in vulnerable ways (being offered too small a gown, too unsteady an examination table), the fat body becomes unerringly familiar with shame as a dominant emotion. Coterminous with shame is disconnection, which

> stimulates the stress-response system producing corticosteroids (cortisol) that feeds back and decreases both endorphin and CRF [cortisol releasing factor] production (CRF stimulates the sympathetic nervous system (SNS) – with less CRF there is less SNS stimulation).
>
> (Banks 2011: 177)

Periods of shame and disconnection leave people feeling inhibited, isolated and alone. Multiple and chronic disconnection can lead to the belief that the individual is to blame for her or his desperate situation, which can motivate the individual to further seek coping strategies that lessen the stress-response system. Eating troubles are one such coping strategy, as Ruth Deery describes in Chapter 1. In relation to the post-natal experience, Banks (2011: 175) describes it thus:

> The bottom line is this, because a child's brain is still developing when he is born, it is imperative for both the individual infant and for the developing human community, that each infant start life in a growth-fostering relationship; one that will shape his brain toward future healthy relationships. Think of the biological uphill battle that exists when whole families, communities, and even nations are formed amidst interpersonal violence. Disconnection can breed chronic disconnections.

Relational resilience is the ability to respond to disconnections in relationships through efforts at reconnection. Relational resilience is accomplished by moving in relationship through connection and disconnection and back to connection. It is accomplished through mutual empathy, reciprocity and trust in growth-fostering relationships (Gingras 2005; see also Kirkham 2010). Due to the plasticity of neural pathways, chronic disconnections, once repaired, can lead to relational reconnection. For someone who is experiencing disconnection due to a non-empowering pregnancy care, the effects are profound and many, but if that person can find another health care provider (perhaps a midwife) that can be vulnerable, open, curious and trustworthy, reconnection is possible. Such a partnership between mother and midwife would be considered growth fostering (Leap 2000; Kirkham 2010).

Miller (1986a) suggests that growth-fostering relationships provide 'five good things': *zest* – when each person feels a greater sense of vitality and energy; *action* – when each person feels more able to act and DOES act; *clarity* – when each person has a more accurate picture of her/himself and the other person and the relationship; *worth* – when each person feels a greater sense of self-worth; and *connection* – when each person feels more connected to the other person and a greater motivation for connections with other people beyond those in the specific client–clinician relationship, i.e. family and community. Importantly, a growth-fostering relationship enables the individuals to enjoy 'moving inward towards social change' (Ellis 2002). This is the power of RCT: that it starts with individuals but soon asserts the possibility of social transformation. It seeks a much wider audience than only the relational dyad, but starts and returns there recurrently.

With this reframing, we encourage the work between the pregnant woman and her midwife to proceed relationally, with each being mutually influenced and moved by the other. RCT provides a way of understanding the shifting power dynamic in practitioner–client relationships introduced by the HAES paradigm. Concomitantly, RCT brings to light the insidious ways in which control discourse thwarts growth-fostering client–practitioner relationships. As Gingras and Brady (2010) explain, control discourse 'inherently delimits possibilities for authenticity and connection in dietitians' relationships with theirs and Others' bodies'. Moving forward relationally, with a view to wisdom discourse, is what we suggest as a suitable means for midwifery practice involving fat women.

What might this mean for midwifery practice?

This section will compare and contrast some of the key Canadian and British guidelines for health professionals who provide pre- and post-natal care to women. It will also explore how a relational-cultural, HAES-based practice might inform a different approach to pregnancy-related care. The pregnancy-related guidelines that we discuss here have been compiled from two key documents: (1) *Prenatal Nutrition Guidelines for Professionals* issued by HC (2010); and (2) the National Institute for Health and Clinical Excellence (NICE) report titled *Dietary Interventions and Physical Activity Interventions for Weight Management Before, During and After Pregnancy* issued by the NHS (NHS/NICE 2010)

The recommendations issued by HC and NHS/NICE concur and diverge at different points in relation to pre-pregnancy, gestational and post-partum nutrition and body weight. Neither the HC nor the NHS/NICE report makes dietary recommendations specific to pre-pregnancy nutrition for women who intend to become pregnant, except to advise that women should take folic acid supplements. Prior to becoming pregnant, nutrition care for most women is based on guidelines outlined in *Eating Well with Canada's Food Guide: A Resource for Educators and Communicators* (HC 2011) in Canada and *The Pregnancy Book* (Department of Health 2009) in the UK. However, both the HC and NHS/NICE reports provide health practitioners with specific guidelines for the antenatal nutrition care of the pregnant woman. First and foremost, both health agencies urge health professionals to advise pregnant women that they should be 'eating "twice as healthy" not "twice as much"' (HC 2010: 8). The aim is to curtail gestational weight gain in order to avoid the long- and short-term complications that are widely believed to be associated with gaining 'too much' weight during pregnancy (Sen, Carpenter, Hochstadt *et al.* 2012). For example, one negative outcome of gaining more than the recommended amount of weight during pregnancy that is highlighted by the HC and NHS/NICE documents is greater post-partum weight retention. What is most troubling about the recommendation that health professionals help women to restrain their eating is that it is given meaning in a particular cultural context in which dieting is normalized. In a dieting culture, eating becomes characterized by a roller-coaster of limiting the amount or type of food eaten in an attempt to manage one's body weight, and later indulging when the dieter is unable to maintain the restriction. In this context women regularly restrict food in order to try to lose weight or maintain a lower weight. The guidelines seem tacitly concerned that pregnancy may be seen as a time during which women may give themselves permission to eat freely and without judgement from themselves or others; against a background of restriction, 'eating freely' may well amount to women eating from defiance, or with abandonment, an experience which may serve to further confuse their attempts at self-care.

What is more, there is a significant degree of disagreement between the NHS/NICE and HC guidelines as to how much extra or when in the pregnancy additional food is required. For singleton pregnancies, HC has it that increased caloric need begins in the second trimester and continues throughout the third in an amount equivalent to approximately two to three additional servings of food from one of the four food groups included in *Eating Well with Canada's Food Guide* (Health Canada 2011b). In contrast, the NHS/NICE guidelines recommend that women be advised that their energy needs do not increase until the third trimester, and then only by about 200 kilocalories per day. The disparity between what are both presented as reliable, evidence-based guidelines belies the exactitude of the science on which they are based and points to the possibility that these guidelines are informed by influences other than science – that is, by weight bias, sexism and a lack of reverence for the pregnant body.

From an RCT-informed, HAES perspective, these guidelines are as interesting for what they omit to say as for what they do say about health, relationships, self-care and the limits of nutrition science. One of the most glaring oversights in both documents is their not addressing the significant role that social injustices, via poverty, sexism, racism etc. play in determining people's health. These guidelines do not address the wider social injustices that bear on the trajectories of women's pregnancies, or women's inequitable access to those resources that might mitigate the impact of social injustices, let alone to those that might proactively support their health throughout pregnancy. While both the HC and NHS/NICE guidelines refer to factors other than 'excessive' weight gain that may have deleterious consequences for the health of their pregnant clients and their unborn children, such as poverty, low income, age under 18 years and immigrant status, there is little to no discussion about how these issues bear on the recommendations given in the remainder of either document. The impact of inequality and oppression, two items that almost certainly are more detrimental to women's pre-natal health than 'excessive' weight gain, is not elaborated upon.

Moreover, recommending a particular quantity of food or calories with which to supplement the diet during pregnancy negates women's body knowledge and further effaces their ability to listen to their bodies' internal cues of hunger and satiety. The discrepancy between the two documents regarding when and by how much pregnant women should increase their food intake belies the precision of these recommendations. The effect of not pointing out the inexactitude of nutrition science is to suggest that the particular amount by which a woman's caloric needs increase can be known, and is known. Regardless of when or by how much an individual woman's energy needs increase during pregnancy, even if a precise caloric need could be determined for each individual, this 'accounting-type' focus on calorie or food-serving counting does nothing to help practitioners to support women in fostering greater self-care, including attuned eating, for their physical and mental well-being. The accounting approach to nutrition management also does not attend to the relational nature of food and its role in women's practices of self-care for their bodies, or its place in maintaining relation-ships between the woman and members of her support network, including her family.

Another interesting similarity between the HC and NHS/NICE guidelines is the recom-mendation that health professionals seize on the opportunity that pregnancy presents to per-manently alter the eating and activity habits of their clients. The rationale is that dietary changes made during pregnancy, a time when women are thought more readily willing to make health behaviour changes, may translate into long-term health improvements for women and their families. Yet, isn't this an unethical, or at least disingenuous, approach to practice? At minimum, attempting to indirectly alter the eating practices of a woman's family is manipulative and makes a number of erroneous assumptions that actually contrib-ute to women's oppression. First, this presumes that pregnant clients take on a particularly gendered role within a heterosexual partnership. This makes heteronormative assumptions about women's reproductive and family lives and their role in food production as nutritional gatekeepers. Ultimately, this approach to practice creates a significant relational disconnec-tion between the practitioner and the client.

With respect to body weight prior to conception, neither the HC nor the NHS/NICE docu-ments provide any specific weight-related guidance for the care of women who fall within the 'healthy' or 'overweight' BMI categories. However, NHS/NICE does give advice for the treatment of women who are 'obese'. The UK guidelines recommend that if a woman has a BMI of 30 or more her healthcare providers should advise her to lose weight equivalent to 5–10% of her body weight or, better, lose enough weight to bring her BMI into the 'healthy' range before becoming pregnant (BMI 18.5–24.9). Basically, the NHS/NICE guidelines rec-ommend that fat people be advised to diet, despite the evidence that dieting not only does not work but is likely harmful to people's mental and physical health. In addition, 'obese' women are disproportionately more likely to be chronic dieters, all too familiar with the health decre-ments of restrained eating and weight fluctuation. Fatter women may indeed have the highest health risk – not due to any metabolic impact of adiposity per se, but because of the direct and indirect effects that weight-based discrimination has on their health via increased stress, diminished access to employment, delay in seeking healthcare and inadequate healthcare provision by practitioners who have misinformed or bigoted ideas about fat people.

Another point of divergence between the HC and NHS/NICE guidelines is on antenatal weight gain. The NHS/NICE guidelines do not specify any particular amount of weight that women, once pregnant, should gain over the course of their pregnancies. Regardless of BMI, the NHS/NICE guidelines indicate that women be advised not to diet while pregnant. Rather, and somewhat paradoxically, health practitioners are told to support clients in prac-tising healthy eating and exercise habits throughout their pregnancies, rather than focus on clients' body weight. However, the guidelines go on to state that the focus on healthy eating and exercise throughout the pre-natal period is in service of post-partum weight loss. While the emphasis on healthy eating and exercise habits in the pre-natal period echoes the focus on intuitive eating and active embodiment in HAES, the underlying intention is still to man-age and control the weight and size of the post-natal body, which fundamentally defies the principles of HAES and RCT.

In contrast to the shift away from pre-natal weight management in the NHS/NICE guide-lines, HC does set out detailed guidelines about how much body weight women should gain, based on their pre-pregnancy BMI and whether they have a singleton or twin pregnancy (see Table 2 and Table 4, Appendix A, in HC 2010). Again, there are a number of reasons for set-ting specific target weight gain ranges. However, it seems to have more to do with managing women's weight postpartum than it does with preventing any deleterious effects that excess weight gain may have on the pregnant woman or her unborn baby.

For women after the birth of their babies, the emphasis in both the NHS/NICE and HC guidelines returns to weight loss, especially for women classified as 'obese'. The NHS/NICE guidelines (p. 15) note:

> Ensure women have a realistic expectation of the time it will take to lose weight gained during pregnancy. Discuss the benefits of a healthy diet and regular physical activity, acknowledging the woman's role within the family and how she can be supported by her partner and wider family. Advice on healthy eating and physical activity should be tailored to her circumstances. For example, it should take into account the demands of caring for a baby and any other children, how tired she is and any health problems she may have (such as pelvic floor muscle weakness or backache).

While the sentiment to take account of the contextual factors that impact on women's lives is clear in this recommendation, the focus is still on weight loss. Although it resists making weight loss an urgent matter, weight loss is still the goal. This recommendation ultimately reiterates a particular gendered idea about weight, health and bodies. What is more, recruiting a woman's support network, whether it include her partner or other support persons, does not support the woman in her relationship with her body, which is undergoing significant changes. Rather, the advice to recruit a woman's partner and family in helping her to juggle the demands of being a new mother while also trying to lose weight not only prioritizes a particularly discriminatory view of fatness, but pits these individuals against her, which will alienate a woman from her support network.

Also in the immediate postpartum period, health professionals are advised to encourage women to breastfeed, in part because it may help them to lose weight gained during their pregnancies. Health professionals are also advised to use conversations about breastfeeding as a means of talking to women about losing weight, which, it is noted, is a sensitive issue. The HC document states:

> Weight gain during pregnancy can be a sensitive topic for many women and health care providers may be reluctant to discuss it. However, health professional advice can influence how much weight a woman gains during pregnancy. By communicating the recommended weight gain ranges early in the pregnancy, health care providers can improve a woman's chances of reaching the recommendations. Engaging women early can also help support their decision to breastfeed.
>
> (p. 6)

To suggest that women partake in breastfeeding their babies for the purposes of losing weight not only perpetuates the ill-informed idea that women should set about losing weight after their birth, but negates the numerous other profound experiences, beliefs, anxieties, concerns, joys, fears, pain, regrets, sorrows and excitement that may emerge in the context of the breastfeeding relationship between the woman and her baby and the woman and her now-lactating body. This is said not as a means to denigrate the mother's decision to bottle feed, which is also a rich attachment experience and should be a decision not based on coercion, guilt, or judgement, since such a decision is not a choice and can be accompanied only by stress and associated poor outcomes.

Creative and critical alternatives to fashioning social action

The active and passive voice allocated to women within maternity service guidelines helps to construct the nature of decision making. The aim of this chapter is to demonstrate that allocating women an active voice within practice guidelines serves the interests of all parties within the healthcare relationship. Clinical guidelines were reviewed and electronic databases and text were searched. The findings indicate that applying the principles of a shared decision making-framework, within clinical practice guidelines, can assist the development of a partnership relationship between midwives and women.

Fasting in Ramadan again draws our attention to the role of context and relationality in supporting women to have healthy pregnancies. Women who are preparing for Ramadan conceptualize not fasting as a social and spiritual risk, while fasting is conceptualized in mainstream healthcare as a risk to mother and baby, with issues such as increased admission for low fetal movement during Ramadan. Supportive responses include providing information to minimize any adverse metabolic effect of fasting (as in diabetes) – for instance, by explaining the benefits of the woman's waking early so as to allow for adequate hydration and knowing how to select foods with sustained energy release and sufficient protein, plus resting if possible (Hui *et al.* 2010).

The Well Rounded Mama website and blog (wellroundedmama.blogspot.ca), written by a childbirth educator and size-acceptance activist is one example of a creative, empowering response to ideologies of maternal obesity. Meredith Nash's book, *Making 'Postmodern' Mothers: Pregnant Embodiment, Baby Bumps and Body Image* (2012,) looks at how women can resist dominant cultural and biomedical readings of fat bodies in motherhood. It provides a multi-disciplinary, empirical account of pregnant embodiment and its place in feminist discourse concerned with gender, bodies, fitness, fatness, celebrity and motherhood.

Although clinical guidelines may not account fully for pregnancy weight gain among fat women, or may do so in a sizeist, non-evidence based manner, practitioners can create spaces where all pregnant women/women's bodies are respected. Some ideas are to include images of pregnant women of all sizes in the midwife's office, seek means to engage women of all sizes in active embodiment, nourishment and acceptance (HAES) and openly discuss the tensions and questions brought about by being fat and pregnant in a social milieu that contests such an outrageously confrontational bodily statement. Create spaces for individuals to participate in social change, since the growth-fostering relationships that both mothers and midwives enjoy together will likely lead to desire for social action.

In extending importance to the brain science underpinning human growth and development, seek ways to bring women together (including midwives) to offer mutual and authentic support to each other, reminding groups of how connection and attachment bathes the babies' brains in pleasure. Work diligently to support women where social forces such as poverty, violence, mental illness, food insecurity and social isolation lead to chronic disconnection. Let those social forces and remedies guide best practices, rather than having a singular focus on adjusting and conforming a new mother's body weight.

References

Aphramor, L. (2010) Health at Every Size, *1st International Wellbeing Conference*, Birmingham City University, 18 July.

Bacon, L. and Aphramor, L. (2011) Weight science: evaluating the evidence for a paradigm shift, *Nutrition Journal*, 10 (9): 1–13. doi: 10.1186/1475-2891-10-9.

Banks, A. (2011) Developing the capacity to connect, *Zygon*, 46 (1): 168–182.

Campos, P., Saguy, A., Ernsberger, P., Oliver, E. and Gaesser, G (2005) The epidemiology of over-weight and obesity: public health crisis or moral panic? *International Journal of Epidemiology*, 35: 55–60.

Cooper, C. (2011) A Queer and Trans Fat Activist Timeline. www.charlottecooper.net/downloads/timelinezine/cooper_queertransfatactivisttimeline_zine_0411.pdf [Accessed 29 May 2013]

Crawford, R. (1980) Healthism and the medicalization of everyday life, *International Journal of Health Services*, 10, 365–388.

Department of Health (2009) *The Pregnancy Book*. http://webarchive.nationalarchives.gov.uk/20130107105354/http://www.dh.gov.uk/prod_consum_dh/groups/dh_digitalassets/@dh/@en/@ps/@sta/@perf/documents/digitalasset/dh_117166.pdf.

Ellis, C. (2002) Being real: moving inward toward social change, *Qualitative Studies in Education*, 15 (4): 399–406.

Freeman, L.M. and Griew, K. (2007) Enhancing the midwife–woman relationship through shared decision making and clinical guidelines, *Women and Birth*, 20 (1): 11–5. Epub 28 November 2006.

Gard, M. and Wright, J. (2005) *The Obesity Epidemic: Science, Morality, Ideology*. New York: Routledge.

Gingras, J.R. (2005) Evoking trust in the nutrition counselor: why should we be trusted? *Journal of Agricultural and Environmental Ethics*, 18: 57–74.

Gingras, J. and Brady, J. (2010) Relational consequences of dietitians' feeding bodily difference. *Radical Psychology*, 8 (1). www.radicalpsychology.org/vol8-1/gingras.html.

HC (Health Canada) (2010) *Prenatal Nutrition Guidelines for Health Professionals* (Cat.: 978-1-100-16831-9), Ottawa, Ontario: Publications, Health Canada. www.hc-sc.gc.ca/fn-an/alt_formats/hpfb-dgpsa/pdf/pubs/guide-prenatal-eng.pdf.

HC (2011) *Eating Well with Canada's Food Guide: A Resource for Educators and Communicators* (HC Pub: 4667 Cat.: H164-38/2-2011E-PDF), Ottawa, Ontario: Publications, Health Canada.

Howard, B.V., Manson, J.E., Stefanick, M.L., Beresford, S.A., Frank, G. *et al.* (2006) Low-fat dietary pattern and weight change over 7 years: the Women's Health Initiative Dietary Modification Trial, *Journal of the American Dietetic Association*, 295: 39–49.

Hui, E., Bravis, V., Hassanein, M., Hanif, W., Malik, R. *et al.* (2010) Clinical review. Management of people with diabetes wanting to fast during Ramadan, *British Medical Journal*, 340: c3053.

Jette, S. and Rail, G. (2012) Ills from the womb? A critical examination of clinical guidelines for obesity in pregnancy, *Health*, 17 (4): 1–15. DOI: 10.1177/1363459312460702.

Katz Rothman, B. (2000) *Recreating Motherhood*, New Jersey: Rutgers University Press.

Kirkham, M. (ed.) (2010) *The Midwife–Mother Relationship*, London: Palgrave Macmillan.

Leap, N. (2000) The less we do the more we give. In: *The Midwife–Mother Relationship*, Kirkham, M. (ed.), Basingstoke: Macmillan.

Marmot, M.G. (2006) Status syndrome: a challenge to medicine. *Journal of the American Dietetic Association*, 295: 1304–1307.

McKibbin, L. (2009) Food for Thought Pyramid. http://food-for-thought-pyramid.com/ [Accessed 29 May 2013].

Miller, J.B. (1986) *Towards a New Psychology of Women* (2nd edn), Boston, MA: Beacon Press.

Miller, J.B. (1986a) What do we mean by relationships? (Work in Progress No. 22), Wellesley, MA: Stone Center Working Paper Series.

Mumford, S.L., Siega-Riz, A.M., Herring, A. and Evenson, K.R. (2008) Dietary restraint and gesta-tional weight gain, *Journal of the American Dietetic Association*, 108 (10): 1646–53.

Nash, M. (2012) *Making 'Postmodern' Mothers: Pregnant Embodiment, Baby Bumps and Body Image* (Genders and Sexualities in the Social Sciences), Basingstoke: Palgrave Macmillan.

NHS/NICE (National Health Service/National Institute for Health and Clinical Excellence (2010) *Dietary Interventions and Physical Activity Interventions for Weight Management Before,*

During and After Pregnancy (N2223). London, UK: NICE Publications. www.nice.org.uk/nicemedia/live/13056/49926/49926.pdf.

Rothblum, E. and Solovay, S. (eds) (2009) *The Fat Studies Reader*, New York: New York University Press.

Schoenfielder, L. and Wieser, B. (eds) (1983), *Shadow on a Tightrope: Writings by Women on Fat Oppression*, USA: Aunt Lute Book Company.

Sen, S., Carpenter, A.H., Hochstadt, J., Huddleston, J.Y., Kustanovich, V. *et al.* (2012) Nutrition, weight gain and eating behavior in pregnancy: a review of experimental evidence for long-term effects on the risk of obesity in offspring, *Physiology and Behavior*, 107: 138–145.

Sheiner, E., Levy, A., Menes, T.S., Silverberg, D., Katz, M. and Mazor, M. (2004) Maternal obesity as an independent risk factor for caesarean delivery, *Paediatric Perinat* al *Epidemiology,* 18 (3): 196–201.

Stavrou, E.P., Ford, J.B., Shand, A.W., Morris, J.M. and Roberts, C.L. (2011) Epidemiology and trends for caesarean section births in New South Wales, Australia: a population-based study, *BMC Pregnancy Childbirth*, 11: 8.

Teicher, M.H., Anderson, S.L., Polcari, A., Anderson, C.M. and Navalta, C.P. (2002) Developmental neurobiology of childhood stress and trauma, *Psychiatric Clinics of North America*, 2: 397–426.

Tormley, C. and Naylor, K.A. (eds) (2009) *Fat Studies in the UK*. York, UK: Raw Nerve Books.

Part IV

PRACTICAL APPLICATION
AND THE WAY FORWARD

14

CONVERSATIONS ABOUT FOOD

Nutritional assessment and counselling in pregnancy

Lorna Davies and Ruth Deery

Introduction

The most significant legacy that a woman can provide for her baby is to give it a nutritionally rich environment by eating well during pregnancy (Davies 2012). Our knowledge and understanding of nutrition in pregnancy has increased exponentially in the last few years and it is widely acknowledged that the role that maternal nutrition plays in terms of health outcomes for the baby is highly significant. This is the case in the short-term, within the perinatal period, and also in the much longer term with regard to lifelong health and well-being (Barker 1997; Gluckman and Hanson 2004; Ramakrishnan *et al.* 2012). This may suggest that, far from being a routine component of healthcare assessment, nutritional assessment needs to be the one, if not primary, assessment within pregnancy.

This chapter aims to provide a platform for discussion around nutritional assessment and counselling[1] in pregnancy for midwives. It will also provide an opportunity to explore how nutritional assessment may be carried out as part of antenatal care and what tools can be used to open up a discussion with the woman about her nutritional status and to plan any resulting actions.

A veterinary physician who was present at a social event that we attended recently made the observation that when people bring their pets to a veterinary appointment, the first thing that the vet usually asks is what the animal is eating and how it is feeding. A medical doctor who was also present responded by saying that although it is understood that nutritional assessment should be a routine component of health assessment, doctors seldom ask the same question of human patients as a first line of action. It would be interesting to reflect on whether midwives feel that they work with the opening gambit of the vet or relate more to the response of the doctor, during their encounters with pregnant women.

Review of the literature

It is being stressed ever more that health professionals, including midwives, need to have a solid foundational knowledge of nutritional requirements (Elias and Stewart 2005; Boland and Gibbons 2009). However, a brief review of the literature might suggest that the main conversations that take place between midwives and women regarding what they eat during pregnancy are concentrated on managing risk in relation to dietary intake. It would not be unreasonable to conclude that the bulk of research associated with diet in pregnancy that has been carried out in the last few years primarily involves obesity, gestational diabetes and food safety, which can be broadly interpreted as 'what not to eat during pregnancy'. A brief review on a midwifery database using the key words 'nutritional assessment' returned 32 results. Most of the listed studies were related to babies and nutritional assessment. When the words 'pregnant' and 'pregnancy' were added, only one study from the 1990s (Sujitor 1994) was retrieved. The search for 'diet in pregnancy' retrieved 54 studies, but none of these related to the role of the midwife in the assessment of women's diet and nutritional status during pregnancy. Perhaps tellingly, the search for 'obesity in pregnancy', which is generally viewed within the literature as a less-than-positive state, led to a deluge of studies and articles, with 93 results. Food safety in pregnancy followed closely behind, with 71 results. There is no clear explanation as to why this focus on the negative takes precedence over discussion about good nutrition. It may be that this is simply an effect of negativity bias. In a literature review titled 'Bad is stronger than good', Baumeister *et al.* (2001) conclude that negativity bias exists as a general principle across a broad range of circumstances. Alternatively, it has been speculated that health professionals are reticent when it comes to talking to patients and clients about their diet because food represents an integral part of our psyche that helps to form both our cultural and personal identities (Barger 2010). Therefore, talking to women about what to eat during pregnancy may feel intrusive and inappropriate. It could also be that our cultural focus on risk management has left us less able or willing to place value on the benefits of proactive behaviours (Van Vuuren 2000). Whatever the reason, it would seem that women who are seeking information about healthy eating during pregnancy are likely to be presented with a mass of information containing mixed messages and conflicting advice (Cheyney and Moreno-Black 2010).

There is no doubt that we need to be up to date with the issues associated with food safety and issues such as obesity and gestational diabetes. Additionally, discussion about foods that women need to be wary of or to avoid during pregnancy, and practices that will help to minimize risk, are key information. However, before pregnancy there is pre-conception care.

Pre-conception care

According to Calleja-Agius (2009), pre-conception care is based on educating women who may be considering pregnancy about issues that can influence neonatal morbidity, in both the short and the long term. Whilst 'educating women' is admirable, there is much discussion in this book that suggests that different approaches to having such encounters with women (see asset-based approach in Chapter 1, HEADDS in Chapter 8 and HAES in Chapter 13) may be more facilitative, engaging and of greater benefit.

We know there is evidence in the literature suggesting a number of lifestyle modifications and interventions that can be of benefit to maternal and neonatal health when applied prior to conception. These include:

- smoking cessation
- supplementation with folic acid
- cessation or moderation of alcohol intake
- improving of diabetic control
- not using recreational drugs
- pre-pregnancy rubella immunization
- seeing a healthcare professional as early in pregnancy as possible.

However, pre-conception care is not widely practised in the UK, despite having been shown to be of benefit to women (Heyes *et al.* 2004) and a huge impact on public health. In

Chapter 13 Jennifer Brady and colleagues point out that reports from neither Health Canada nor NICE in the UK make dietary recommendations specific to pre-pregnancy nutrition for women who intend to become pregnant, except to advise that women should take folic acid supplements.

Many women may not be aware of the importance of pre-conception nutrition and supplementation, nor even have access to nutrition information (Gardiner *et al.* 2008). Given adequate resources and time, midwives are in an ideal position to be able to discuss pre-conception nutrition with women. A Dutch study in 2006 concluded that although midwives appeared enthusiastic about playing an active role in the provision of pre-conception care, there was a mismatch between this willingness and the provision of appropriate education to support it (Van Heesch *et al.* 2006). There seems to have been little research in this area, in spite of the growing body of evidence that many of the most significant determinants of birth outcomes may be present before conception takes place. An increase in the commitment to providing good quality pre-conception care, with a strong emphasis on diet and nutrition, may serve to support (if not reframe) a public health approach aimed at the further improvement of birth outcomes (Wise 2008).

Food safety

Women in pregnancy are in an immunocompromised state and are therefore more susceptible to food-borne infection than are the general population (Tam *et al.* 2010; Lund and O'Brien, 2011). Additionally, the potential consequences for the fetus can be devastating (Table 14.1), which means that we need to share such information with pregnant women (Cox and Phelan 2009; Ockenden 2013) (Table 14.1 and Box 14.1). Pregnant women also need to be aware that if they experience flu-like symptoms or gastrointestinal symptoms such as diarrhoea, they should seek medical advice as soon as possible, as the symptoms may be indicative of a food-borne illness (Tam *et al.* 2010). In general, during pregnancy, as at any other time in life, women need to ensure that their food is obtained from reliable sources and stored, handled and cooked well and in a timely manner.

Attitudinal change

Pregnancy may be viewed by many women as a period in their lives when they are open to change, and non-judgemental support could potentially mitigate or even prevent complications related to diet (Cheyney and Moreno-Black 2010). Discussion about food safety, for example, may provide education that will serve the woman and her family well for the rest of their lives. However, too heavy an emphasis on the negative may be counter-productive, resulting in feelings of fear and guilt instead of prompting an informative and empowering dialogue, as discussed in Chapters 12 and 13. We also need to bear in mind that food and eating are emotion-laden areas of life for many women. As Lydia Turner identifies in Chapter 6, many women have less-than-healthy relationships with food. In many ways we are stepping into unknown territory when we engage in a discussion about food and diet, and we need to address the area with both objectivity and sensitivity. We need to use our finely honed communication skills to the greatest effect in order to avoid triggering any feelings of judgement on the part of the woman, regardless of what she says about her food and diet, and regardless of her body shape and size. An alarmist approach may fail to address the fact that, by changing habits and behaviours in relation to food, even to a small extent, women could

Table 14.1 Foods that present potential sources of risk during pregnancy

Food	Pathogens	Effect	Advice
Soft cheeses made from unpasteurized milk, including Brie, feta, Camembert. Soft-veined blue cheese.	E-coli or listeria	Miscarriage Preterm birth Still birth or perinatal death	Avoid.
Pâté Ready-to-eat meats	Listeria	Miscarriage Preterm birth Still birth or perinatal death	Avoid pâté. Some countries advise pregnant women not to eat cold meats or smoked fish. Check local guidelines.
Unpasteurized milk/products	Campylobacter E. coli Listeria Salmonella	Miscarriage Preterm birth Still birth or perinatal death	If only raw or green-top milk is available, it should boiled first.
Raw egg/soft-cooked egg Undercooked meat and poultry	Listeria E. coli Campylobactor Salmonella	Miscarriage Preterm birth Still birth or perinatal death	*Avoid raw egg products such as mayonnaise. Use a food thermometer to check the internal temperature of meat when cooking.*
Unwashed raw fruit and vegetables	Toxoplasmosis	Early miscarriage Vision and hearing loss Impaired cognitive development Seizures	Wash carefully before eating.
Liver	Over-consumption of vitamin A	Birth defects	
Hummus/tahini	Salmonella	Infection in fetus Perinatal death	
Raw sushi or ceviche	Vibrionaceae and Salmonella and protozoan species	Perinatal death Parasitic infection of the fetus	Avoid.
Swordfish Shark Marlin	High methylmercury levels	Neurological effects	Avoid. However. low-mercury alternatives such as salmon, crab and prawns can be consumed more regularly.
Tuna	High methylmercury levels	Neurological effects	Limit to 1 or 2 times a week.
Honey	Has been associated with botulism		Unless there is gastrointestinal pathology, women do not need to avoid during pregnancy.

Sources: Ministry of Health New Zealand (2009); Lund and O'Brien (2011); Tam *et al.* (2010); NHS Choices website.

make a significant difference to health outcomes for their babies and benefit their own health and well-being as well. Therefore, midwives also need to communicate information about the benefits of good nutrition for both mothers and babies, and about how women can best provide a nutritionally rich environment for their babies and themselves during pregnancy. We have to incorporate a discussion about the benefit of good nutrition into any encounters

---

Box 14.1 General food safety precautions during pregnancy

- Wash hands regularly, but particularly after using or cleaning the bathroom, handling dirty towels or linens and touching animals or their environments.
- Food should be safely handled, stored and protected from cross-contamination.
- Cooked food and ready-to-eat foods should be kept separate from raw and unprocessed foods, to avoid cross-contamination.
- Freshly cooked foods should be eaten as soon as possible after cooking.
- Cooked or prepared foods should be stored in a refrigerator and eaten within two days.
- Cooked food should be reheated thoroughly so that it is hot (about 70°C).
- Special attention should be paid when heating food using microwave ovens.
- Raw vegetables and fruit should be washed thoroughly.
- Hands, utensils and chopping boards should be washed before using for a different food.
- Pregnant women should avoid eating raw eggs.
- Drinking water should be obtained from a well-maintained and controlled supply system.
- Canned food should be eaten immediately after opening the can. Any leftovers should be removed from the can for storage in the refrigerator and eaten within two days.
- Unpasteurized milk and fruit juices should be avoided during pregnancy.

Source: Adapted from Ministry of Health New Zealand (2009).

---

that we have with women during pregnancy; it is too important to leave this to chance. This is an on-going conversation that doesn't start and end with the handing over of a few leaflets on food safety during the booking appointment.

Introducing nutrition

The ways in which midwives and other health care practitioners present the subject of nutrition to women during pregnancy could be viewed as a useful area of study helping us to evaluate the potential impact of nutrition-related intervention on birth outcomes and for the health status of mothers and babies. However, there would seem to be very limited information advising how midwives can best raise the subject of food, diet and nutrition with women during pregnancy. A 2011 US study surveyed 187 women about diet and exercise during pregnancy. Most of the women who responded claimed that they were not informed as to how much food they should be eating during pregnancy and had not been made aware of their own personal healthy gestational weight-gain targets (Ferraro *et al.* 2011). The few authors that have addressed the preparation of student midwives and midwives to carry out nutritional assessment and counselling have concluded that education on applied evidence-based nutrition needs to be incorporated into all midwifery curricula (Mulliner *et al.* 1995; Elias and Stewart 2005). It would be very difficult to establish how comprehensively this recommendation is borne out in practice, but the fact that this subject is significantly absent from the midwifery literature may suggest that it is not yet considered to be a mainstream subject in midwifery education or practice. Furthermore, there is no clear indication as to the availability of tools that might assist women to review what they eat, and it is uncertain how frequently midwives carry out a nutritional assessment with women during their professional relationship. In summary, we have little knowledge of where discussion about nutrition takes place within the midwife–woman interface, what form such discussion actually takes and, most significantly, whether midwife/health professional intervention as it stands actually makes a difference.

Nutritional assessment

A good nutritional assessment may help to ascertain the nutritional status of the woman, and thus assist in identifying an individualized approach to her dietary needs. It can also serve as a benchmark and therefore needs to take the shape of an on-going process and conversation throughout pregnancy. However, it would normally commence through the gathering and evaluation of data from a comprehensive nutritional assessment during the booking appointment. The information needs to be collected by using skillful communication to incorporate the type of questions outlined in Box 14.2. These are only suggested questions and the list is far from being definitive.

Box 14.2 Questions to gather information for nutritional assessment

What are the woman's normal patterns of eating?

- What she is eating?
- When she is eating?
- Why is she eating?
- How much she is eating?
- How often she is eating?

What are her food beliefs?
Are any of these affected by cultural norms?
What is her knowledge around making food purchases?
What are her skills in preparing food?
Is she taking any supplements?
Does she have any medical conditions that may affect her nutritional status?
What does she do for a living?

The questions needs to be framed in a way that makes them acceptable and non-judgemental. A general discussion about nutrition may arise from asking about whether the woman has any food cravings (pica) or whether she is a vegetarian or a meat eater. The question of supplements can arise from a discussion around taking folic acid or iodine early in pregnancy. Religious beliefs may open the door for discussion about what steps a Muslim woman will take during Ramadan to ensure that her nutritional status will not be compromised. A woman's disclosure that she works in a flower shop may offer the chance for a conversation about how to avoid exposure to pesticides. The questions do not need to be asked in a questionnaire format in order to gather the information. The answers to questions may lead the way to an opportunistic 'teaching moment'.

Minor problems of pregnancy

The so called 'minor' problems of pregnancy that relate to food and diet may also provide a window of opportunity to discuss nutrition. If the woman can relate the discomfort in some way to the fact that her body is behaving normally, then it may make it easier for her endure. For example if the woman complains of heartburn, a discussion about the effects of progesterone on smooth muscle may give her a greater degree of understanding of the physiology of pregnancy, which may help to some degree. Instead of reaching for the antacid, she could be encouraged to try some of the dietary-related solutions that might help, such as avoiding eating fatty or spicy foods that may decrease gastric motility. She could be advised to eat little and often, with snacks throughout the day, rather than three big meals, and to avoid eating and drinking at the same time, which may lead to an increase in intragastric pressure and stomach volume. Similar advice could help with morning sickness, for which the use of ginger products offers some relief. Although the evidence for the effectiveness of ginger is said to be limited (Matthews *et al*. 2010), anecdotally, it does seem to help some women. All of the above provide a good way in to the subject of nutrition without the need for a formalized approach.

Similarly, if the woman finds that she is constipated, dietary adaptations that may help to relieve the problem can be discussed. These may include increasing the amount of wholegrain cereals, fruit and vegetables and legumes in the diet and ensuring a good fluid intake. All of these tips may help to improve the nutritional intake of the woman and her family in addition to improving the peristalsis of her bowel.

The ABCD of nutritional assessment

It would probably be fair to assume that, when considering the concept of nutritional assessment, we generally think of talking to the woman about her food intake as the primary mode of assessment. However, although food intake is probably the principal determinant of nutritional status, it is not the only one. Nutritionists talk about direct and indirect nutritional assessment. The direct methods deal with the individual and measure objective criteria in relation to a person, whilst indirect methods use community health indices that reflect nutritional influences (Gibson 2005).

The methods used in the direct method are the one that the midwife is more likely to use with women in pregnancy. The acronym ABCD is used to represent the four recognized components of the method, namely anthropometric, biochemical, clinical and dietary. These are outlined in Table 14.2. Midwives already incorporate anthropometric and biochemical testing as part of a general assessment without necessarily thinking of these as being part of a nutritional assessment. For example, we may request the woman's body mass index (BMI) for several reasons, or obtain routine blood tests for screening purposes. Likewise, information may be gathered during a general health assessment at the booking appointment. This might include, for example, whether the woman smokes, which may affect micronutrient absorption; whether she has food allergies, or may be exposed to pesticides or herbicides in the work environment.

Table 14.2 The ABCD of nutritional assessment

Component	Used to assess
Anthropometric	Anthropometry measures all physical aspects of the human body. Simple measurements include height and weight. This means gathering information that relates to the woman's physical being, such as height, weight, BMI etc.
Biochemical	Biochemical tests are used to measure nutrients or metabolites in the body. Either blood or urine tests can be used to identify conditions such as anaemia or hyperglycemia.
Clinical/general health	This is the routine health assessment that is carried out during the booking visit generally, where the medical history of the woman is carried out, sometimes with a preliminary physical assessment.
Dietary	The dietary element is the most commonly used component of the assessment. It is used to determine the food intake of the woman, which can then be converted into nutrient components for evaluating. It also allows for the cross-referencing of intake with reference values and recommendations. A range of tools are designed for this particular activity.

Anthropometric assessment

Some of the anthropometric assessments are quite technical and fall beyond the remit of the midwife. If a woman needs an assessment that requires a range of measurements such as skin-fold thickness, head circumference and head:chest ratio, then she will almost certainly be referred to a dietician or a nutritionist for a more specialist consultation. There are also shortcomings in some of the measurement values. For example, if a woman is being seen by different midwives there is scope for inter-observer errors. There are no universal standards, which may lead to confusion if a woman moves from one place to another during pregnancy, and it is argued that the statistical cut-offs for abnormal levels are quite arbitrary (United Nations University 2013). For example, a measurement such as the waist:hip ratio clearly has limited value in pregnancy. Interestingly, though, it is suggested in the current NICE guidelines on weight management in pregnancy (NICE 2010). For many years it was argued that weighing women during pregnancy was unnecessary because it was felt to have poor predictive value for outcomes such as low birth weight (Dawes *et al.* 1992; Thompson *et al.* 1997). However, the current concerns about the correlation of low birth weight and its associated health-related problems for the baby (RCOG 2013) have led to a refocus on weighing the woman during pregnancy. Although 'it is no longer recommended that women are routinely weighed during pregnancy' (NICE 2010; RCOG 2013), it is recommended instead that health professionals encourage women to check their weight from time to time, or get them to think about the fit of their clothes (which may be a little difficult in pregnancy). It is recommended that a BMI is obtained for a number of reasons, which are discussed further in this chapter. This means that midwives have to be prepared for finding an effective way of eliciting the weight (and height) of women that feels comfortable (both midwife and woman) and with full informed consent from the woman.

How do we weigh women?

The weighing of an individual could never be considered to be a precise science, but if the woman consents to having her weight recorded, it is important that it is benchmarked and monitored as accurately as possible, with due care and consideration given to the discussion that precipitates this action. For example, do we, in the knowledge that people are notoriously inaccurate when asked for their weight measurement (HSE 2011), accept the woman's own verbal weight estimate? Or do we weigh her using our own scales? How do we address, this if she is a large bodied woman, such that she does not see it as a judgement (see Chapters 12 and 13), or communicate effectively with a teenage woman who may take umbrage at being asked her weight (see Chapter 8)? For a BMI, we need to measure the woman's height as well as her weight. How can we accurately measure the height of a woman if she herself does not know it? Some guidelines are presented in Box 14.3, which address the practicalities of performing these measurements. What this seemingly small and insignificant act does is to throw up a whole raft of practical and ethical issues of the sort that can make the tools of nutritional assessment a thorny area in practice. The advice in Box 14.3 may be practical in a clinic setting, where the equipment is relatively stationary, but it may not be so practical where the woman is receiving visits at home from a community midwife.

Box 14.3 **Measuring weight and height in pregnancy**

Measuring weight

Use a regularly calibrated electronic or balanced-beam scale.
The woman should be wearing light clothes with no shoes.
Read the weight to the nearest 100gm (0.1kg)

Measuring height

The woman should be standing erect and bare footed on a stadiometer with a movable headpiece.
The headpiece is levelled with skull vault and the height is recorded to the nearest 0.5cm.

Measuring BMI

The validity of BMI as a reliable form of measurement is challenged in Chapter 12, where it is pointed out that weight distribution within the individual has more bearing than does BMI. A cautionary tale lies in reports of rugby players and other sportspeople who fall into the obese category by virtue of their dense muscle mass (Duthie 2005). However, in spite of its shortcomings, as we previously suggested, it is a measurement that appears to be used increasingly in practice. Current evidence suggests that a woman with a high BMI (>35) is at greater risk of having a baby that incurs intra-uterine growth restriction, or is subject to intra-uterine death or stillbirth (Gardosi *et al.* 2013; RCOG 2013). As a result, we have seen the introduction of customized growth charts that require a recorded BMI for accuracy in producing the individualized chart for the woman. The BMI of a woman is also said to be necessary for screening purposes such as maternal serum screening tests, as it would seem that an inaccurate weight assessment may invalidate the assayed result (Reynolds *et al.* 2006). As a tool in combination with other forms of assessment, the BMI may have some, albeit limited, value. Nonetheless, it should always be viewed as one tool of many, and never be used in isolation. Midwives and other health professionals therefore need to know how to 'do the math' related to the practice. Although there are many online BMI calculators and 'apps' for smartphones, tablets and other devices, it is always useful to be able to work out the measurement manually working. The formula for working out a BMI is provided in Box 14.4.

Box 14.4 **Calculating BMI**

To work out a BMI:

- Divide the woman's weight in kilograms (kg) by her height in metres (m).
- Then divide the answer by height again, to get the BMI.

For example:

- If the woman's weight is 70kg and she is 1.75m tall: divide 70 by 1.75. The answer is 40.
- Then divide 40 by 1.75. The answer is 22.9. This is the woman's BMI.

BMI classifications

- BMI <18.5 = Underweight
- BMI 18.5–24.5 = Healthy weight range
- BMI 25–30 = Overweight

There are three different classes of obesity:

- BMI >30–34.9 = Obese (Class 1)
- BMI >35–39.9 = (Class 2)
- BMI >40 = (Class 3 or morbidly obese)

Sources: Adapted from NICE (2010) and CMACE/RCOG (2010)

Biochemical assessment

A biochemical assessment can range from something as simple as using multistix to screen for glycosuria to more exacting laboratory work for more definitive diagnostic results. These measures may help to detect nutrient deficiencies before anthropometric measures identify significant change or before clinical signs or symptoms appear.

A blood test, in addition to offering insight into the nutritional status of the woman by identifying some of the more common nutritionally related conditions of pregnancy such as anaemia, may highlight other associated underlying medical conditions, such as hyperthyroidism or Type 1 diabetes, both of which will have an impact on what the woman will be advised to eat and drink during pregnancy.

Clinical/general health assessment

Our nutritional status is incontrovertibly affected by the quality and quantity of what we eat, but it is far more complex than that. Many other factors may affect how our body deals with the nutrients that it receives. Taking a general health history may uncover some of these factors, and without additional effort they may become part of a nutritional assessment. Some of these are related to medical conditions, such as Type 1 diabetes, Crohn's disease and hypocalcaemia. We should also consider any medications that the woman is taking, as these may have a significant effect on her relationship with food, or may lead to interactions with food that influence what she eats. A well-known example of a food that interacts with many drugs is grapefruit. Grapefruit, and particularly grapefruit juice, contain a group of compounds called furanocoumarins that exert inhibitory action on the metabolism of many drugs, including the combined oral contraceptive (Bailey *et al.* 2012)

Observation

Like all practice-based appraisals, the nutritional assessment needs to begin with observation. By simply surveying a woman, it will be possible to obtain some information about her nutritional status. It is not difficult to recognize if a woman is overweight or underweight, or to ascertain whether she is 'blooming' or jaded, and this observation may offer insight into her dietary behaviours. If she has thin, sparse hair, this may indicate protein or zinc deficiency (Daniells and Hardy 2010). A sore and fissured tongue may indicate a lack of vitamin B6 or niacin (Downey n.d.). Anaemia is associated with spooning of the nails, and transverse lines visible on the nails may signify a protein deficiency (James *et al.* 2005). Signs of bruising may point to a shortage of vitamin K, but equally may suggest a deficiency of vitamin C and folic acid (Hampl *et al.* 2004). By being cognizant of such signs and symptoms, the midwife is in a position to initiate a discussion with the woman about nutrition.

Psychological and social factors

Psychosocial, cultural and spiritual factors play a significant role in our relationships with food and nutrition, and this is discussed at length in many of the chapters in this book, including Chapters 5, 6, 12 and 13. It is important that the context of the woman's life is taken into account if an individualized approach is to be taken. For example, it may be futile to encourage a family living on a limited budget to consider using expensive foodstuffs, but there is always scope for exploring the use of seasonal fruit and vegetables, which are generally less expensive (see Chapter 10). Equally, a woman who may not be able to eat certain foods for religious reasons may welcome ideas for receiving the nutrients from other food sources.

Stress

Recognising when stress is affecting the life of a woman is important on many levels. From a nutritional perspective, stress has an influence on both how and what we eat. It can make us pay less attention to our food intake and ignore our nutritional status, and this may in turn lead to a further increase in stress levels. Stress effects are, arguably, even more significant during pregnancy because of the added risks for the baby. Severe psychological stress in pregnancy can result in miscarriage, preterm birth and low birth weight (Reis *et al.* 1999; Nepomnaschy *et al.* 2006; Poggi-Davis and Sandman 2006). However, it would seem that elevated basal cortisol, which would normally be a cause for concern, is not necessarily abnormal in pregnancy (McLean and Smith 1999). Research indicates that increased stress hormone levels in pregnancy may help to prime a maternal instinct in women and initiate brain development and lung maturation in the baby. However, at extreme levels (which may vary for individuals), hypercortisolism can interfere with the biochemistry of the body and have significant effects on how food is digested and metabolized. Stress can also lead to increased reliance on agents such as alcohol and caffeine. However, even when stress is not a significant factor in the life of a woman, she may well wish to receive information about the effects of both caffeine and alcohol (see Boxes 14.5 and 14.6).

Assessing nutritional intake

The final section of this chapter introduces a variety of different tools/resources that may be used to assist in the assessment of diet and nutritional status during pregnancy. The tools can be used to: assist the woman in modifying her diet or reassure her that she is eating well; help to streamline the process of optimizing the identification of nutritional status (an important consideration in our busy lives); and highlight the need for referral to a nutritionist or dietician for more specialized support (Widen and Siega-Riz 2010). These methods may not appeal to all health practitioners, but they do provide another mode of assessment and some women might enjoy using tools and resources of this type, so it is always good to keep an open mind.

Box 14.5 Caffeine

- Caffeine is found in a wide range of foods and beverages, including coffee, tea, chocolate, cola and energy drinks.
- The half-life of caffeine may be up to 11 hours in women during pregnancy, and up to 100 hours in babies (Klebanoff *et al.* 1999).
- There are associations between caffeine and miscarriage, congenital abnormalities, intrauterine growth restriction and low birth weight (Signorello and McLaughlin 2004; CARE Study Group 2008; Peck *et al.* 2010; Brent *et al.* 2011; Sengpiel *et al.* 2013).
- Current UK and New Zealand recommendations suggest a daily caffeine intake of less than 200mgs a day, which approximately equates to two cups of coffee a day (FSAUK 2008; FSANZ 2011).

Instant coffee	75mg per 190ml cup
Brewed coffee	100–125mg per 190ml cup
Decaffeinated coffee (brewed or instant)	3–9mg per 190ml cup
Tea	75mg per 190ml cup
Green tea	50mg per 190ml cup
Drinking chocolate	1.1–8.2mg per 200ml cup
Cola (regular and diet)	11–70mg per 330ml can
Energy drinks (with added caffeine and/or guarana)	28–87mg per 250ml can
Milk chocolate	Up to 25mg per 50g bar
Caffeine tablets	200mg per tablet

Source: Adapted from FSAUK (2004).

Box 14.6 **Alcohol**

- In the UK, alcoholic drinks are measured in units and each unit corresponds to 7.9 grams (g) or 10 millilitres (ml) of ethanol. However one unit does not necessarily tally with the measure served, and different methods are used to define standard measurements in other parts of the world.
- Alcohol is a well-known teratogen that may continue to affect the fetus beyond the early embryonic stages of development. Alcohol crosses the barrier of the placenta, producing equivalent concentrations in fetal circulation (Randall 1987; Spagnolo 1993).
- The effects of alcohol on the fetus vary according to the stage of pregnancy and the frequency of consumption (Randall 1987; Spagnolo 1993).
- Alcohol consumption in pregnancy has been related to low birth weight and pre-term birth (Henderson *et al.* 2007; Bakker *et al.* 2010; Patra *et al.* 2011).
- If a woman consumes alcohol throughout pregnancy, this may lead to fetal alcohol spectrum disorder (FASD) in the baby. Approximately 8,000 new cases of FASD are diagnosed annually in the UK.
- FFASD represents a continuum of disorders that result from the excessive consumption of alcohol during pregnancy. These include Fetal Alcohol Syndrome (FAS), Partial Fetal Alcohol Syndrome (PFAS), Alcohol-Related Birth Defects (ARBD) and Alcohol-Related Neurodevelopmental Disorder (ARND) (NOFAS-UK 2013).
- Two units of alcohol daily during late pregnancy may increase the risk of low birth weight (NOFAS-UK 2013).
- Alcohol use and abuse is more common where women have mental health problems or are in abusive relationships (Maloney *et al.* 2011).
- Recent studies may have created conflicting impressions about safe levels of alcohol during pregnancy. However, the current UK advice is that it is safer not to drink at all during the first three months of pregnancy and that if women choose to drink alcohol, they should limit consumption to between one and two units once or twice a week.
- In many countries the official guidelines on this matter work on the premise that, since there is no current consensus on the threshold of maternal consumption, abstinence would be advised during pregnancy (ICAP 2013).

Nutritional intake can be assessed in several different ways, including a 24-hour dietary recall, a food and diet questionnaire or a food diary. It needs to be acknowledged that these tools are primarily used for research purposes, but there is no reason why they cannot be modified to be used as practice-based tools which has been done extensively in many different fields. There is also a focus in the literature on the pre-conceptual period (Coad 2003; Salima *et al.* 2011), but it is recognized that a large percentage of pregnancies are unintended (Cheng *et al.* 2009), and it is unknown how many women with unplanned pregnancies have sought pre-conceptual support from a healthcare provider.

24-hour dietary recall method

The dietary recall method works by getting the woman to recollect verbally what she has eaten in the last 24 hours. It is a reasonably quick and easy-to-use method but it does rely on the memory of the woman. It also relies on a specific 24-hour period of reporting that may not represent what the woman normally eats and drinks (Polusna *et al.* 2009). It involves the woman recalling all that she has eaten in the previous 24 hours. Once the information has been gathered the midwife and the woman can engage in a dialogue, tailored to the woman's individual needs, about her diet and nutritional intake.

Nutrition and lifestyle questionnaire

A nutrition and lifestyle questionnaire is another tool that can be used to elicit information. This method is slightly more detailed and involves a series of questions about what the woman's food intake looks like. An advantage is that it can include questions about the woman's social circumstances and broader health and lifestyle. Questions may be asked about whether the woman feels that she can afford to eat as well as she would like to, or about what access she has to cooking and storage facilities. Distinct dietary patterns in pregnancy have been identified within socio-economic groups that may have a significant bearing on both the short- and long-term health of both mother and the baby. The ALSPAC study (Northstone *et al.* 2008) identified that social factors need to be accounted for in planning for dietary changes. The tool could be used as a non-threatening lead-in to a discussion on such socially related issues. Questions that give an indication of the woman's understanding of food safety and establish whether or not she has animals in the house can be included. They may also touch on lifestyle factors such as special dietary needs, work–life balance and the use of alcohol. The advantage of this approach is that it is not too time consuming and can cover many different bases. If appropriate, it can be given to the woman to complete and return for discussion at a subsequent meeting, or it can be filled in with the woman at the time of the appointment. The respective disadvantages of either of these approaches are that it requires a good level of literacy if the woman is going to fill it in on her own, and it is relatively time consuming to complete. An example of a questionnaire, adapted from the questionnaire designed by Elizabeth Widen (Widen and Siega-Riz 2010), is provided at the end of this chapter as Appendix 1. It is user friendly and may be particularly useful, as, in addition to the questions, it contains tips and ideas to improve nutrition. It would sit quite comfortably within a woman's hand-held notes. It can be altered to address the particular circumstances of the woman if necessary.

The food diary

A food diary can be used if the food questionnaire identifies a potential problem, or it can be used independently. The woman is asked to keep a record of everything that she eats and drinks for three to five days. She writes down the food and drink at the times that she takes it, in order to ensure that all food and drink is recorded. Pictures can be used where literacy presents a problem. For more specialized monitoring, she may additionally be requested to include the amount (including weights) of food (Wrieden *et al.* 2003). However, as midwives would be principally interested in the intake of types food it would probably be better to keep things as simple as possible and not keep a record of the amounts of all foods consumed.

Asking for this level of detail could be quite challenging, and it would seem that if the instructions were too demanding, women might not record as accurately and, in particular, might under-report their consumption (Rennie *et al.* 2007). The woman may be happy to provide an estimated weight in the form of 'a cup of milk' or a 'fist-sized piece of fish'. It may be better, however, to aim for an overview of her nutritional intake. A US study followed up the completion of food diaries in a population of pregnant women with a telephone call for a debriefing session. This appeared to result in increased awareness of both macro- and micronutrient intake on the part of women (Crozier *et al.* 2008). It would be interesting to see if support from a midwife had a similar effect. The diary could then be used for comparison with guidelines for nutrition in pregnancy, examples of which can be found in the further resources section at the end of this chapter. A sample 3-day food diary is provided in Appendix 2.

An example of a healthy diet may be a useful tool to share with the woman. They are quite easy to do and can be very creative to make. It would be possible to create a healthy three-day diet plan for a limited budget, or for a woman with not much time for food preparation, or for a woman who is vegan. This is perhaps the sort of activity that women could do for themselves during preparation for childbirth and parenting sessions. In the same vein, and thinking laterally, if a venue with a kitchen were available, perhaps 'Food for a healthy pregnancy' sessions could be held for locally based pregnant women. A midwife might facilitate the sessions and the group members could take turns to present a healthy recipe which the group could then cook and eat together as a shared meal. Dieticians, gardeners and nutritionists could be invited as guest speakers. Might it be possible that such an arrangement could lead to better birthing outcomes than do the regular 'menu of choice' antenatal education sessions that are currently largely prevalent? Food for thought, indeed.

Conclusion

If we believe that negative birth outcomes can be reduced by improving the nutrition of women in pregnancy – and there seems to be a body of evidence to support this assumption – then we need to be effective in what we do and how we do it, and to have a real commitment to spending more time engaging with women on the topic of food.

Back in 2001, Annie Anderson wrote that 'giving written advice (which is the most widespread method of giving information) can influence knowledge about healthier eating, but does not seem to alter attitudes, or indeed behaviour' (Anderson 2001).

A decade on, anecdotally at least, it would seem that we are still relying heavily on printed or, increasingly, web-based forms of information about diet and nutrition in pregnancy. The support of oral information has been long advocated as a crucial component in information giving. Pamphlets, leaflets, books and articles and, we would add, web pages and social networking sites, are of far less value without the follow-up discussion with a trusted and well-informed health professional. Yet, it would seem that in our increasingly complex world there is less time than ever for talking. Pregnancy would also seem to be a good time for addressing dietary and lifestyle changes as part of a life-based skill and knowledge set, thus meeting our role as health promoters and educators. However, as we have identified, the subject needs to be approached with skill and sensitivity, and this requires time to talk, to discuss the issues arising and ask and answer questions. It calls for a conversation about food.

Appendix 1: Food and lifestyle questionnaire

Would you like to make some changes to your diet during pregnancy? Please tick the response that applies to you:

- I am ready to make some changes and would appreciate support.
- I'm not sure if I am ready to change but I am happy to start the conversation.
- I don't think that I am ready to make any changes at the moment.

How well do you eat? Please circle the answer that applies to you.	**Tips to help you eat well**
How many servings of fruit and vegetables do you eat each day?	Aim for five or more servings of fruit and vegetables a day. If possible, 5 servings of vegetables and 2 servings of fruit is ideal. These can be fresh, frozen or canned. Try to eat a fruit or vegetable at every meal. Raw fruit and vegetables are easy snacks.
2 or less 3–4 5 or more	
How many times a week do you eat fried food?	Try to use cold-pressed oils such as olive oil wherever possible for frying. Baking and grilling are good substitutes to cut down on frying food. Eat less fast food. If you do eat fast food, keep it simple and regular sized, and try to eat it with a salad.
Less than 1 1–3 4 or more	
How many soft carbonated or sweetened drinks do you have each day?	Drink water as your first choice. Limit fizzy and sweetened drinks to one a day.
Less than 1 1–2 3 or more	
How many times a week do you eat chicken, fish or beans (like kidney beans or chickpeas)?	Beans and lentils are a great and cheap substitute for meat. Try to keep tuna and swordfish to 2 servings a week. White fish and salmon are great substitutes. Eat baked or broiled chicken and fish.
Less than 1 1–2 3 or more	
How many times a week do you eat crisps or crackers?	Popcorn is a good substitute for crisps and crackers. Eat a couple of tablespoons of almonds or walnuts or a couple of brazil nuts for a tasty and nutritious snack.
Less than 1 1–3 4 or more	
How many times a week do you eat cakes and biscuits?	Try to eat fruit or yogurt instead of cakes and biscuits, where possible. Have stewed or baked fruit for a change. Sorbet is a good dessert choice. Eat fruit bread or have a small serving of dried fruit to curb sweet cravings.
Less than 1 1–3 4 or more	

Question / Statement	Suggestion
How much butter, lard and animal fat (visible fat in red meat, chicken skin) do you eat? Very little Some A lot	Use plant-based oils such as olive oil. Use butter, but not too much: 1 tsp (5g) on a slice of bread. Season food with salt to taste, and with herbs and spices.
How much tea and coffee do you drink each day Less than 1 1–3 4 or more	Try to stick to no more than 2 cups of coffee or 3 cups of tea a day. Drink decaffeinated tea and coffee. Try herbal or fruit teas as an alternative.
How much alcohol do you drink each week? None at all 1–2 units 3 or more units	The current recommendation is that no level of alcohol is known to be safe. You are advised to try to avoid drinking alcohol in pregnancy. Try drinking sparkling mineral water or soda water with ice and lemon, or elderflower cordial for a special occasion. Try to find other ways of relaxing if you use alcohol to unwind. Go for a walk. Watch a nice movie or try some meditation.
How do you feel about food? Do you agree with any of the statements below?	**You may want to try these suggestions**
Healthy foods cost too much.	Eat less meat and more beans and lentils. Eat canned and frozen foods. Eat at home instead of going out or having takeaways. Cook your own food instead of pre-prepared meals. Bulk-buy foods. Grow your own food wherever possible. Even a balcony will hold pots for growing herbs and salad greens. Eat foods that are in season they are usually cheaper.
Healthy food doesn't taste as good as junk food.	Don't give up your favourite snacks and less-healthy favourites – just try to cut down. Try new recipes and ideas for food.
I eat when I am tired, bored or depressed.	Find something else to do to distract you. Go for a walk. Do something with your hands, or knitting or reading. Call a friend. Have a supply of healthy snacks available.
It's hard to eat out and eat healthily.	Avoid 'all that you can eat' restaurants and cafes. Order grilled food or low-fat sandwiches. Ask for half-sized or child portions. Ask for a doggy bag and take some home.
I eat too much at social events.	Eat a healthy snack before you go to fill up. Choose a few things that you really enjoy and savour them.
I tend to pick when I am cooking or clearing away food.	Chew gum as you cook. Ask someone to throw the food away while you do something like washing the dishes.

I tend to snack throughout the day and eat my meals in front of the television.	Make time for regular meals. Sit at the table with a glass of water and lemon juice with your family or even on your own. Eat slowly, chew your food well and enjoy the experience of focusing on your food.

Making a plan

What goals do you want to set for yourself now that you have completed the questionnaire? Before my next appointment I am going to . . .
Examples:
Aim to eat 5 fruit and vegetable a day. Prepare healthy snacks to eat.

Source: Adapted from Widen and Siega-Riz (2010).

Appendix 2: Sample 3-day food diary

Day 1	Day 2	Day 3
Breakfast	*Breakfast*	*Breakfast*
Wholegrain breakfast cereal/porridge with banana or berries Skimmed or semi-skimmed milk Wholemeal toast with peanut butter Decaffeinated/herb tea	Well-boiled egg Wholemeal toast with butter Piece of fruit Decaffeinated/herb tea	Fruit smoothie made from banana, skimmed milk, small pot yogurt, handful frozen berries Decaffeinated/herb tea
Snack	*Snack*	*Snack*
Bran and apple muffin Tea or coffee	Mixed nuts and dried fruit Tea or coffee	Small piece of Edam cheese with crackers. Tea or coffee
Lunch	*Lunch*	*Lunch*
Baked beans on wholemeal toast Piece of fruit Water	Wholemeal pitta bread with hummus and vegetable sticks Small fruit yoghurt Fruit juice	Lentil, tomato and carrot soup Wholemeal bread, cheese and ham toastie Piece of fruit Water
Snack	*Snack*	*Snack*
Hummus and vegetable sticks Decaffeinated/herb tea	Slice of fruit loaf Decaffeinated/herb tea	Small fruit yoghurt Decaffeinated/herb tea
Dinner	*Dinner*	*Dinner*
Chicken and vegetable stir-fry Brown rice Baked apple and scoop of ice-cream	Baked fillet of fish Broccoli and carrots Fruit smoothie	Bean and vegetable casserole Jacket potato Banana
Snack	*Snack*	*Snack*
Milky drink	Milky drink	Milky drink

Note

1 Counselling is defined in this context as a supportive process within a face-to-face situation, where the pregnant woman can be supported to identify ways in which she might benefit from considering aspects of her attitude and behaviour in response to food, diet and nutrition.

References

Anderson, A. (2001) Nutritional adaptation to pregnancy and lactation. Pregnancy as a time for dietary change? *Proceedings of the Nutrition Society Scottish Section and the Reproduction and Development Group of the Nutrition Society University of Dundee*, 28–29 March 2001

Bailey, D., Dresser, G., and Arnold, J.M.O. (2012) Grapefruit-medication interactions: Forbidden fruit or avoidable consequences? *Canadian Medical Association Journal* (Canadian Medical Association), 185 (4): 309–16.

Bakker, R., Pluimgraaff, L.E., Steegers, E.A., Raat, H., Tiemeier, H. *et al.* (2010) Associations of light and moderate maternal alcohol consumption with fetal growth characteristics in different periods of pregnancy: The Generation R Study. *International Journal of Epidemiology*, 39 (3): 777–89.

Barker, D.J.P. (1997) Maternal nutrition, fetal nutrition, and disease in later life. *Nutrition*, 13: 807.

Barger, M.K. (2010) Maternal Nutrition and Perinatal Outcomes. *The Journal of Midwifery & Women's Health*, 55: 502–511.

Baumeister, R.F., Bratslavsky, E., Finkenauer, C. and Vohs, K.D. (2001) Bad is stronger than good. *Review of General Psychology*, 5 (4): 323.

Boland, R. and Gibbons, M. (2009) The cost of healthy eating for pregnant and breastfeeding women in Otago. *NZ College of Midwives Journal*, 41: 26–28.

Brent, R.L., Christian, M.S. and Diener, R.M. (2011) Evaluation of the reproductive and developmental effects of caffeine. *Birth Defects Research Part B, Developmental and Reproductive Toxicology Teratology Society*, 92 (2): 152–87. Epub 2 March 2011.

Calleja-Agius, J. (2009) Pre-conception care: Essential advice for women, *British Journal of Midwifery*, 17 (1): 38–44.

CARE Study Group (2008) Maternal caffeine intake during pregnancy and risk of fetal growth restriction: A large prospective observational study. *British Medical Journal*, 337: a2332. DOI: 10.1136/bmj.a2332.

Cheyney, M. and Moreno-Black, G. (2010) Nutritional counseling in midwifery and obstetric practice. *Ecology of Food and Nutrition*, 49: 1–29.

Cheng, D., Schwartz, E.B., Douglas, E. and Horon, I. (2009) Unintended pregnancy and associated maternal preconception, prenatal and postpartum behaviors. *Contraception*, 79 (3): 194–8.

Coad, J. (2003) Pre and peri-conceptual nutrition. In: Morgan, J. and Dickerson, J.W.T. (eds) *Nutrition in Early Life* (pp. 39–71), Chichester: Wiley.

Cox, J. and Phelan, S. (2009) 'What can I eat, doctor?' Food safety in pregnancy . . . part 2. *Contemporary OB/GYN*, 54 (12): 24, CINAHL with Full Text, EBSCO*host* [accessed 26 May 2013].

Crozier, S.R., Inskip, H.M., Godfrey, K.M. and Robinson, S.M. (2008) Dietary patterns in pregnant women: a comparison of food-frequency questionnaires and 4 day prospective diaries. *British Journal of Nutrition*, 99: 869–75.

Daniells, S. and Hardy, G. (2010) Hair loss in long-term or home parenteral nutrition: Are micronutrient deficiencies to blame? *Current Opinion in Clinical Nutrition & Metabolic Care* 13 (6): 690–7.

Davies, L. (2012) Sitting next to Nellie: Food for thought: nutrition in pregnancy. *Essentially MIDIRS* 3 (9): 40–4.

Dawes, M.G., Green, J. and Ashurst, H. (1992) Routine weighing in pregnancy. *British Medical Journal*, 304 (6825): 487–9.

Downey, M. (n.d.) B Vitamins. (*Online*) Available at http://vitalitymagazine.com/article/b-vitamins [accessed 24 May 2012].

Duthie, G.M. (2005) High Body Mass Index is not a barrier to physical activity: Analysis of international rugby players' anthropometric data. *European Journal of Sport Science*, 5 (2): 77.

Elias, S. and Stewart, S. (2005) Developing nutrition within the midwifery curriculum. *British Journal of Midwifery*, 13: 456–60.

Ferraro, Z., Rutherford, J., Keely, E. *et al.* (2011) An assessment of patient information channels and knowledge of physical activity and nutrition during pregnancy. *Obstetric Medicine* (1753–495X) 4: 59–65.

FSANZ (Food Safety Agency Australia and New Zealand) (2011) Caffeine. (*Online*) Available at: www.foodstandards.gov.au/consumer/whatsin/caffeine/pages/default.aspx [accessed 21 April 2013].

FSAUK (Food Standards Agency UK) (2004) Survey of Caffeine Levels in Hot Beverages. Food Survey Information Sheet 53/04. (*Online*) Available at: www.food.gov.uk/multimedia/pdfs/fsis5304.pdf.

FSAUK (2008) High Caffeine Energy Drinks and other Foods Containing Caffeine. (*Online*) Available at www.food.gov.uk/policy-advice/additivesbranch/energydrinks#.UavclevRx40 [accessed 18 April 2013].

Gardiner, P.M., Nelson, L., Shellhaas, C.S., Dunlop, A.L., Long, R. (2008) The clinical content of preconception care: Nutrition and dietary supplements. *American Journal of Obstetrics and Gynecology*, 199 (6): S345–S356.

Gardosi, J., Madurasinghe, V. and Williams, M. (2013) Maternal and fetal risk factors for stillbirth: Population based study. *British Medical Journal*, 346: f108.

Gibson, R. (2005) *Principles of Nutritional Assessment*. New York: Oxford University Press.

Gluckman, P. and Hanson, M. (2004) *The Fetal Matrix: Evolution, Development and Disease*. Cambridge: Cambridge University Press.

Hampl, J.S., Taylor, C.A. and Johnston, C.S. (2004) Vitamin C deficiency and depletion in the United States: The third national health and nutrition examination survey, 1988 to 1994. *Journal Information*, 94: 5.

Health Survey England (HSE) (2011) Health Survey for England – 2011, Health, social care and life-styles. (*Online*) Health and Social Care Information Centre. Available at: www.hscic.gov.uk/catalogue/PUB09300 [accessed 23 May 2013].

Henderson, J., Gray, R. and Brocklehurst, P. (2007) Systematic review of effects of low–moderate prenatal alcohol exposure on pregnancy outcome. *British Journal of Obstetrics and Gynaecology*, 114 (3): 243–52.

Heyes, T., Long, S. and Mathers, N. (2004) Preconception care practice and beliefs of primary care workers. *Family Practice*, 21 (1): 22–7.

ICAP (International Center for Alcohol Policy) (2013) International Guidelines on Drinking and Pregnancy. *(Online)* Available at: www.icap.org/Table/InternationalGuidelinesOnDrinkingAndPregnancy [accessed 12 May 2012].

James, W., Berger, T. and Elston, D. (2005) *Andrews' Diseases of the Skin: Clinical Dermatology* (10th edn). Philadelphia: Saunders.

Klebanoff, M.A., Levine, R.J., Dersimimonian, R., Clemens, J.D., Wilkins, D. *et al.* (1999) Maternal serum paraxanthine, a caffeine metabolite, and the risk of spontaneous abortion. *The New England Journal of Medicine*, 341: 1639–1644, 1688–1689.

Lund, B.M. and O'Brien, S.J. (2011) The occurrence and prevention of foodborne disease in vulnerable people. *Foodborne Pathogens and Disease*, 8: 961–73.

Maloney, E., Hutchinson, D., Burns, L., Mattrick, R.R. and Black, E. (2011) Prevalence and predictors of alcohol use in pregnancy and breastfeeding among Australian women. *Birth*, 38 (1): 3–9. DOI: 10.1111/j.1523–536X.2010.00445.x.

Matthews, A., Dowswell, T., Haas, D.M., Doyle, M. and O'Mathúna, D. (2010) Interventions for nausea and vomiting in early pregnancy. *Cochrane Database System Review*, 8 (9): CD007575.

McLean, M. and Smith, R. (1999) Corticotropin-releasing hormone and human parturition. *Reproduction*, 121: 493–501.

Ministry of Health New Zealand (2009) Food and nutrition guidelines for healthy pregnant and breast-feeding women: a background paper (first published 2006), www.health.govt.nz/publication/food-and-nutrition-guidelines-healthy-pregnant-and-breastfeeding-women-background-paper.

Mulliner, C., Spilby, H. and Fraser, R. (1995) A study exploring midwives' education in, knowledge of and attitudes to nutrition in pregnancy. *Midwifery*, 11: 37–41.

NICE (National Institute of Health and Care Excellence) (2010) PH27. Weight management before, during and after pregnancy. (*Online*) Available at: http://publications.nice.org.uk/weight-management-before-during-and-after-pregnancy-ph27/recommendations#weight-management-a-definition [accessed 21 May 2013].

Nepomnaschy, P.A., Welch, K.B. and McConnell, D.S. (2006) Cortisol levels and very early pregnancy loss in humans. *Proceedings of the National Academy of Science USA*, 103: 3938–42.

NOFAS-UK (National Organisation for Foetal Alcohol Syndrome UK) (2013) No Alcohol No Risk – FASD Information for Midwives (*Online*) Available at: www.nofas-uk.org/ [accessed 1 June 2013].

Northstone, K., Emmett, P., and Rogers, I. (2008) Dietary patterns in pregnancy and associations with socio-demographic and lifestyle factors. *European Journal of Clinical Nutrition*, 62 (4): 471–9, Academic Search Complete, EBSCO*host* [accessed 29 May 2013].

Ockenden, J. (2013) Midwifery basics: diet matters (3): Obesity in pregnancy. *Practising Midwife*, 10 (11): 39–40.

Patra, J., Bakker, R. and Irving, H. (2011) Dose-response relationship between alcohol consumption before and during pregnancy and the risks of low birthweight, preterm birth and small for gestational age (SGA): a systematic review and meta-analyses. *British Journal of Obstetrics and Gynaecology*, 118 (12), 1411–21.

Peck, J.D., Leviton, A. and Cowan, L.D. (2010) A review of the epidemiologic evidence concerning the reproductive health effects of caffeine consumption: a 2000–2009 update. *Food and Chemical Toxicology*, 48 (10): 2549–76.

Poggi-Davis, E. and Sandman, C.A. (2006) Prenatal exposure to stress and stress hormones influences child development. *Infants and Young Children*, 19 (3): 246–59.

Poslusna, K., Ruprich, J., de Vries, J.H.M., Jakubikova, M. and van Veer, P. (2009) Misreporting of energy and micronutrient intake estimated by food records and 24 hour recalls, control and adjustment methods in practice. *The British Journal of Nutrition*, 101: S73–85.

Ramakrishnan, U., Grant, F., Goldenberg, T., Zongrone, A. and Martorell, R. (2012) Effect of women's nutrition before and during early pregnancy on maternal and infant outcomes: A systematic review. *Paediatric and Perinatal Epidemiology*, 26: 285–301.

Randall, C.L. (1987) Alcohol as a teratogen: a decade of research in review. *Alcohol*, Suppl. 1: 125–32.

RCOG (2013) Green Top Guideline No. 31 (2nd edn) The Investigation and Management of the Small-for-Gestational-Age Fetus. (*Online*) Available at: www.rcog.org.uk/files/rcog-corp/22.3.13GTG31SGA.pdf [accessed 31 May 2013].

Reis, F.M., Faldati, M., Florio, P. and Petraglia, F. (1999) Putative role of placental corticotrophin-releasing hormone in the mechanisms of human parturition. *Journal of the Society for Gynecologic Investigation,* 6 (3): 109–19.

Rennie, K.L., Coward, A. and Jebb, S.A. (2007) Estimating under-reporting of energy intake in dietary surveys using an individualised method. *British Journal of Nutrition*, 97 (6): 1169–76.

Reynolds, T.M., Vranken, G. and Van Neuten, J. (2006) Weight correction of MoM values: which method? *Journal of Clinical Pathology*, 59 (7): 753–58.

Salima, T., Mounira, K. and Nadjia, D. (2011) Assessment of nutritional status of pregnant women attending the city Tebessa PMI (Algeria). *National Journal of Physiology, Pharmacy and Pharmacology,* 1 (2): 97–105.

Sengpiel, V., Elind, E., Bacelis, J., Nilsson, S., Grove, J. *et al.* (2013) Maternal caffeine intake during pregnancy is associated with birth weight but not with gestational length: results from a large prospective observational cohort study. *BMC Medicine*, 11 (1): 42.

Signorello, L.B. and McLaughlin, J.K. (2004) Maternal caffeine consumption and spontaneous abortion: a review of the epidemiologic evidence. *Epidemiology*, 15 (2): 229–39.

Spagnolo, A. (1993) Teratogenesis of alcohol. *Annali dell'Istituto Superiore di Sanita*, 29 (1): 89–96.

Sujitor, C.W. (1994) Nutritional assessment of the pregnant woman. *Clinical Obstetrics and Gynecology*, 37 (3): 501–14.

Tam, C., Erebara, A. and Einarson, A. (2010) Food-borne illnesses during pregnancy. *Canadian Family Physician*, 56: 341–3.

Thompson, M.L., Theron, G.B. and Fatti, L.P. (1997) Predictive value of conditional centile charts for weight and fundal height in pregnancy in detecting light for gestational age births. *European Journal of Obstetrics and Gynecology and Reproductive Biology*, 72 (1): 3–8.

United Nations University (2013) Anthropometric Reference Data. http://unu.edu/unupress/food/V182e/ch12.htm.

Van Heesch, P.N.A.C.M., De Weerd, S., Kotey, S. and Steegers, E.A.P. (2006) Dutch community midwives' views on preconception care. *Midwifery*, 22: 120–4.

Van Vuuren, W. (2000) Cultural influences on risks and risk management: Six case studies. *Safety Science*, 34: 31–45.

Widen, E. and Siega-Riz, A.M. (2010) Prenatal nutrition: a practical guide for assessment and counseling. *Journal of Midwifery & Women's Health*, 55: 540–9.

Wise, P.H. (2008) Transforming preconceptional, prenatal, and interconceptional care into a comprehensive commitment to women's health. *Women's Health Issues*, 18: S13–S18.

Wrieden, W., Gregor, A. and Barton, K. (2008) Have food portion sizes increased in the UK over the last 20 years? *Proceedings of the Nutrition Society*. (Presented at the Scottish Section Nutrition Society meeting, 27–28 March 2008; abstract available at: www.nutritionsociety.org/files/uploads/0080218ScottishMeetingOriginalCommunications.pdf)

Online resources

Resources for health professionals

Food and nutrition guidelines
New Zealand guidelines for food and nutrition in pregnancy and during lactation
www.health.govt.nz/publication/food-and-nutrition-guidelines-healthy-pregnant-and-breastfeeding-women-background-paper
Dietary deficiencies
McGraw-Hill (publisher's) website that presents widely recognized symptoms of nutrient deficiency, excess, and toxicity in each major body system
www.mhhe.com/hper/nutrition/nutriquest/body.mhtml

Religions and food practices

Internet FAQ Archives page on religion and food practices. Doesn't specifically relate to pregnancy but gives a good overview of a host of religious practice
www.faqs.org/nutrition/Pre-Sma/Religion-and-Dietary-Practices.html

Alcohol in pregnancy

No Alcohol No Risk – video about the effects of FAS
www.nofas-uk.org/

Resources for women

UK NHS Choices website. Advises women on healthy food choices in pregnancy
www.nhs.uk/conditions/pregnancy-and-baby/pages/healthy-pregnancy-diet.aspx
Alcohol in pregnancy
www.nhs.uk/chq/Pages/2270.aspx?CategoryID=54#close
Food safety
www.nhs.uk/conditions/pregnancy-and-baby/pages/foods-to-avoid-pregnant.aspx#close
Food allergy and intolerance
www.patient.co.uk/health/food-allergy-and-intolerance
Caffeine intake
Archived but still current advice on caffeine in pregnancy
http://webarchive.nationalarchives.gov.uk/20120206100416/http:/food.gov.uk/news/newsarchive/2008/nov/caffeinenov08
More generic information on caffeine intake
www.nutritionfoundation.org.nz/nutrition-facts/nutrition-a-z/Caffeine

INDEX

Note: In page references, '*b,*' '*f,*' 'n' and '*t*' refer to boxes, figures, notes and tables.